THE NEUROLOGIC EXAMINATION

Scientific Basis for Clinical Diagnosis

Hiroshi Shibasaki, MD, PhD

EMERITUS PROFESSOR

KYOTO UNIVERSITY GRADUATE SCHOOL OF MEDICINE

KYOTO, JAPAN

Mark Hallett, MD

CHIEF

HUMAN MOTOR CONTROL SECTION

NATIONAL INSTITUTION OF NEUROLOGICAL DISORDERS AND STROKE

NATIONAL INSTITUTE OF HEALTH

BETHESDA, MARYLAND;

PRESIDENT

INTERNATIONAL FEDERATION OF CLINICAL NEUROPHYSIOLOGY

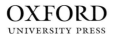

OXFORD

UNIVERSITY PRESS

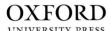

Oxford University Press is a department of the University of Oxford. It furthers
the University's objective of excellence in research, scholarship, and education
by publishing worldwide. Oxford is a registered trade mark of Oxford University
Press in the UK and certain other countries.

Published in the United States of America by Oxford University Press
198 Madison Avenue, New York, NY 10016, United States of America.

Library of Congress Cataloging-in-Publication Data
Names: Shibasaki, Hiroshi, 1939– , author. | Hallett, Mark, 1943– , author.
Title: The neurologic examination : scientific basis for clinical diagnosis/by Hiroshi Shibasaki and Mark Hallett.
Description: Oxford ; New York : Oxford University Press, [2016] | Includes
    bibliographical references.
Identifiers: LCCN 2015048147 | ISBN 9780190240974 (alk. paper)
Subjects: | MESH: Neurologic Examination—methods | Nervous System
    Diseases—diagnosis | Medical History Taking—methods | Neurologic
    Manifestations
Classification: LCC RC386.6.N48 | NLM WL 141 | DDC 616.8/0475—dc23
LC record available at http://lccn.loc.gov/2015048147

9 8 7 6 5 4 3 2

Printed by Sheridan Books, Inc., United States of America

Dedication

To Shinobu, Judy, and our families for their constant support, and to the many patients we have examined who have taught us about the neurologic examination.

CONTENTS

List of Boxes   *xi*

Preface   *xiii*

Explanatory Notes   *xv*

1. DIAGNOSIS OF NEUROLOGIC DISEASES
   (GENERAL PRINCIPLE)   1
   1. Anatomical Diagnosis   1
   2. Etiological Diagnosis   2
   3. Clinical Diagnosis   4

2. HISTORY TAKING   5
   1. The Present Age and the Age at Onset   5
   2. Sex   5
   3. Chief Complaints   5
   4. History of the Present Illness   7
   5. Past Medical History   7
   6. Social History   7
   7. Family History   8

3. PHYSICAL EXAMINATION   9
   1. General Physical Examination
      and Neurologic Examination   9
      A. General Physical Examination at the Initial
         Clinical Evaluation   9
      B. General Physical Findings and Neurologic
         Findings   19
   2. Steps of Neurologic Examination   20

4. EVALUATION OF CONSCIOUSNESS   23
   1. Anatomical Basis of Consciousness   23
   2. Mechanisms of Disturbances of Consciousness   24
   3. Observation of the State of Consciousness   24
   4. Modes of Consciousness Disturbance and
      the Coma Scale   25
   5. Conditions That Should Be Distinguished
      from Clouding of Consciousness   26

5. BRAINSTEM AND CRANIAL NERVE TERRITORIES   29
   1. Brainstem   29
   2. Common Structures of Cranial Nerves   29
   3. Cranial Nerves Related to Somatosensory
      Function   31
   4. Cranial Nerves Related to Autonomic
      Nervous Function   31

   5. Location of the Cranial Nerve Nuclei in
      the Brainstem   32

6. OLFACTORY SENSATION   35
   1. Structures and Neurotransmitters of
      the Olfactory System   35
   2. Examination of Olfactory Sensation   35

7. VISUAL FUNCTIONS   37
   1. Anatomy and Function of the Visual System   37
      A. Retina   37
      B. Optic Nerve and Optic Chiasm   38
      C. Lateral Geniculate Body and Optic Radiation   40
      D. Visual Cortex   42
      E. Blood Supply to the Visual Pathway   42
      F. Cytoarchitecture of the Visual System
         and Higher Cortical Functions   42
   2. Examination of Visual Functions   44
      A. Visual Acuity   44
      B. Visual Field   44
      C. Ophthalmoscopic Examination of Ocular Fundus   46

8. PUPILS AND ACCOMMODATION   49
   1. Nerve Innervation of Intraocular Muscles   49
      A. Light Reflex and Convergence Reflex   49
      B. Sympathetic Nervous System
         and Horner Syndrome   51
      C. Accommodation and Its Abnormality   52
   2. Examination of Intraocular Muscles   53
      A. Oculomotor Nerve Palsy and Horner Syndrome   53
      B. Examination of the Light Reflex and
         Its Abnormality   54
      C. Special Abnormal Findings of Pupils   55
      D. Examination of the Convergence Reflex   55
      E. Examination of Accommodation   55

9. EXTRAOCULAR MUSCLES, GAZE, AND EYE MOVEMENTS   57
   1. Nerve Innervation of Extraocular Muscles   57
      A. Third Cranial Nerve (Oculomotor Nerve)   57
      B. Fourth Cranial Nerve (Trochlear Nerve)   60
      C. Sixth Cranial Nerve (Abducens Nerve)   60
   2. Neural Control Mechanism of Gaze   61
      A. Central Control Mechanism of Gaze   61

B. Lateral Gaze and Lateral Gaze Palsy 62

C. Vertical Gaze and Vertical Gaze Palsy 62

D. Convergence and Convergence Palsy 62

3. Medial Longitudinal Fasciculus and Internuclear Ophthalmoplegia 63

4. Central Control Mechanism of Eye Movements 63

A. Central Control Mechanism of Saccades 64

B. Central Control Mechanism of Smooth Pursuit 64

C. Roles of Cerebellum and Basal Ganglia in Eye Movements 65

5. Examination of Extraocular Muscles, Gaze, and Eye Movements 65

A. Ptosis 66

B. Examination of Extraocular Muscles 66

C. Examination of Fixation, Gaze, and Eye Movements 68

D. Involuntary Movements of Eyes 70

10. TRIGEMINAL NERVE 75

1. Structures and Functions 75

A. Somatosensory Pathway 75

B. Cortical Reception of Somatosensory Input from Face 76

C. Nerve Innervation of Masticatory Muscles 76

D. Reflex Pathway of Jaw Jerk 77

E. Neural Pathway of Corneal Reflex 78

2. Examination of Functions Related to the Trigeminal Nerve 78

A. Motor Nerve 78

B. Sensory Nerve 79

C. Jaw Jerk (Masseter Reflex) 80

D. Corneal Reflex 80

E. Primitive Reflexes 81

11. FACIAL NERVE 83

1. Structures and Functions 83

A. Motor Nerve 83

B. Somatosensory Nerve 84

C. Taste Sense 85

D. Lacrimation and Salivation 85

E. Parasympathetic Innervation of Facial Skin and Mucosa 86

2. Examination of Functions Related to the Facial Nerve 86

A. Motor Function 86

B. Somatosensory Function 88

C. Taste Sense 88

D. Lacrimation and Salivation 88

E. Facial Skin and Mucosa 88

12. AUDITORY FUNCTION 89

1. Structures of the Auditory Pathway 89

2. Examination of Auditory Function 90

13. SENSE OF EQUILIBRIUM 93

1. Structures and Functions of the Pathways Related to Equilibrium 93

2. Examination of the Sense of Equilibrium 94

14. SWALLOWING, PHONATION, AND ARTICULATION 97

1. Innervation of Swallowing, Phonation, and Articulation 97

A. Glossopharyngeal Nerve and Vagus Nerve 97

B. Hypoglossal Nerve 97

C. Cortical Innervation of Bulbar Muscles 98

D. Involvement of the Cranial Nerves Innervating Bulbar Muscles 99

2. Somatosensory Innervation of Pharynx and Larynx 100

3. Taste Sense 100

4. Salivation 101

5. Autonomic Innervation of Visceral Organs 101

6. Afferent Pathway from the Visceral Organs 102

7. Examination of Swallowing, Phonation, and Articulation 102

A. Examination of the Tongue 103

B. Examination of the Soft Palate and Swallowing 103

C. Bulbar Palsy and Pseudobulbar Palsy 104

15. NECK AND TRUNK 105

1. Examination of the Neck 105

A. Postural Abnormality of the Neck 105

B. Examination of Muscles Innervated by the Accessory Nerve 105

C. Cervical Spondylosis 106

D. Meningeal Irritation 106

2. Examination of the Trunk 106

16. MOTOR FUNCTIONS 109

1. Final Common Pathway of the Motor System 109

A. Motor Cortex and Corticospinal Tracts 109

B. Structure and Function of Spinal Cord 112

C. Anterior Horn Cells and Peripheral Motor Nerves 113

D. Neuromuscular Junction and Muscle 115

2. Central Control of Voluntary Movement 115

A. Higher Functions of Motor Cortices 115

B. Basal Ganglia 116

C. Cerebellum 125

3. Examination of Motor Functions 132

A. Posture 132

B. Muscle Atrophy and Fasciculation 132

C. Muscle Strength 134

D. Muscle Tone 142

E. Muscle Spasm and Cramp 145

F. Myotonia 147

G. Coordination 147

17. TENDON REFLEXES AND PATHOLOGICAL REFLEXES ... 153

    1. Physiological Mechanism of the Tendon Reflex ... 153

    2. Examination of Tendon Reflexes ... 153

    3. Pathological Reflexes and Their Generating Mechanisms ... 156

    4. Loss of Superficial Reflex as a Pyramidal Sign ... 157

18. INVOLUNTARY MOVEMENTS ... 159

    1. Examination of Involuntary Movements ... 159

    2. Tremor ... 159

    3. Chorea ... 166

    4. Ballism ... 167

    5. Athetosis ... 167

    6. Dystonia ... 167

    7. Dyskinesia ... 172

    8. Myoclonus ... 172

    9. Motor Stereotypies ... 178

    10. Involuntary Movements That Can Be Suppressed Momentarily ... 179

    11. Involuntary Movements of Peripheral Nerve Origin ... 181

19. SOMATOSENSORY FUNCTION ... 185

    1. Structure and Functions of the Somatosensory System ... 185

      A. Somatosensory Receptors ... 185

      B. Peripheral Somatosensory Nerves ... 185

      C. Somatosensory Pathway in the Spinal Cord ... 186

      D. Nociceptive Pathway ... 187

      E. Proprioceptive Pathway ... 188

      F. The Third Sensory Neuron and Cortical Receptive Areas ... 188

    2. Examination of Somatosensory Function and Abnormal Findings ... 188

      A. Examination of Somatosensory Function ... 189

      B. Somatosensory Symptoms/Signs ... 190

      C. Impairment of the Somatosensory Nervous System and Distribution of the Sensory Symptoms ... 191

20. AUTONOMIC NERVOUS SYSTEM ... 199

    1. Structure and Function of the Autonomic Efferent System ... 199

      A. Sympathetic Nervous System ... 199

      B. Parasympathetic Nervous System ... 199

      C. Disorders of the Peripheral Autonomic Nerves ... 201

      D. Cortical Center of the Autonomic Nervous System ... 201

      E. Neural Control of Urination ... 202

    2. Structure and Function of the Autonomic Afferent System ... 202

    3. Examination of the Autonomic Nervous Function ... 202

      A. Autonomic Symptoms of Skin ... 202

      B. Micturition and Sexual Functions ... 203

      C. Gastrointestinal Symptoms ... 203

      D. Orthostatic Hypotension ... 203

21. POSTURE AND GAIT ... 205

    1. Central Control Mechanism of Gait ... 205

    2. Examination of Gait ... 205

      A. Spastic Gait ... 205

      B. Parkinsonian Gait ... 206

      C. Ataxic Gait ... 206

      D. Waddling Gait and Steppage Gait ... 207

22. MENTAL AND COGNITIVE FUNCTIONS ... 209

    1. Examination of Mental/Cognitive Functions ... 209

      A. Orientation ... 209

      B. Memory ... 210

      C. Calculation ... 213

      D. Common Knowledge and Judgment ... 215

      E. Emotion and Character ... 215

      F. Illusion, Hallucination, and Delusion ... 215

      G. State of Daily Living ... 216

    2. Dementia ... 216

      A. Alzheimer Disease and Related Disorders ... 216

      B. Frontotemporal Lobar Degeneration ... 217

      C. Leukoencephalopathy ... 218

23. APHASIA, APRAXIA, AND AGNOSIA ... 223

    1. Neural Circuits Related to Language, Praxis, and Recognition ... 223

      A. Language ... 223

      B. Praxis ... 227

      C. Recognition ... 229

    2. Examination of Language, Praxis, and Recognition ... 231

      A. Examination of Language and Aphasia ... 231

      B. Examination of Praxis and Apraxia ... 232

      C. Examination of Recognition and Agnosia ... 233

      D. Use of Simple Test Battery ... 233

24. PAROXYSMAL AND FUNCTIONAL DISORDERS ... 237

    1. Epilepsy and Convulsion ... 237

      A. Classification of Epileptic Seizures ... 237

      B. Diagnosis of Epilepsy ... 241

    2. Headache and Migraine ... 242

      A. Classification of Headache ... 242

      B. Migraine and Related Disorders ... 243

      C. Tension-Type Headache ... 244

3. Sleep Disorders 244
    A. Obstructive Sleep Apnea-Hypopnea Syndrome 244
    B. Central Sleep Apnea-Hypopnea Syndrome 245
    C. REM Sleep Behavior Disorders 245
    D. Narcolepsy and Related Disorders 246
    E. Periodic Limb Movement in Sleep 246
    F. Kleine-Levin Syndrome 246
    G. Fatal Familial Insomnia 246

25. ION CHANNEL DISORDERS 249
  1. Hereditary Channelopathies 249
    A. Hereditary Channelopathies of the Central Nervous System 249
    B. Hereditary Channelopathies of the Peripheral Nervous System 252
    C. Hereditary Channelopathies of Muscles 252
  2. Autoimmune Channelopathies 253
    A. Myasthenia Gravis 254
    B. Lambert-Eaton Syndrome 254
    C. Isaacs Syndrome (Neuromyotonia) 254

26. PSYCHOGENIC NEUROLOGIC DISEASES 257
  1. Psychogenic Motor Paralysis 257
  2. Psychogenic Sensory Loss 257
  3. Psychogenic Constriction of Visual Field 258
  4. Common Features of Psychogenic Neurologic Diseases 258

27. THALAMUS 259
  1. General Structure of the Thalamus 259
  2. Ventral Posterior Nucleus as the Sensory Relay Center 259
  3. Ventral Anterior Nucleus and Ventrolateral Nucleus as the Motor Thalamus 261
  4. Medial Dorsal Nucleus as a Relay Center to the Prefrontal Cortex 261
  5. Anterior Nucleus and Memory 262
  6. Pulvinar as a Relay Center to the Parietal Lobe 262
  7. Intralaminar Nucleus as a Relay Center of the Ascending Reticular Activating System 262
  8. Relay Nucleus for the Visual and Auditory System 262

28. HYPOTHALAMUS AND NEUROENDOCRINOLOGY 265
  1. Structure and Function of the Hypothalamus 265
  2. Neuroendocrinology 265
    A. Anterior Lobe of the Pituitary Gland (Adenohypophysis) 265
    B. Posterior Lobe of the Pituitary Gland (Neurohypophysis) 266

3. Adjustment to the External Environment and Control of the Internal Milieu 267
    A. Control of Circadian Rhythm 267
    B. Control of Feeding 267
    C. Control of Body Temperature 267
    D. Homeostasis 267

29. NEUROLOGIC EMERGENCY 269
  1. Disorders with Respiratory Paralysis 269
    A. Crisis of Myasthenia Gravis 269
    B. Guillain-Barré Syndrome 270
    C. Acute Anterior Poliomyelitis 270
    D. Acute Brainstem Lesion 270
    E. Amyotrophic Lateral Sclerosis 270
  2. Disorders with Disturbance of Consciousness 270
  3. Status Epilepticus 272
  4. Conditions Expected to Have Poor Functional Recovery Unless Appropriately Treated at Early Clinical Stage 272
    A. Acute Compression of Spinal Cord 273
    B. Progressive Ischemic Cerebrovascular Diseases 273
  5. Examination of Coma 273
    A. Degree of Coma (Coma Scaling) 274
    B. Presence or Absence of Asymmetry in Neurologic Signs 274
    C. Examination of Brainstem Functions 274
    D. Meningeal Irritation 278
  6. Judgment of Brain Death 278

30. DISABILITY, FUNCTIONAL RECOVERY, AND PROGNOSIS 281
  1. Assessment of Disability Scale 281
  2. Mode of Tissue Damage, Functional Disability, and Its Recovery 281
  3. Mechanisms of Functional Recovery 282

31. HOW TO PLAN LABORATORY TESTS 285
  1. Functional Neuroimaging Studies and Electrophysiological Studies 285
  2. Lumbar Puncture 285
  3. Use of Laboratory Tests for Prevention of Diseases 287

Afterword: For Those Who Wish to Study Neurology 289
Index 291

LIST OF BOXES

1. Onset of neurologic symptoms in cerebrovascular diseases 4

2. Risk factors for vascular diseases in young population 6

3. Lacunar infarction 7

4. Clinical neurology from a wide viewpoint 9

5. Inflammatory diseases of the nervous system 16

6. Subclavian steal syndrome 24

7. Causes of syncope 25

8. Locked-in syndrome 27

9. Clinical features of demyelinating diseases: Is the Uhthoff phenomenon due to physical exercise or increase in body temperature? 39

10. Weber syndrome 59

11. Top of the basilar artery syndrome 60

12. Saccadic eye movement and smooth pursuit eye movement 65

13. Miller Fisher syndrome 68

14. Marcus Gunn phenomenon 79

15. Raeder (paratrigeminal) syndrome 80

16. Forced grasping 81

17. Head retraction reflex and opisthotonus 81

18. Orbicularis oris muscle and orbicularis oculi muscle 86

19. Crocodile tears syndrome 86

20. Bilateral facial paralysis 87

21. Wallenberg syndrome and related conditions 98

22. Why the tongue deviates on protrusion even in a unilateral hemispheric lesion 99

23. Named syndromes related to brainstem and cranial nerves 100

24. Frey syndrome 101

25. Mirror movement 111

26. Nonmotor symptoms/signs in Parkinson disease 122

27. Pedunculopontine nucleus 124

28. Neurodegeneration with brain iron accumulation (NBIA) 126

29. Conditions other than Parkinson disease in which L-dopa may improve the parkinsonian symptoms 126

30. Bassen-Kornzweig disease 130

31. Hereditary disorders characterized by cerebellar ataxia, spastic paralysis, and cataract 130

32. Inclusion body myositis 133

33. Bulbospinal muscular atrophy 133

34. Juvenile muscular atrophy of unilateral upper extremity (Hirayama disease) 137

35. Neuromyelitis optica spectrum disorders 142

36. Acute disseminated encephalomyelitis (ADEM) versus multiple sclerosis (MS) 143

37. Degenerative disorders of upper motor neurons 143

38. Adrenomyeloneuropathy 143

39. HTLV-I-associated myelopathy/tropical spastic paralysis (HAM/TSP) and subacute myelo-optico-neuropathy (SMON) 144

40. Malignant syndrome and malignant hyperthermia 145

41. What can occur in Parkinson patients during L-dopa treatment? 145

42. Significance of finger flexor reflex 156

43. Achilles tendon reflex and peripheral nerve lesions 156

44. Complete motor paralysis of toes and Babinski sign 157

45. Abdominal reflex and abdominal muscle reflex 157

46. Why is the resting tremor in Parkinson disease suppressed by voluntary movement? 163

47. Asymmetry of tremor 163

48. Involuntary movements suppressed by ethanol intake 163

49. Tremor caused by midbrain lesion 165

50. Fragile X-associated tremor/ataxia syndrome 166

51. Genotype and phenotype of Huntington disease 166

52. Generating mechanism of dystonia 169

53. Hereditary myoclonus-dystonia syndrome 172

54. Hereditary paroxysmal dyskinesia 172

55. Unverricht-Lundborg disease 174

56. Benign adult familial myoclonus epilepsy 175

57. Mitochondrial encephalomyopathy and abnormality of mitochondrial functions 175

58. Unilateral asterixis due to thalamic lesion 176

59. Transient myoclonic state with asterixis in elderly patients 176

60. Palatal tremor and Guillain-Mollaret triangle 176

61. Startle reflex in progressive supranuclear palsy 178

62. Prion disease 179

63. Pain associated with herpes zoster 191

64. Carpal tunnel syndrome 191

65. Thalamic pain and Dejerine-Roussy syndrome 192

66. Fabry disease 192

67. Impairment of dorsal root ganglion cells 193

68. Familial amyloid polyneuropathy 201

69. Diagnostic criteria of multiple system atrophy 204

70. How does paradoxical kinesia occur? 206

71. Idiopathic normal-pressure hydrocephalus 207

72. Intermittent claudication 207

73. Transient global amnesia 211

74. Wernicke encephalopathy 212

75. Subacute and fluctuating behavioral abnormality 213

76. Change of emotion and character by a lesion of the right temporal lobe 215

77. Dementia pugilistica (chronic traumatic encephalopathy) 217

78. HIV-related neurologic disorders 218

79. Progressive supranuclear palsy and corticobasal degeneration 218

80. Vanishing white matter disease 219

81. Nasu-Hakola disease 219

82. Progressive multifocal leukoencephalopathy (PML) 219

83. Kanji (morphogram) and kana (syllabogram) of Japanese language 226

84. Syndrome of Alice in Wonderland 229

85. Amusia 229

86. Savant syndrome 230

87. Ventriloquist effect and cocktail party effect 230

88. Williams syndrome 230

89. Landau-Kleffner syndrome 232

90. Balint syndrome 234

91. Gelastic epilepsy (ictal laughter) 240

92. Cerebrovascular diseases and epilepsy 242

93. Post-lumbar puncture headache 243

94. Could sleep apnea syndrome cause cognitive disturbance? 245

95. Limbic encephalitis 255

96. Hoover sign 258

97. Acute poisoning causing respiratory paralysis 270

98. Reye syndrome 272

99. Acute meningoencephalitis 273

PREFACE

A number of books related to neurology and neurologic diagnosis have been published and are currently available in updated editions, but most of them are disease oriented or anatomy oriented, and only few are function oriented. As a consequence of recent advances in laboratory testing including electrophysiology and neuroimaging, the importance of history taking and physical examination in neurologic diagnosis tends to be neglected. However, the correct interpretation of symptoms and signs based on modern scientific knowledge is of utmost importance in the diagnosis of neurologic diseases. In this regard, this book is organized in terms of functional anatomy of the nervous system and aims at providing a bridge from the basic sciences such as anatomy, physiology, pharmacology, and molecular biology to neurologic symptoms and signs. As one of the unique features of this book, about 100 boxes are included in order to discuss some specific topics of current interest and some clinical issues that the authors have been particularly interested in.

This book is primarily aimed at neurology residents and registrars, but it is hoped that it will be also useful for neurologists in general practice, pediatric neurologists, neurosurgeons, psychiatrists, physical therapists, technicians of clinical neurophysiology and neuroimaging, and medical students.

One of the authors, Hiroshi Shibasaki, learned clinical neurology from a number of senior neurologists, including Dr. Yoshigoro Kuwoiwa and Dr. Shukuro Araki of Japan, Dr. A. B. Baker and Dr. John Logothetis (currently in Greece) of the United States, and Dr. A. M. Halliday and Dr. Ian McDonald of the United Kingdom. He also received a profound impact from Dr. Jun Kimura while they worked together in Kyoto University. He has also collaborated with Dr. Mark Hallett who is a coauthor of this book and Dr. Hans O. Lüders of the United States for many years. By integrating all the information collected from those distinguished neurologists and based on his own vast clinical experience, he has created his own concept of neurologic diagnosis. He published a book titled *Diagnosis of Neurological Diseases* in Japanese from Igaku-Shoin

in Tokyo, the first edition in 2009 (Shibasaki, 2009) and the second edition in 2013 (Shibasaki, 2013). Since those books have been widely accepted among Japanese neurologists, he decided to publish an updated English version for international readers and asked Mark Hallett to help.

Mark Hallett learned his clinical neurology in Boston from Drs. Raymond Adams, C. Miller Fisher, H. Richard Tyler, and Norman Geschwind. The neurologic examination in Boston in those days was heavily influenced by Dr. Derek Denny-Brown, who himself was influenced by Dr. Gordon Holmes. Like Dr. Shibasaki, Dr. Hallett spent time in London and was influenced there by Dr. C. David Marsden. Dr. Hallett notes that while he and Dr. Shibasaki had the good fortune to be originally trained by giants in the field, the examination does continue to evolve and we appreciate all our neurologic colleagues over our years of practice.

Since the two authors have had their main interests in the field of human motor control, movement disorders, involuntary movements, and clinical neurophysiology, the number of references cited for each chapter have been influenced, leading to a relatively larger number of literature citations for the chapters related to those specialty fields.

We are grateful to Professor Per Brodal of Oslo for allowing us to use many of the neuroanatomy figures from his book *The Central Nervous System* (Brodal, 2010). HS expresses his thanks to Dr. Masao Matsuhashi of Kyoto University for his valuable help in computer processing. Finally we acknowledge the efficient help of Mr. Craig Allen Panner and Ms. Emily Samulski of Oxford University Press; Mr. Saravanan Kuppusamy, Ms. Divya Vasudevan and the team at Newgen KnowledgeWorks in preparing this book.

BIBLIOGRAPHY

Brodal P. The Central Nervous System: Structure and Function. 4th ed. Oxford University Press, New York, 2010.

Shibasaki H. Diagnosis of Neurological Diseases. Igaku-Shoin, Tokyo, 2009 (in Japanese).

Shibasaki H. Diagnosis of Neurological Diseases. 2nd ed. Igaku-Shoin, Tokyo, 2013 (in Japanese).

EXPLANATORY NOTES

Regarding the use of medical terminology, the following principles are adopted in this book.

Symptom: subjective condition determined from the complaints of a patient during the history taking.

Sign: objective finding identified by the physician during the physical examination.

Lesion: site of the nervous system affected by pathology or functionally impaired.

Disturbance: abnormality of nervous functions.

Rostral (applied to the brainstem and spinal cord): superior, or directed toward the cranium.

Caudal (applied to the brainstem and spinal cord): inferior, or directed toward the feet. (In the brain, "anterior" and "posterior" are used to describe front and back, respectively.)

Ventral: inferior in the brain, and anterior in the brainstem and spinal cord.

Dorsal: superior in the brain, and posterior in the brainstem and spinal cord.

1.

DIAGNOSIS OF NEUROLOGIC DISEASES (GENERAL PRINCIPLE)

In order to make the diagnosis of neurologic diseases in a systematic way, it is practical and useful to make a three-step diagnosis; anatomical diagnosis, etiological diagnosis, and clinical diagnosis in this order. It is effective to adopt this principle through all steps of neurologic diagnosis from the history taking to the neurologic examination, before choosing the necessary laboratory tests.

1. ANATOMICAL DIAGNOSIS

While taking the history and carrying out the neurologic examination, it is essential to consider whether the lesion involves the central nervous system, the peripheral nervous system, or the muscular system, or more than one of these systems. Furthermore, within each of these systems, the sites of lesion should be estimated as precisely as possible. This is a special feature of neurology because any site of the nervous system, if affected, presents with symptoms and signs that are specific for that particular site. In the cerebrum, for example, whether the lesion involves the superficial gray matter (cortex), the deep gray matter such as the thalamus and basal ganglia, or the intermediate white matter should be considered. Furthermore, it is possible to estimate the precise location of the lesion within each site of the cerebral hemisphere. As for the peripheral nervous system, whether the lesion involves a particular nerve, more than one nerve, or all the nerves diffusely can be estimated. In addition, the precise location of the lesion, as to whether it is the proximal or the distal part of the nerve fibers, can be also estimated. Furthermore, careful clinical examination allows us to estimate the kind of nerve fibers affected, whether motor, sensory, or autonomic nerve fibers, or even whether the axon or the myelin sheath.

For example, when the patient complains of muscle weakness in one hand, it is useful to systematically take into account the motor cortex, the corticospinal tract

through the cerebral white matter, internal capsule and brainstem to the cervical cord, the anterior horn cells, and then the α motor fibers, neuromuscular junction, and finally muscles in this order. Of course, this process can be done in the opposite order from the periphery to the motor cortex. For another example, if the patient complains of numbness in one hand, it is practical to consider the responsible site of lesion first in the peripheral nerve innervating that region of the skin, then the brachial plexus, dorsal root ganglion, dorsal root, gray matter of the cervical cord, somatosensory fibers in the cervical cord and brainstem, relay nucleus in the thalamus, thalamocortical fibers, and finally the hand area of the contralateral somatosensory cortex. This process is often possible even during the history taking, if carefully done.

Distribution of the Lesion at the Tissue Level

For neurologists, it is not enough to just estimate the location of lesion at the level of gross neuroanatomy. They are expected to be able to consider the more precise distribution of pathology at the tissue level. The mode of distribution of the tissue damage is important not only to make correct diagnosis but also to predict the severity and prognosis of the symptoms and signs caused by the lesion.

Five forms of representative distribution of tissue damage are illustrated in Figure 1-1, taking the localized lesion in the cervical cord as an example. In a **diffuse** lesion, the tissue is homogeneously damaged throughout. A typical example of this case is transverse myelitis of the cervical cord, in which the patient is expected to show severe quadriplegia at least in the acute stage. In a **disseminated** lesion, the lesion is scattered as if seeds were spread on the ground. Pathologically it is characterized by perivascular cell infiltration. An example is disseminated myelitis as seen in neuromyelitis optica spectrum disorders (Takahashi et al, 2007; Sato et al, 2014; Wingerchuk et al,

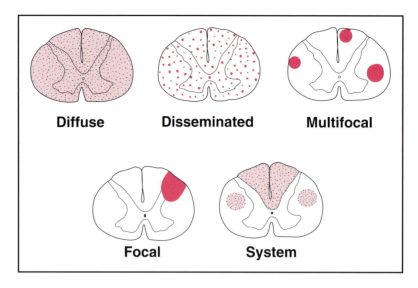

Figure 1-1 Schematic illustration of the distribution of lesions in a transverse section of the cervical cord.

2015), acute disseminated encephalomyelitis (ADEM), neuro-Behçet, and HTLV-I associated myelopathy (HAM/TSP) (Osame, 2002, for review). In this condition, the lesion usually also extends longitudinally over a relatively long distance in the spinal cord. In contrast with acute transverse myelitis, which usually manifests quadriplegia (paraplegia in case of thoracic cord lesion) of severe degree below the affected segment, the disseminated cord lesion typically presents with severe spasticity of lower extremities while muscle strength is relatively spared, and it is especially so in the chronic stage.

A **focal** lesion is localized to an area in the central nervous system and is typically seen in vascular ischemic disease or tumor. Multiple sclerosis and metastatic tumors typically show **multifocal** lesions. **System** involvement is characteristically seen in neurologic diseases, and it affects a group of neurons or a neuronal network that has specific function(s). Its typical examples are neurodegenerative diseases such as Parkinson disease, motor neuron disease, and Alzheimer disease. Intoxication due to heavy metals and drugs also belongs to this group.

Selective Vulnerability

This is the basic concept for explaining system involvement of the nervous system due to heavy metal or drug intoxication. A typical example is organic mercury poisoning (**Minamata disease**), which is clinically characterized by dysarthria and ataxia due to cerebellar damage, constriction of the peripheral visual field due to involvement of the occipital cortex, and hearing difficulty (**Hunter-Russell syndrome**) (see Chapter 7-2B).

Negative versus Positive Neurologic Symptoms/Signs

Neurologic symptoms and signs can be divided into two types: negative and positive. The negative neurologic symptoms/signs are neurologic deficits caused by impairment or loss of functions of the nervous system, and the positive neurologic symptoms/signs are caused by over-excitation of the nervous system or loss of its inhibition. Examples of negative symptoms/signs are unconsciousness, memory loss, aphasia, visual field defect, motor paralysis, bradykinesia, freezing of gait, sensory deficit, and orthostatic hypotension. Examples of positive symptoms/signs are convulsion, involuntary movements, spasm/cramp, pain, and dysesthesia. Psychiatric symptoms like hallucination and delusion may also be interpreted as positive symptoms. As positive phenomena are not always present during the physical examination, it often depends on the patient's description or situations reported by observers. Most of the negative signs are observable by physical examination, but intermittent or paroxysmal negative phenomena like transient ischemic attacks and periodic paralysis have to be confirmed by careful history taking.

2. ETIOLOGICAL DIAGNOSIS

The information as to how the neurologic symptoms started (**mode of onset**) and how they have changed after the onset (**clinical course**) provides the most useful clue to the cause or pathogenesis of the disease. The mode of onset is classified into four types: sudden, acute, subacute, and insidious (Figure 1-2).

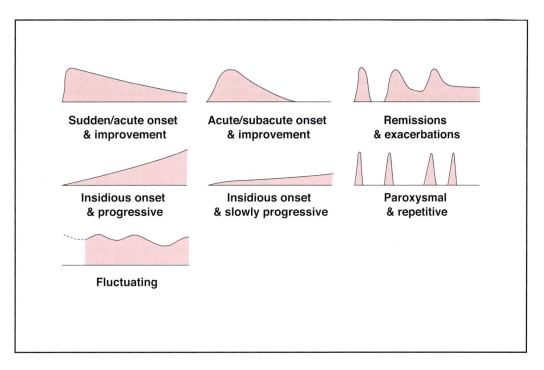

Figure 1-2 Mode of onset and the following clinical course of neurologic symptoms. The time course is shown on the horizontal axis, and the degree of symptoms/signs is shown on the vertical axis.

When the symptom reaches the maximal degree within a week, its mode of onset is defined as **acute**. Acute onset is commonly encountered in vascular diseases, inflammatory diseases, and acute poisoning. When the symptom occurs abruptly, its mode of onset is defined as **sudden**, which is commonly seen in embolism and subarachnoid hemorrhage. The conditions that start acutely tend to be followed by some **improvement** if properly diagnosed and treated. The prognosis of the conditions that start suddenly depends on the severity of the pathology. When the symptom reaches the maximum over a period of more than a week but less than four weeks after the clinical onset, its mode of onset is classified as **subacute**. This is commonly seen in inflammatory diseases or metabolic/toxic diseases. The above definition of categories for indicating the mode of onset is rather arbitrary, and it is actually important to describe the exact time in the medical history (Box 1).

When the symptom begins gradually and reaches the maximum over a period of more than a month, its mode of onset is called **insidious**. The following clinical course in this case is either **progressive** as seen in brain tumors, or **slowly progressive** as seen in neurodegenerative diseases. A **polyphasic** clinical course with **remissions and exacerbations** is typically seen in inflammatory demyelinating diseases such as multiple sclerosis. Repetition of short episodes

with intervals of variable length is seen in **paroxysmal** disorders such as epilepsy and migraine. Ion channel disorders such as periodic paralysis and episodic ataxia may also show this pattern of clinical course. A **fluctuating** clinical course is commonly seen in metabolic or endocrine encephalopathy. In the disorders showing paroxysmal or repetitive clinical course, the onset of each attack or each episode is usually sudden or acute.

When describing the history of the present illness, it is sometimes practical and useful to illustrate the mode of onset and the clinical course in a diagram showing the severity of each symptom in the vertical axis along the horizontally drawn time course, as shown in Figure 1-2. Since more than one symptom may appear in many diseases, illustration of the time course for each individual symptom will help in understanding the temporal relationship among different symptoms.

As described above, neurologic symptoms are either negative or positive. When indicating the severity of each symptom in the vertical axis of the illustration (Figure 1-2), a negative symptom or a neurologic deficit is usually correlated with the severity of the lesion or the tissue damage, but that is not necessarily the case for positive symptoms. This is because the positive symptoms may result from excessive excitation of the nervous system or loss of inhibition. Furthermore, some positive symptoms such as pain

ONSET OF NEUROLOGIC SYMPTOMS IN CEREBROVASCULAR DISEASES

Cerebral infarction is classified into atherothrombosis, lacunar infarction (see Box 3), and cardiogenic embolism. The type of infarctions can often be estimated from the clinical symptoms. In **cardiogenic embolism**, the initial neurologic symptom is completed suddenly all at once. Moreover, if the functions of cerebral regions supplied by different arteries are simultaneously impaired, this supports the diagnosis of cardiogenic embolism. **Atherothrombosis** is further classified into three types: thrombotic, embolic, and hemodynamic. The **hemodynamic** form tends to occur in the borderzone territory supplied by two large arteries, especially when the blood pressure drops (**watershed infarction**). Therefore, this form of infarction tends to be completed over a period of a few hours during sleep at night. The **embolic form of atherothrombosis** occurs when a blood clot is detached from the wall of a large artery and flows into its smaller branch to form an embolic infarction there. A typical example is occlusion of the ophthalmic artery by a blood clot originating from atherothrombosis of the internal carotid artery.

Intracerebral hemorrhage is sudden in onset, and the symptoms rapidly progress to cause loss of consciousness and headache. Hemorrhages are common in the putamen, thalamus, pons, and cerebellum, and subcortical hemorrhages are not uncommon. Lobar intracerebral hemorrhage is often caused by **amyloid angiopathy**. In this condition, there are β amyloid deposits in the wall of small arteries in the cortex and leptomeninges (Biffi & Greenberg, 2011, for review). Cerebral amyloid angiopathy may also be associated with MRI findings of lobar cerebral microbleeds, cortical superficial siderosis, and white matter hyperintensities (Charidimou et al, 2015). **Subarachnoid hemorrhage** is characterized by sudden onset of severe headache rapidly followed by loss of consciousness.

In cases of atypical stroke presenting with headache, disturbance of consciousness, and convulsion, **venous sinus thrombosis** has to be kept in mind. Small juxtacortical hemorrhages on CT image are characteristically seen in cerebral venous thrombosis (Coutinho et al, 2014).

and involuntary movements may also result from plastic changes of the nervous system during the process of functional restoration following an acute insult, as is typical following a stroke (see Chapter 30-3).

3. CLINICAL DIAGNOSIS

By considering the anatomical diagnosis and the etiological diagnosis throughout the process of history taking and neurologic examination as described above, the most likely sites of lesion and the most likely cause of the lesion can be combined together, which will help in reaching the most reasonable clinical diagnosis. In addition, a few additional conditions might emerge as candidates for the **differential diagnosis**. Of course, a number of conditions may come to mind as candidates for differential diagnosis during the history taking, but if the history is adequately obtained, the differential diagnosis is typically expected to be limited to two or three at most at the end of the history taking. An excessive list of differential diagnoses is not practical and may even disturb the smooth proceeding of neurologic examination and laboratory testing.

BIBLIOGRAPHY

Biffi A, Greenberg SM. Cerebral amyloid angiopathy: a systematic review. J Clin Neurol 7:1–9, 2011. (review)

Charidimou A, Linn J, Vernooij MW, Opherk C, Akoudad S, Baron JC, et al. Cortical superficial siderosis: detection and clinical significance in cerebral amyloid angiopathy and related conditions. Brain 138:2126–2139, 2015.

Coutinho JM, van den Berg R, Zuurbier SM, VanBavel E, Troost D, Majoie CB, et al. Small juxtacortical hemorrhages in cerebral venous thrombosis. Ann Neurol 75:908–916, 2014.

Osame M. Pathological mechanisms of human T-cell lymphotropic virus type I-associated myelopathy (HAM/TSP). J Neurovirol 8:359–364, 2002. (review)

Sato DK, Callegaro D, Lana-Peixoto MS, Waters PJ, de Haidar Jorge FM, Takahashi T, et al. Distinction between MOG antibody-positive and AQP4 antibody-positive NMO spectrum disorders. Neurology 82:474–481, 2014.

Takahashi T, Fujihara K, Nakashima I, Misu T, Miyazawa I, Nakamura M, et al. Anti-aquaporin-4 antibody is involved in the pathogenesis of NMO: a study on antibody titre. Brain 130:1235–1243, 2007.

Wingerchuk DM, Banwell B, Bennett JL, Cabre P, Carroll W, Chitnis T, et al. International consensus diagnostic criteria for neuromyelitis optica spectrum disorders. Neurology 85:177–189, 2015.

2.

HISTORY TAKING

History taking, if appropriately done, is expected to provide the most important information for reaching the correct neurologic diagnosis. Usually the history is obtained from the patient directly, but if the patient is unconscious, demented, aphasic, or uncooperative, the history has to depend on information obtained from the patient's family or accompanying persons. The information to be obtained when taking the medical history includes the present age, gender, chief complaints, the age at onset of symptoms, history of the present illness, past medical history, social history, and family history. When describing the medical history in the record or when presenting it in the medical conferences, it is customary and convenient to describe the information in the above order, but when actually taking the history, one does not always have to follow this sequence.

1. THE PRESENT AGE AND THE AGE AT ONSET

Each neurologic disease occurs in the population of a certain age range (Figure 2-1). However, as a consequence of recent advances in the understanding of pathogenesis and with change in the environment, it is increasingly recognized that there are exceptions to the age predilection. For example, ischemic cerebrovascular diseases that are common in the aged population can also occur in the young population (Box 2). Likewise, the paroxysmal disorders or the hereditary degenerative diseases that were thought to be common in children and young adults may occur for the first time in adults.

2. SEX

Many diseases are more common in one sex than in the other. The sex of the patient is usually obvious from his/her appearance and from the medical record, but if any uncertainty exists, it should be confirmed during the history taking. Sex is the biological designation of male/female, while "gender" refers to self identification.

3. CHIEF COMPLAINTS

Some physicians might believe that the chief complaints are symptoms the patient mainly complains of, but that is not always correct. A patient might mainly complain of a particular symptom at the time of the history taking, but that symptom might not be directly related to the neurologic disease that the patient is actually suffering from. It is important to determine the most important complaint(s) of that particular patient during the process of history taking. In this sense, to identify the chief complaint for a patient is to find what the main problem is for that patient, and thus it is a process of **problem-finding**. In the medical record or when presented in conferences, the chief complaint is usually described or reported before the history of the present illness, but in clinical practice, the most appropriate chief complaint(s) can be chosen after completing the history taking.

It is of utmost importance to find out what the real problem is for the patient and what he/she really means. For this purpose, it is not always advisable to describe exactly what the patient complains of; it is often necessary to interpret the patient's words with reference to medical knowledge. For example, a patient complaining of "numbness" in the hand usually means a sensory abnormality such as tingling or pinprick sensation, but some patients may use the word "numb" to express weakness. In this case, it is not sufficient to record just "numb" in the medical record; it should be further described as "weak." Patients commonly complain of dizziness, but some patients use the word "dizzy" when they feel like fainting,

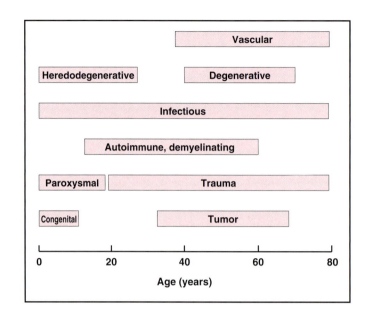

Figure 2-1 Common age at onset of neurologic diseases. Most neurologic diseases occur in the population of certain age range, but exceptional cases are not rare.

whereas others may use it to describe feeling unsteady with real vertigo. Thus, these two should be distinguished as much as possible by taking the history carefully (see Chapter 13-2).

When describing symptoms on the first page of the medical record, it is better not to use medical terminology. For example, when a patient complains of difficulty in speaking, it is not advisable to describe it as either "dysarthria" or "aphasia"; rather, it is much better to call it "speech disturbance." This is because the first impression might have to be changed later as a result of neurologic examination. However, when reporting in medical conferences or when writing a case report later, it

BOX 2 RISK FACTORS FOR VASCULAR DISEASES IN YOUNG POPULATION

Recently strokes in young populations have become increasingly common (Larrue et al, 2011; Aarnio et al, 2014). In addition to the common risk factors for vascular diseases such as diabetes mellitus, hypertension, hyperlipidemia, increased blood viscosity, obesity, and heavy smoking, special conditions have to be considered for young populations. Those are congenital heart disease, among others the patent foramen ovale associated with aneurysm of the atrial septum, atrial myxoma, positive antiphospholipid antibody, migraine with aura, use of contraceptives, eclampsia, systemic lupus erythematosus, Behçet disease, malignant atrophic papulosis, Degos disease, fibromuscular dysplasia, homocystinuria, Fabry disease (see Box 66), pseudoxanthoma elasticum, moyamoya disease, and mitochondrial encephalomyopathy (see Box 57) (see Chapter 3-1 for some of the skin abnormalities). **Homocystinuria** is due to lack of cystathionine synthetase and is inherited via autosomal recessive transmission. Clinically it is characterized by dislocation of lens and arachnodactylia similar to Marfan syndrome. **Moyamoya disease** is characterized by an extensive network of abnormal collaterals associated with occlusion of the proximal cerebral arteries (Albrecht et al, 2015; Al-Yassin et al, 2015). It causes ischemic attacks or convulsion in children and subarachnoid hemorrhage in adults. Physiologically, hyperventilation causes marked, prolonged slowing in EEG. **Mitochondrial encephalomyopathy, lactic acidosis and stroke-like episodes (MELAS)** is known to cause strokes at young ages (see Box 57). This condition also shows convulsions, migraine attacks, and mental retardation. Lactic acid is increased in the serum and cerebrospinal fluid, and ragged red fibers are seen on muscle biopsy. Recent use of drugs such as cocaine has drawn a particular attention to this behavior as a risk factor for strokes in the young population (Sordo et al, 2014).

THE NEUROLOGIC EXAMINATION

is reasonable to use the medical terminology. The chief complaint may not be single, and more than one symptom can be listed as chief complaints as necessary.

4. HISTORY OF THE PRESENT ILLNESS

When taking the history of the present illness, it is important to know how the symptom started and how it has changed since its onset. Patients may certainly have more than one symptom. Regardless of whether those symptoms are caused by a single disease or multiple diseases, mode of onset and clinical course should be carefully described for each individual symptom. In this case, it is convenient to illustrate the time course of each symptom in a diagram as shown in Figure 1-2.

For each symptom, it is also important to obtain information as to what time of the day, what season of the year, or in what kind of conditions it tends to occur or to worsen. Furthermore, it is useful to identify any precipitating factor that might bring up or increase the symptom or any factor that may help ameliorate the symptom.

If a patient reports that he/she has experienced a neurologic symptom in the past, it should be described in the history of the present illness if judged to be related to or a phase of the present illness, but it can be described in the past medical history if judged to be unrelated to the present illness. Likewise, if the present neurologic condition was judged to be caused by or to be a part of a systemic condition such as hypertension and diabetes mellitus, those systemic conditions should be described also in the history of the present illness. Other systemic conditions can be listed in the past medical history.

5. PAST MEDICAL HISTORY

Regarding the past medical history, how much detail is to be described in the medical record depends on the clinical situation, but all medical histories have to be recorded if they are judged to be related to the present illness. As a patient does not necessarily tell the physician all the past medical history, it may be necessary to ask specific questions to make sure certain topics are covered. For example, when the history of the present illness suggests a possibility of strokes, information about **risk factors for vascular diseases** including diabetes mellitus, hypertension, hyperlipidemia, history of cardiovascular diseases, and history of heavy smoking should be obtained as much as possible. Among cardiac arrhythmias, atrial fibrillation is known to be a leading cause of recurrent stroke. In particular, paroxysmal atrial fibrillation, which is also an important risk factor, may be detected only by a long-term ECG monitoring (Gladstone et al, 2014).

It is noteworthy that some infections might cause neurologic disorders a long time afterward. Typical examples are the occurrence of subacute sclerosing panencephalitis in adults following measles virus infection in childhood, and occurrence of myelitis as long as years after varicella zoster virus infection (**postherpetic myelitis**). In these cases, confirmation of the past medical history is important for the correct diagnosis.

6. SOCIAL HISTORY

The social history includes information about the patient's occupation, allergies, smoking, drinking, hobby, sports, and environmental situations at home and at the work place. Just like the past medical history, the necessary information of the social history depends on the history of the present illness. Since **handedness** is an important factor for higher cortical functions, it can be confirmed when taking the social history, although it may also be confirmed while carrying out the physical examination.

BOX 3 LACUNAR INFARCTION

A small infarction (less than 15 mm) in the territory supplied by a **penetrating arterial branch** in the deep cerebral hemisphere is called lacunar infarction. It mainly occurs in the corona radiata, internal capsule, thalamus, basal ganglia, and brainstem. Typical clinical manifestations are **pure motor hemiplegia** or **hemianesthesia without motor paralysis**, but it can be asymptomatic. An infrequent manifestation caused by lacunar infarction in the internal capsule or pons is "**dysarthria-clumsy hand syndrome**" (Arboix et al, 2004). An underlying pathology of lacunar infarction was believed to be lipohyalinosis of the penetrating arteries, which is commonly seen in hypertensive patients, but atherothrombosis at the bifurcation of a penetrating arterial branch from a main cerebral artery (**branch atheromatous disease**) has drawn more recent attention (Caplan, 1989). The latter condition in the internal capsule causes repetitive transient hemiparesis (capsular warning syndrome), and a similar condition of the lenticulostriatal artery and anterior pontine artery also causes progressive motor disturbance (Yamamoto et al, 2011).

7. FAMILY HISTORY

As many neurologic diseases are inherited, and as the background or precipitating factors might be genetically determined, information about the family is quite important in the history taking. Occurrence of similar diseases among the family members is important, and the history about consanguineous marriage in the patient's parents or in the grandparents is also important. When there is a possibility of familial conditions, it is useful to draw a family tree with the patient's permission.

BIBLIOGRAPHY

Aarnio K, Haapaniemi E, Melkas S, Kaste M, Tatlisumak T, Putaala J. Long-term mortality after first-ever and recurrent stroke in young adults. Stroke 45:2670–2676, 2014.

Albrecht P, Blasberg C, Lukas S, Ringelstein M, Müller A-K, Harmel J, et al. Retinal pathology in idiopathic moyamoya angiopathy detected by optical coherence tomography. Neurology 85:521–527, 2015.

Al-Yassin A, Saunders DE, Mackay MT, Ganesan V. Early-onset bilateral cerebral arteriopathies. Cohort study of phenotype and disease course. Neurology 85:1146–1153, 2015.

Arboix A, Bell Y, Garcia-Eroles L, Massons J, Comes E, Balcells M, et al. Clinical study of 35 patients with dysarthria-clumsy hand syndrome. J Neurol Neurosurg Psychiatry 75:231–234, 2004.

Biffi A, Greenberg SM. Cerebral amyloid angiopathy: a systematic review. J Clin Neurol 7:1–9, 2011. (review)

Caplan LR. Intracranial branch atheromatous disease: a neglected, understudied, and underused concept. Neurology 39:1246–1250, 1989.

Charidimou A, Martinez-Ramirez S, Shoamanesh A, Oliveira-Filho J, Frosch M, Vashkevich A, et al. Cerebral amyloid angiopathy with and without hemorrhage. Evidence for different disease phenotypes. Neurology 84:1206–1212, 2015.

Gladstone DJ, Spring M, Dorian P, Panzov V, Thorpe KE, Hall J, et al. Atrial fibrillation in patients with cryptogenic stroke. New Eng J Med 370:2467–2477, 2014.

Larrue V, Berhoune N, Massabuau P, Calviere L, Raposo N, Viguier A, et al. Etiologic investigation of ischemic stroke in young adults. Neurology 76:1983–1988, 2011.

Sordo L, Indave BI, Barrio G, Degenhardt L, de la Fuente L, Bravo MJ. Cocaine use and risk of stroke: a systematic review. Drug and Alcohol Dependence 142:1–13, 2014. (review)

Yamamoto Y, Ohara T, Hamanaka M, Hosomi A, Tamura A, Akiguchi I. Characteristics of intracranial branch atheromatous disease and its association with progressive motor deficits. J Neurol Sci 304:78–82, 2011.

3.

PHYSICAL EXAMINATION

1. GENERAL PHYSICAL EXAMINATION AND NEUROLOGIC EXAMINATION

Even in the specialty clinic of neurology, **general physical examination** is as important as **neurologic examination**, mainly because all health aspects are important for the patient and also because neurologic symptoms are often related to systemic diseases in terms of clinical manifestation and pathogenesis (Box 4).

The general physical examination and neurologic examination can be carried out separately in this order, but it is often more practical to carry out the two kinds of examination together. Otherwise, a series of examinations from the top of the head to the toes has to be repeated, which is not practical particularly when the time spent for each patient is limited in an outpatient clinic. Thus, when examining eyes, for example, we can check the cornea,

palpebral conjunctiva, bulbar conjunctiva, and ocular bulb first, and then we can examine the visual acuity, visual field, pupils, extraocular muscles, ocular movements, and ocular fundi if necessary. When examining the oral cavity, for another example, we check the mucosa of oral cavity and pharynx, teeth, tongue, and tonsils first, and then check the presence or absence of muscle atrophy and fasciculation, and movement of the tongue, position and movement of the soft palate, gag reflex if necessary, and voice, speech, and swallowing. This way, we do not have to come back to eyes or mouth after having completed the general physical examination. This approach is more efficient not only for neurologists but also for the patient's convenience.

A. GENERAL PHYSICAL EXAMINATION AT THE INITIAL CLINICAL EVALUATION

When examining each patient for the first time, the general physical examination usually includes observation of head, hair and facial skin, eyes (eyelids, cornea, palpebral and bulbar conjunctivae, and iris), ears and nose, oral mucosa, pharynx and tongue, neck (lymph nodes, thyroid, and vascular bruit if necessary), arterial pulse and blood pressure, chest (skin, respiration, percussion and auscultation of heart, and breast as necessary), abdomen (skin, percussion, palpation and percussion of liver, and bowel sound as necessary), and extremities (skin, joints, and edema) in this order. Pulsation of arteries is to be checked at the radial arteries bilaterally, and the dorsalis pedis arteries should also be palpated as necessary.

Skin Abnormalities Seen in Congenital or Hereditary Neurologic Diseases

Observation of skin is especially important when examining the patients with possible congenital neurologic diseases, because both the nervous system and the skin

---

BOX 4 CLINICAL NEUROLOGY FROM A WIDE VIEWPOINT

It is important to take a wide view throughout the diagnostic procedure of neurologic diseases. That is because the neurologic symptoms in question might be a manifestation of a systemic disease, like Crow-Fukase syndrome (polyneuropathy, organomegaly, endocrinopathy, M-protein and skin changes, PO-EMS). The neurologic symptom might be a complication of a systemic disease, like diabetic polyneuropathy. The neurologic symptom might have resulted from a systemic disease, like cerebrovascular diseases as a result of hypertension, hyperlipidemia and cardiac diseases. The neurologic disease might have common pathogenesis with a systemic disease, like paraneoplastic syndrome (Box 5). In bulbospinal muscular atrophy, as another example of this last category, the genetic abnormality of the androgen receptor might be related to the involvement of anterior horn cells (see Box 33). Approach to neurologic conditions with a wide view has contributed to discovery of some new neurologic diseases or to elucidation of their pathogenesis.

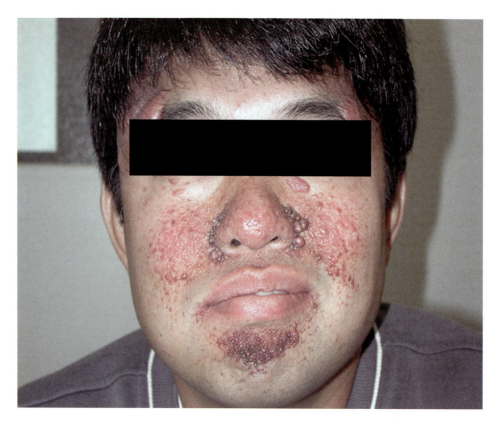

Figure 3-1 Facial angiofibroma seen in a patient with tuberous sclerosis. (Courtesy of Dr. Akio Ikeda, Kyoto University)

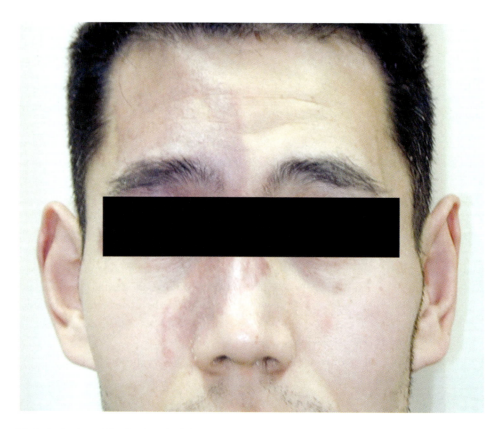

Figure 3-2 Port wine stain in the territory of the first branch of the right trigeminal nerve in a patient with Sturge-Weber syndrome. (Courtesy of Dr. Akio Ikeda, Kyoto University)

tissues are embryologically derived from the ectodermal cells. In **tuberous sclerosis**, a common cause of epilepsy in children, **facial angiofibroma** (adenoma sebaceum) is characteristic (Figure 3-1), but it is not seen at birth and appears later in infancy. In addition, the depigmented nevi, shagreen patch, and periungual fibroma may also be seen. Port wine stain in the territory of the first branch of the trigeminal nerve is seen in **Sturge-Weber syndrome**, which is also called encephalotrigeminal angiomatosis (Figure 3-2).

This condition may be associated with atrophy and calcification in the occipital cortex and angioma in the retina and meninges, and clinically it presents with convulsions. Xanthoma in the neck and axilla is seen in **pseudoxanthoma elasticum** (Grönblad-Strandberg syndrome), which may be associated with angioid streaks in the retina and cardiovascular disorders (Figure 3-3). **Ichthyosis** on the anterior aspect of lower legs may be associated with mental retardation and spastic gait (**Sjögren-Larsson**

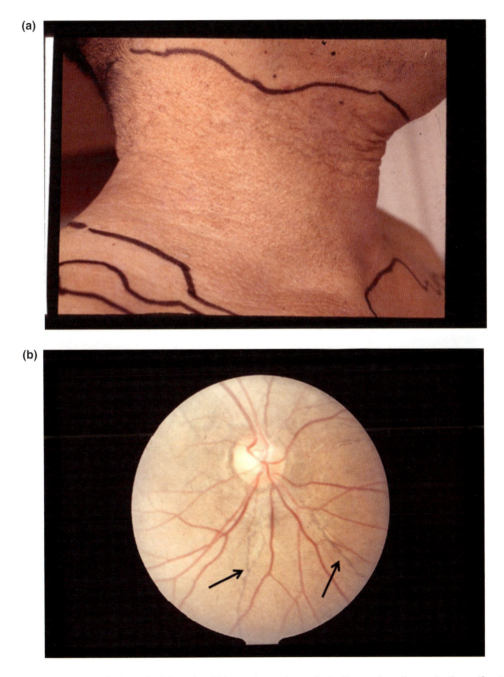

(a)

(b)

Figure 3-3 Cervical skin lesion (a) and angioid streak of the retina (b) (arrows) seen in a patient with pseudoxanthoma elasticum. (Courtesy of Department of Neurology, Kyushu University)

syndrome), and it is also a cardinal symptom of **Refsum disease**, which is characterized by sensory ataxia due to polyneuropathy, retinal pigment degeneration, and sensorineural deafness.

Neurofibromatosis is an autosomal dominant hereditary disease that is characterized by neurofibroma and café-au-lait spots (Figure 3-4). Neurofibromatosis is grouped into two types. NF-1 is called **von Recklinghausen disease**, and NF-2 is often associated with acoustic neurofibroma and multiple meningiomas. **Fabry disease** is a lipidosis due to X-linked deficiency of α-galactosidase and presents with angiokeratoma, anhidrosis, severe pain induced by exercise and fever, clouding of cornea and lens, and various kinds of vascular disorders (Lenders et al, 2015; Löhle et al, 2015) (see Box 66). In this condition, angiokeratoma may be seen only in the scrotum.

Livedo reticularis (livedo racemosa) (Figure 3-5) and acrocyanosis may be seen in patients with positive serum antibody against phospholipid, and it may cause transient ischemic attack and ischemic strokes (**Sneddon syndrome**) (Bottin et al, 2015). **Ehlers-Danlos syndrome** is a hereditary disease characterized by hyperelasticity of skin and hyperexensibility of joints due to abnormality of collagen fibers in the skin, blood vessels, and joint capsules (Figure 3-6). The mode of inheritance is variable, and it may also be associated with abnormalities in the peripheral nerves and muscles (Voermans et al, 2009).

Skin Abnormalities Seen in Inflammatory Neurologic Diseases

Some inflammatory diseases of the nervous system are associated with characteristic inflammatory diseases of the skin. Infection of the geniculate ganglion with varicella/zoster virus causes vesicular skin rash in the external auditory meatus and may be associated with facial nerve palsy (**geniculate zoster, Ramsay Hunt syndrome**) (Figure 3-7). Swelling of ear lobes is also seen in **relapsing polychondritis,** which may be associated with meningoencephalitis (see Box 95). **Behçet disease** is characterized by uveitis, painful oral ulcer (aphtha) and genital ulcer, and may also be associated with erythema nodosum (Figure 3-8) and purulent dermatitis at the site of needle injection. This disease is neurologically important because it may cause recurrent meningitis or encephalitis, or both. Uveitis, meningitis, and hearing loss may also be seen in Vogt-Koyanagi-Harada disease, but there is no skin lesion in this condition. **Sweet disease** is characterized by painful purulent erythema (Figure 3-9),

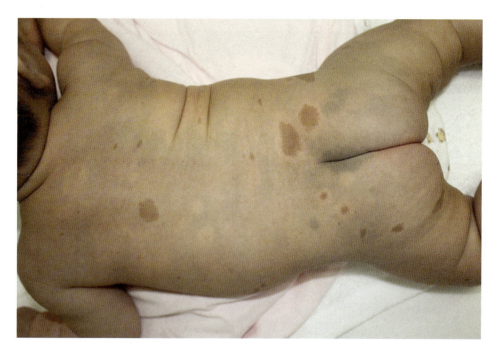

Figure 3-4 Café-au-lait spots seen in a patient with neurofibromatosis type 1. (Courtesy of Dr. Yumi Matsumura, Department of Dermatology, Kyoto University)

THE NEUROLOGIC EXAMINATION

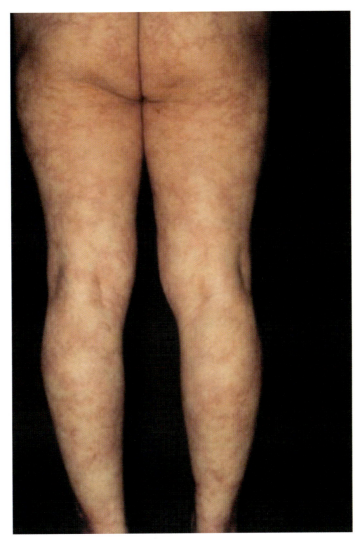

Figure 3-5 Livedo reticularis seen in a patient with Sneddon syndrome. (Courtesy of Dr. Yumi Matsumura, Department of Dermatology, Kyoto University)

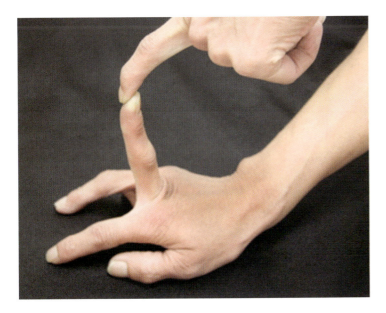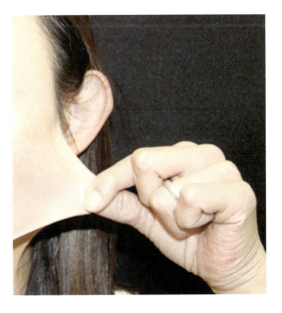

Figure 3-6 Hyperextensibility of joint and hyperelasticity of skin seen in a patient with Ehlers-Danlos syndrome. (Courtesy of Dr. Yumi Matsumura, Department of Dermatology, Kyoto University)

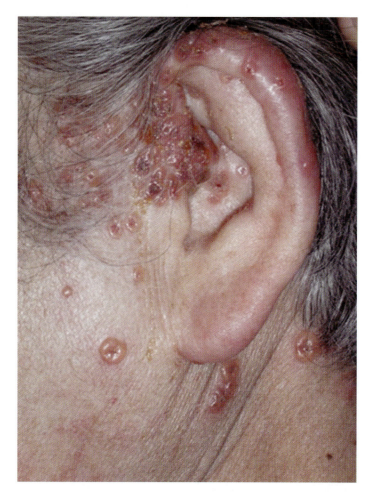

Figure 3-7 Geniculate zoster seen in a patient with Ramsay Hunt syndrome. (Courtesy of Dr. Yumi Matsumua, Department of Dermatology, Kyoto University)

fever, joint pain, leukocytosis, and elevated erythrocyte sedimentation rate. This condition is also known to cause recurrent meningoencephalitis or cerebral vasculitis (Charlson et al, 2015). About 25% of the patients with this condition have been reported to develop leukemia, lymphoma, or cancer. **Degos disease** (malignant atrophic papulosis) is characterized by red necrotic papules in the trunk and extremities, which will evolve to be white in color and squamous. This condition can be associated with thrombosis in the skin, gastrointestinal tract, and central nervous system. Polymyositis (see Chapter 16-3C) might be associated with various erythema over the dorsum of the fingers, and the bony parts of the shoulders, elbows, and legs (**dermatomyositis**).

Brownish discoloration of skin, hypertrichosis, and edema are seen in association with osteosclerotic plasmacytoma, and this condition is known as **polyneuropathy, organomegaly, endocrinopathy, M-protein, and skin changes (POEMS, Crow-Fukase syndrome)** (Figure 3-10). In this condition, vascular endothelial growth factor (VEGF) is markedly elevated in the serum. Significant improvement of neurologic symptoms by peripheral blood stem cell transplantation has been reported in this condition (Kuwabara et al, 2008; Karam et al, 2015) (Box 5).

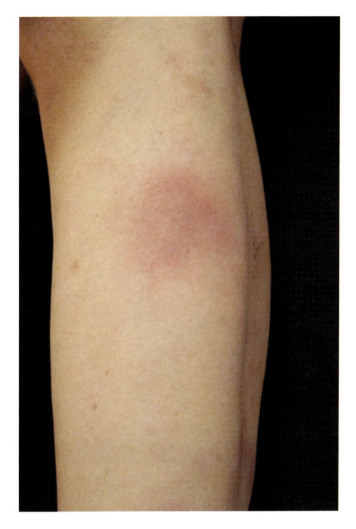

Figure 3-8 Erythema nodosum seen in a patient with myelodysplastic syndrome. (Courtesy of Dr. Yumi Matsumura, Department of Dermatology, Kyoto University)

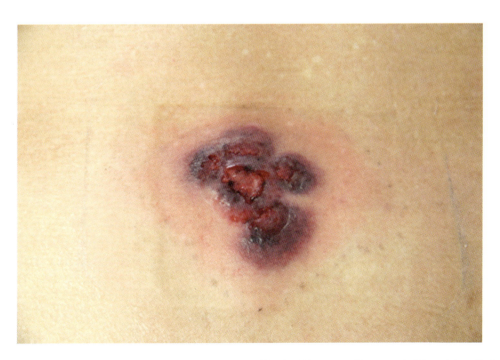

Figure 3-9 Purulent erythema seen in a patient with Sweet disease. (Courtesy of Dr. Yumi Matsumura, Department of Dermatology, Kyoto University)

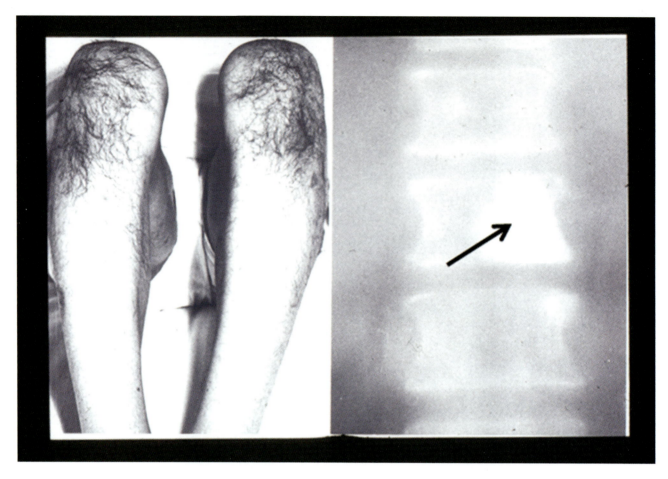

Figure 3-10 Hypertrichosis (left) and osteosclerotic plasmacytoma of the spine (right, see arrow) seen in a patient with POEMS. (Courtesy of Department of Neurology, Kyushu University)

INFLAMMATORY DISEASES OF THE NERVOUS SYSTEM

Causes of inflammatory diseases of the nervous system are grouped into **infection** and **autoimmunity** for both the central and peripheral nervous systems. The infectious group is caused by direct infection of the nervous system by bacteria or virus. Most of the autoimmune inflammatory disorders of the nervous system are caused by the nervous tissue itself as the antigen, but some of them are caused by the connective tissue as the antigen, as in vasculitis. In the former group, the symptoms occur in association with infections (**parainfectious**), or they occur a week or two after the infections (**postinfectious**), as in acute disseminated encephalomyelitis (ADEM) and Guillain-Barré syndrome. A special group of autoimmune neurologic diseases is the **paraneoplastic syndrome,** which is not due to direct invasion of the nervous system by a tumor but due to an autoimmune process against the neoplastic tissue, which is thought to share a common antigen with the nervous system. Clinically a paraneoplastic syndrome is manifested as inflammation like limbic encephalitis and dermatomyositis, neurodegeneration, or ion channel disorders (see Chapter 25-2).

Skin Abnormalities Seen in Toxic Neurologic Diseases

Intoxication with some heavy metals shows characteristic skin changes. Alopecia is characteristically seen in **thallium poisoning**, which results from oral ingestion of an organophosphate insecticide thallium and causes unconsciousness due to strong inhibition of cholinesterase in the acute phase and polyneuropathy mainly involving the autonomic nervous system in the chronic phase (Figure 3-11-a). Keratosis of skin, pigmentation, and white horizontal line on the nail (**Mees line**) are seen in intoxication with thallium and **arsenic** (Figure 3-11-b).

Sunlight Photosensitivity of Skin

In this condition, skin rash is either induced or worsened by exposure to sunlight. It is seen in systemic diseases including systemic lupus erythematosus, porphyria, niacin deficiency (pellagra), xeroderma pigmentosum, and Cockayne disease. **Xeroderma pigmentosum** is an autosomal recessive hereditary disease that clinically manifests marked sunlight

THE NEUROLOGIC EXAMINATION

(a)

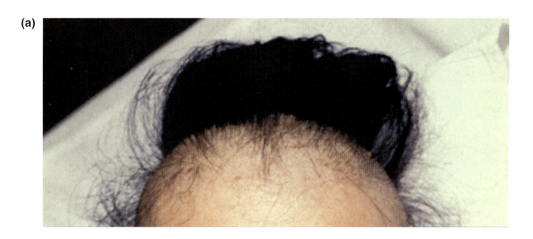

(b)

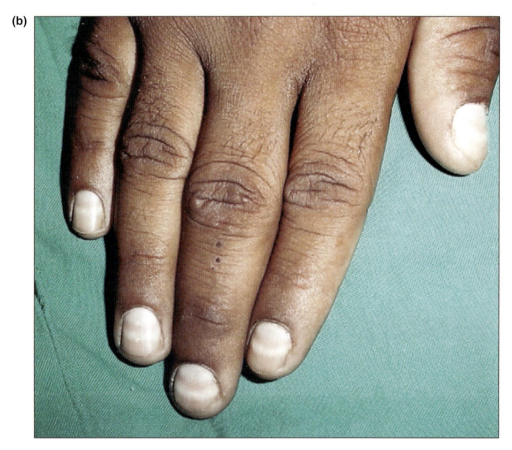

Figure 3-11 (a) Alopecia seen in a patient with thallium poisoning (Courtesy of Department of Neurology, Kyushu University) and (b) Mees line seen in the finger nails (reproduced from Chauhan et al, 2008 with permission).

photosensitivity of skin from infancy (Figure 3-12). It is associated with progressive decline of intellectual and other neurologic functions (**De Sanctis-Cacchione syndrome**). In this condition, abnormality of a repairing mechanism of the damaged DNA has been reported (Anttinen et al, 2008). **Cockayne disease** is also an autosomal recessive hereditary disease, and it is clinically characterized by dwarfism, micrognathia, retinal pigment degeneration, marked sunlight photosensitivity, mental retardation, deafness, and progressive

spastic and ataxic gait, which start appearing before the age of 2 years.

Abnormalities of Oral Cavity Seen in Neurologic Diseases

In case there is any possibility of **Behçet disease**, the oral cavity should be carefully checked for **aphtha**, typically white small ulcers (Figure 3-13). In the patients

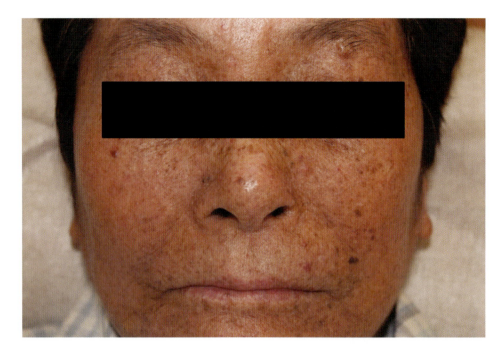

Figure 3-12 Sunlight photosensitivity of skin in a patient with xeroderma pigmentosum. (Courtesy of Dr. Yumi Matsumura, Department of Dermatology, Kyoto University)

with **pellagra** due to niacin deficiency, ruby erythema of tongue is seen in addition to diarrhea, dermatitis, dementia, and polyneuropathy. Abnormally enlarged tongue (**macroglossia**) is seen in Down syndrome, primary amyloidosis, and acromegaly. If there is any scar on the tongue due to a bite, it suggests the presence of vigorous involuntary movements, convulsion involving the mouth, or self-mutilation. **Tongue bite** due to severe choreic movements is seen in **neuroacanthocytosis** (chorea-acanthocytosis, Levine-Critchley syndrome) (Figure 3-14). Typical example of tongue self-mutilation is **Lesch-Nyhan syndrome,** which shows hyperuricemia

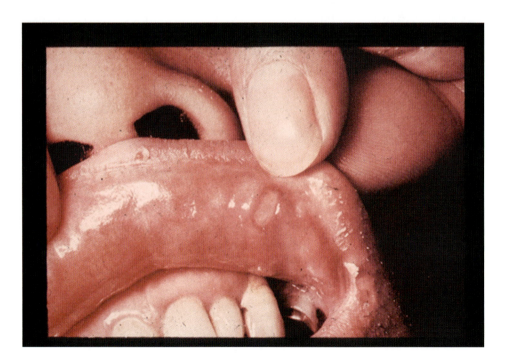

Figure 3-13 Aphthous ulcer of oral mucosa seen in a patient with Behçet disease. (Courtesy of Department of Neurology, Kyushu University)

THE NEUROLOGIC EXAMINATION

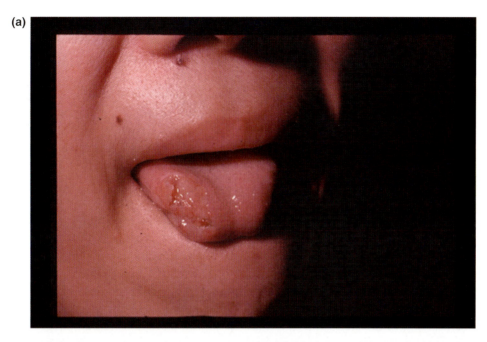

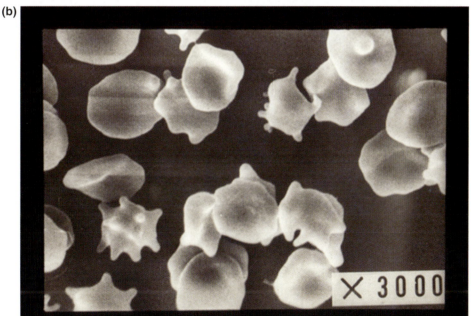

Figure 3-14 Tongue bite (a) and acanthocytes (b) seen in a patient with neuroacanthocytosis. (Courtesy of Department of Neurology, Kyushu University)

and gout due to the inherited (X-linked) lack of hypoxanthine phosphoribosyltransferase.

B. GENERAL PHYSICAL FINDINGS AND NEUROLOGIC FINDINGS

As explained at the beginning of this chapter, it is practical to carry out the general physical examination and the neurologic examination as a single block of physical examination. However, when describing those findings in the medical record, reporting in case reports or presenting in medical conferences, it is useful to describe the general physical findings first and then the neurologic findings. In this regard, it is important to keep in mind that the general physical findings are not just those dealt with in internal medicine, but it is necessary to include all findings related to other specialties such as ophthalmology, otorhinolaryngology, oral and dental health, dermatology, orthopedics, urology, and gynecology.

2. STEPS OF NEUROLOGIC EXAMINATION

Neurologic findings are usually described or reported in the following order: consciousness; mental or intellectual functions; aphasia, apraxia, and agnosia, if any; brainstem and cranial nerve territories; neck; trunk; motor system of extremities; tendon reflexes and pathological reflexes; somatosensory functions; posture and gait; autonomic nervous functions; and disturbance of daily activities. When we perform the neurologic examination, however, we do not have to follow this order. In many cases, it is more convenient and practical to adjust to the actual situation with flexibility.

In any case, it is useful to start with evaluation of consciousness. In most cases, disturbance of consciousness, mental or intellectual abnormalities, and language abnormality, if any, can be suspected during the history taking. If any abnormality in the higher cortical functions is suspected, they may be tested in detail after completing the physical examination. In the ordinary situation, it is more practical to do the physical examination first and to test the higher cortical functions later in the course of examination, mainly because it is rather embarrassing for the patient to go through a series of questions about intelligence and language from the beginning and also because it spends a relatively long time before carrying out the physical examination. Furthermore, abnormalities of the higher cortical functions are usually noticed during the physical examination, because verbal communication with the patient is necessary for the physical examination. Moreover, a more comfortable relationship can be established between the patient and the physician through the course of physical examination. In this book, therefore, the following chapters are arranged in the actual order of the physical neurologic examination, starting from the consciousness and immediately moving to the brainstem and cranial nerve functions, and the examination of mental and higher cortical functions will be described after all the chapters related to the physical examination. Furthermore, examination of patients with coma will be described toward the end of the book because the knowledge about the whole physical examination is necessary for the physical examination of comatose patients.

If the history is effectively taken, responsible sites of lesion, possible pathogenesis or etiology, and the most likely clinical diagnosis can be estimated before starting the physical examination. Therefore, although the neurologic examination is executed in the order as described above, an emphasis is placed on certain aspects depending on the above information obtained from the history taking (**hypothesis-driven neurologic examination**) (Kamel et al, 2011).

When carrying out the neurologic examination of extremities and trunk, the order of examination can be freely chosen depending on the circumstances. When a patient is examined in the supine position, it is more practical to examine the functions of all four extremities at once. By contrast, when a patient is examined in the sitting position, the upper extremities and the lower extremities may be examined separately. At any rate, stressful burden and uncomfortable maneuvers for the patient should be limited to the minimum necessary.

As structure and function of the nervous system are symmetrically formed between the left and right with exception of some higher cortical functions and the peripheral autonomic nervous system, it is important to pay attention to **symmetry** of neurologic signs throughout the neurologic examination. However, there may be some asymmetry in the homologous muscles in volume and strength depending on the occupation of or sports played by the patient.

The purpose of the neurologic examination is to confirm the neurologic condition that was thought to be most likely based on the careful history taking, and to exclude the candidate diagnoses listed as the differential diagnosis. Finally, it is of utmost importance to judge the level of **activities of daily living** and to estimate possible prognosis of the present condition.

BIBLIOGRAPHY

Anttinen A, Koulu L, Nikoskelainen E, Portin R, Kurki T, Erkinjuntti M, et al. Neurological symptoms and natural course of xeroderma pigmentosum. Brain 131:1979–1989, 2008.

Bottin L, Francès C, de Zuttere D, Boëlle P-Y, Muresan I-P, Alamowitch S. Strokes in Sneddon syndrome without antiphospholipid antibodies. Ann Neurol 77:817–829, 2015.

Charlson R, Kister I, Kaminnetzky D, Shvartsbeyn M, Meehan SA, Mikolaenko I. CNS neutrophilic vasculitis in neuro-Sweet disease. Neurology 85:829–830, 2015.

Chauhan S, D'Cruz S, Singh R, Sachdev A. Mees' lines. Lancet 372:1410, 2008.

Kamel H, Dhaliwal G, Navi BB, Pease AR, Shah M, Dhand A, et al. A randomized trial of hypothesis-driven vs screening neurologic examination. Neurology 77:1395–1400, 2011.

Karam C, Klein CJ, Dispenzieri A, Dyck PJB, Mandrekar J, D'Souza A, et al. Polyneuropahy improvement following autologous stem cell transplantation for POEMS syndrome. Neurology 84:1981–1987, 2015.

Kondo T, Fukuta M, Takemoto A, Takami Y, Sato M, Takahashi N, et al. Limbic encephalitis associated with relapsing polychondritis responded to infliximab and maintained its condition without recurrence after discontinuation: a case report and review of the literature. Nagoya J Med Sci 76:361–368, 2014.

Kuwabara S, Misawa S, Kanai K, Suzuki Y, Kikkawa Y, Sawai S, et al. Neurologic improvement after peripheral blood stem cell transplantation in POEMS syndrome. Neurology 71:1691–1695, 2008.

Lenders M, Karabul N, Duning T, Schmitz B, Schelleckes M, Mesters R, et al. Thromboembolic events in Fabry disease and the impact of factor V Leiden. Neurology 84:1009–1016, 2015.

Löhle M, Hughes D, Milligan A, Richfield L, Reichmann H, Mehta A, et al. Clinical prodromes of neurodegeneration in Anderson-Fabry disease. Neurology 84:1454–1464, 2015.

Voermans NC, van Alfen N, Pillen S, Lammens M, Schalkwijk J, Zwarts MJ, et al. Neuromuscular involvement in various types of Ehlers-Danlos syndrome. Ann Neurol 65:687–697, 2009.

4.

EVALUATION OF CONSCIOUSNESS

Consciousness is defined as the state of waking with subjects being aware of self and the environment. Namely, when subjects are fully conscious, they can pay attention to the external environment, accept the information and respond by language or behavior. Regarding the response by language or behavior, however, cases suffering from neurological deficits such as aphasia and motor paralysis are exceptions. A typical example is the locked-in syndrome, which is described later in this chapter.

1. ANATOMICAL BASIS OF CONSCIOUSNESS

It is generally believed that a critical center for the production of consciousness is in the **brainstem reticular formation**. The brainstem reticular formation is a poorly demarcated gray matter structure situated in the dorsal part of the brainstem extending longitudinally through the whole length of the brainstem. Which parts of the reticular formation are most critical is not known. The brainstem reticular formation is formed by a large number of neurons and their projections. It receives inputs from various ascending afferent fibers and projects ascending fibers to the intralaminar thalamic nucleus and then widely to the cerebral cortex through **the diffuse thalamocortical projection system** (Figure 4-1). This **ascending reticular activating system** activates activities of the cerebral cortex. Therefore, if the reticular formation is damaged, the cerebral cortex becomes unable to be activated; as a result, it is unable to pay attention to or receive the external information and to respond by language or behavior (**unconsciousness**). The brainstem reticular formation also sends fiber projections to the spinal cord, various nuclei of the brainstem, and the cerebellum for controlling muscle tone and postural adjustment. Multiple neurotransmitters,

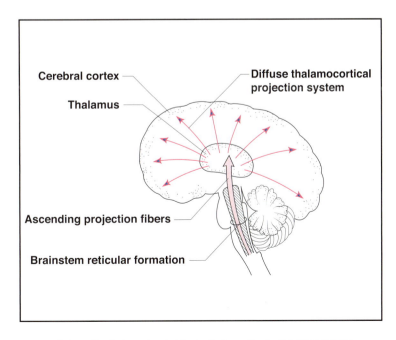

Figure 4-1 Schematic diagram showing the brainstem reticular formation and the thalamocortical activating system.

including acetylcholine, noradrenalin, dopamine, and serotonin, are known to take part in the activities of the reticular formation.

2. MECHANISMS OF DISTURBANCES OF CONSCIOUSNESS

Consciousness is impaired as the result of functional loss of neurons of the reticular formation through two mechanisms. One is the loss of excitability of the neurons due to a decrease or loss of excitatory postsynaptic potentials (EPSP) resulting in inability to generate action potentials. The other is a loss of neuronal activity due to their excessive discharge or hyperexcitability. An example of the first mechanism is tissue damage of the reticular formation due to ischemia, hemorrhage, inflammation, mechanical/traumatic injury, and cerebral herniation, and a typical example of the second mechanism is epilepsy.

As regards ischemic damage of the brainstem reticular formation, unconsciousness may result from two different types of ischemia. One is a decrease or loss of blood flow due to ischemia of the vertebrobasilar artery territory that directly supplies arterial blood to the reticular formation (Box 6). The other is a decreased supply of blood or oxygen to the whole brain due to cardiac or respiratory failure or a sudden decrease in blood pressure (shock). Loss of consciousness due to the latter mechanism is called **syncope**. Thus, **transient loss of consciousness** is caused by transient ischemic attack in the vertebrobasilar artery territory, syncope due to hypoperfusion or hypoxia, or epileptic attacks.

Syncope

Syncope is known to occur in at least six specific conditions (Table 4-1). Therefore, precise history taking is critical for the correct diagnosis (Box 7). Usually the attack of syncope starts with loss of ability to think clearly, followed by fixation of eyes in the midline, loss of facial expression, constriction of the visual field, blackout, inability to hear, and finally loss of consciousness (Wieling et al, 2009). The whole process may be completed within several seconds. In general, patients with hypoxia due to chronic pulmonary diseases or with anemia due to hematological diseases tend to suffer from syncope, and this is especially so for elderly patients.

3. OBSERVATION OF THE STATE OF CONSCIOUSNESS

Usually, the state of consciousness can be accurately evaluated while taking the history from the patient. Actually, evaluation of the patients with consciousness disturbance starts from the time when the examiner approaches the patient. If the patient pays attention to the examiner and greets verbally or behaviorally, the consciousness level is considered to be alert or only mildly impaired. In case the patient does not pay attention to the examiner, his/her attention should be aroused by calling his/her name or by giving various stimuli (see the next section). Since the consciousness level tends to change from moment to moment, it is important to observe the patient repeatedly along the

---

BOX 6 SUBCLAVIAN STEAL SYNDROME

A **steal phenomenon** is a cause of transient ischemic attack due to stealing of blood flow from a large artery supplying the nervous system into the contracting muscles, and the subclavian steal syndrome is its typical example. In this condition, the patient develops vertigo, unsteadiness, and clouding of consciousness when he/she moves an upper limb. In the background of this particular condition, there is stenosis or occlusion of the subclavian artery proximal to the bifurcation of the vertebral artery, and the muscle activity of the upper limb supplied by the subclavian artery steals its blood supply from the vertebral artery territory, causing poor perfusion in the brainstem supplied by the vertebral artery. The subclavian steal syndrome is more common in association with the movement of the left upper limb, because the left vertebral artery bifurcates from the left subclavian artery after the latter bifurcates directly from the aortic arch while the right vertebral artery bifurcates from the right subclavian artery soon after it bifurcates from the brachiocephalic artery. Some form of intermittent claudication is also caused by a steal mechanism (see Box 72).

TABLE 4-1 ETIOLOGICAL CLASSIFICATION OF SYNCOPE

1. Cardiac syncope
2. Orthostatic hypotension
3. Vasovagal syncope
4. Carotid sinus hypersensitivity
5. Micturition syncope
6. Cough syncope

Syncope is caused by six different conditions (Table 4-1). **Cardiac syncope**, also called **Stokes-Adams syndrome**, is due to transient loss of blood flow due to arrhythmia or cardiac arrest. In this condition, clonic movements might be seen, which necessitates distinction from epileptic attacks. Although cardiac arrest might occur as a result of epilepsy, the distinction is not difficult from the past history and the EEG. **Orthostatic hypotension** is a common cause of syncope, which will be explained in relation to the autonomic nervous system (Chapter 20). **Vasovagal syncope** is caused by a sudden reflex elevation of vagal nerve function resulting in hypotension. This condition may be encountered even in healthy subjects when, for example, exposed to severe pain. **Carotid sinus hypersensitivity** is seen in patients whose baroreceptors of the carotid sinus are pathologically sensitive. In this condition, a mechanical stimulus like massage to the anterior neck tends to cause hypotension (Chapter 20).

Micturition syncope occurs during or immediately after micturition due to a sudden decrease of intra-abdominal pressure followed by a reflex decrease of cardiac output. This phenomenon may be seen even in healthy subjects after heavy drinking, but the repetitive occurrence of this condition suggests abnormality of the autonomic nervous system. **Cough syncope** occurs after vigorous coughing, which causes a sudden increase of the intrathoracic pressure, like the Valsalva maneuver, and reflex excitation of the vagal nerve causing hypotension.

clinical course. In elderly patients in particular, it should be kept in mind that the consciousness level tends to change depending on general conditions like hydration, nutrition, blood count, and respiratory function.

4. MODES OF CONSCIOUSNESS DISTURBANCE AND THE COMA SCALE

Disturbances of consciousness can be classified into two types. One is a decrease in the level of consciousness (**clouding of consciousness**) and the other is manifested as a language or behavioral abnormality (**alteration of consciousness**). Clouding of consciousness is grouped into four categories according to degree.

Somnolence: The consciousness level is decreased if the patient is left alone.

Stupor: The patient can be aroused by strong stimulus and moves for a short period of time.

Semicoma: The patient can respond to a strong stimulus only with simple movements.

Coma: No response at all, even to strong stimulus.

There are various ways for grading the level of consciousness disturbance; the Glasgow Coma Scale and Japan Coma Scale are presented here. In the Glasgow Coma Scale (Table 4-2), the alert condition (normal) is graded 15 and deep coma is graded 3. In the Japan Coma Scale (Table 4-3), disturbance of consciousness is graded into 9 degrees, ranging from score 1 (mildly impaired) to score 300 (deep coma).

Alteration of Consciousness and Delirium

When alteration of consciousness is associated with psychomotor agitation, hallucination, and delusion in addition to the clouding of consciousness, the condition is called **delirium**. Delirium of acute onset is often seen in **acute confusional states**. The state of delirium is often

TABLE 4-2 THE GLASGOW COMA SCALE

EYE OPENING	
Open spontaneously	4
Open only to verbal stimuli	3
Open only to pain	2
Never open	1
BEST VERBAL RESPONSE	
Oriented and converses	5
Converses, but disoriented, confused	4
Uses inappropriate words	3
Makes incomprehensible sounds	2
No verbal response	1
BEST MOTOR RESPONSE	
Obeys commands	6
Localizes pain	5
Exhibits flexion withdrawal	4
Decorticate rigidity	3
Decerebrate rigidity	2
No motor response	1

TABLE 4-3 THE JAPAN COMA SCALE

GRADE I SPONTANEOUSLY AROUSED
1. Slightly unclear.
2. Poorly oriented in time, place, or person.
3. Unable to tell the patient's own name and date of birth.

GRADE II AROUSED BY STIMULUS
10. Opens eyes easily by verbal call.
20. Opens eyes in response to loud call or shaking body.
30. Barely opens eyes by painful stimulus plus repetitive calling.

GRADE III NOT AROUSED EVEN BY STIMULUS
100. Responds to painful stimulus by throw off.
200. Responds to painful stimulus by small movements or facial grimacing.
300. No response to painful stimulus.

TABLE 4-4 ETIOLOGICAL CLASSIFICATION OF ACUTE ENCEPHALOPATHY

1. Toxic encephalopathy
1. Ethanol and its related disorders
Wernicke encephalopathy (Box 74)
Alcoholic pellagra encephalopathy
2. Pharmaceutical drugs
Intoxication due to sleeping drugs
Serotonin syndrome
3. Carbon monoxide intoxication
4. Heavy metal intoxication: arsenics, lead
5. Intoxication due to organic solvents: trichloroethylene
6. Insecticide poisoning: organophosphate
2. Metabolic encephalopathy: hyperglycemia, hypoglycemia, hepatic failure, renal failure, electrolyte abnormalities
3. Anoxic encephalopathy
4. Hypertensive encephalopathy

associated with tremulous or fumbling movements of hands (**delirium tremens**). This condition is commonly seen in acute ethanol poisoning, drug intoxication, and metabolic encephalopathy. In this regard, it is quite important to draw a blood sample from a patient in the acute stage and save it for a later laboratory test to measure the blood level of possible drugs. As the selective serotonin reuptake inhibitors (SSRIs) are often used for the treatment of depression, **serotonin syndrome** is not infrequently seen. The serotonin syndrome manifests shaking of the legs, restlessness, fever, confusion, visual hallucinations, excessive sweating, and tachycardia.

The state of acute clouding or alteration of consciousness without any gross organic lesion in the brain is called **acute encephalopathy**. As this condition is due to a number of different causes, as listed in Table 4-4, careful history taking and the general physical examination play an important part in its diagnosis.

5. CONDITIONS THAT SHOULD BE DISTINGUISHED FROM CLOUDING OF CONSCIOUSNESS

Some special conditions may resemble disturbance of consciousness and need to be distinguished. Those are deep sleep, advanced stage of dementia, akinetic mutism, catatonic stupor, and locked-in syndrome. Needless to say, the patient under general anesthesia induced for the medical purpose is comatose.

Deep Sleep

Usually it is not difficult to distinguish sleep from coma, but in some cases, especially after sleep deprivation or after taking sleeping drugs, deep sleep may be confused with disturbance of consciousness. The subject in ordinary sleep can be completely aroused by verbal calling or other stimuli, and can maintain the aroused state for some time, but the subject under special conditions may easily fall back to sleep soon after being awakened. On the other hand, even a patient with mild consciousness disturbance may remain foggy at least for a minute or so after being aroused. This condition is called **lethargy**. The electroencephalogram (EEG) might help distinguish between sleep and disturbance of consciousness. The EEG activities specific for sleep, like vertex sharp waves (V waves) and sleep spindles, may be seen during sleep, and the subject shows the posterior dominant rhythm of α frequency after being aroused. In contrast, those sleep-specific EEG activities are not seen in patients with consciousness disturbance, and the background EEG activity is abnormal even when the patient appears awake. Observation of daily activities provides useful information for the diagnosis of consciousness disturbance.

Advanced Stage of Dementia

The patient with marked dementia due to diffuse cerebral damage of severe degree cannot pay attention to the external environment and is unable to accept information and respond. This condition corresponds to a state of **inattention** and **apathy**, and is encountered in the recovery phase from acute encephalitis or anoxic encephalopathy of severe degree, and at the terminal stage of Creutzfeldt-Jakob disease and Alzheimer disease. Distinction of this condition from consciousness disturbance is not difficult from the information about the clinical course and other neurologic findings, and the laboratory tests including EEG and neuroimaging will provide supplementary information. The sleep-wakefulness cycle is usually maintained in the patient with severe dementia, whereas it is lost or disrupted in the patient with consciousness disturbance. Furthermore, in patients with severe brain lesions, motor abnormalities such as spastic quadriplegia, dystonia, and Gegenhalten (Chapter 16-3D) are commonly seen.

Akinetic Mutism

In this condition, the eyes are open and blinks and spontaneous ocular movements are seen during the daytime, but the patient cannot direct his/her gaze to, recognize, or respond to even familiar persons. Spontaneous movements are almost absent or very few. However, the patient usually can chew and swallow food once it is put into the mouth. The sleep-wakefulness cycle is relatively well preserved, and functions of the autonomic nervous system and the endocrine system are normally preserved. Thus, the prolonged state of this condition is called **vegetative state**.

Akinetic mutism was originally reported by Cairns et al. in 1941 in a patient with an epidermoid cyst of the third ventricle (Cairns et al, 1941), but akinetic mutism is more commonly encountered in association with diffuse cortical lesions or diffuse white matter lesions that functionally disconnect the cerebral cortex from the deep gray matter. These conditions correspond to the decorticate state or **apallic syndrome** (German: das apallisches Syndrom). The **decorticate state** is often associated with decorticate rigidity and spastic quadriplegia. In **decorticate posture**, the upper limbs are flexed due to increased muscle tone in the flexors and the lower limbs are extended due to increased muscle tone in the extensors. In akinetic mutism due to lesions around the third ventricle, the cerebral cortex is considered to be disconnected from the limbic cortex, and physical signs like spastic quadriplegia are few if any. Akinetic mutism might be transiently seen in the recovery phase from anoxic encephalopathy, but this condition should be distinguished from the vegetative state.

It is often claimed that akinetic mutism has been mistaken as brain death, but the distinction is not difficult as far as brain death is correctly defined. Namely, brainstem functions are fully intact in akinetic mutism, whereas all neurons including the brainstem neurons are irreversibly damaged in brain death (Chapter 29-6).

Catatonic Stupor

This condition is similar to akinetic mutism in that the patient keeps the eyes open and there are no spontaneous movements or response to verbal call or stimuli. It is characterized by the fact that, once the upper limb is passively lifted, the patient maintains that posture (**catatonia, waxy flexibility**). Furthermore, the patient may recall some of the events that have happened during the unresponsive episode, if asked later. Catatonic stupor usually occurs during the clinical course of psychosis or during neuroleptic medication, but in some cases its cause is undetermined. In contrast with akinetic mutism, catatonic stupor is not associated with any organic lesion in the brain even on conventional neuroimaging. Usually it spontaneously improves over a period of several days, but some patients may respond to

---

BOX 8 **LOCKED-IN SYNDROME**

Locked-in syndrome is totally different from clouding of consciousness or akinetic mutism, because the patient under this condition is just unable to express him/her-self because of the total motor paralysis in spite of the intact mental functions. A typical example of this condition is complete tetraplegia due to an infarction of the bilateral pontine basis as a result of the basilar artery occlusion, which interrupts the corticobulbar and corticospinal tracts bilaterally. However, as the vertical gaze center and the oculomotor nucleus in the midbrain are spared in most cases, the patient can still elevate the upper eyelid and move the eyes vertically (see Chapter 9-1, 9-2). Horizontal eye movements are lost because the horizontal gaze center is located in the pontine tegmentum. Furthermore, as the functions of the brainstem tegmentum including the reticular formation and the ascending sensory pathways are preserved in this condition, the patient can understand the environment and spoken language.

In fact, locked-in syndrome may also occur in the advanced stage of motor neuron disease and in the acute phase of severe Guillain-Barré syndrome, in which all the voluntary muscles including the extraocular muscles may be completely paralyzed.

benzodiazepine administration. Among the organic brain lesions, catatonic stupor has been reported in patients with multiple sclerosis showing diffuse demyelinating lesions in the cerebral white matter. This case, however, must be distinguished from akinetic mutism.

Locked-in Syndrome

This condition is totally different from the conditions already described, such as clouding of consciousness and akinetic mutism, but it may cause misunderstanding on the side of the patient's family and even the physician. In this condition, consciousness is entirely clear, and sensory and cognitive functions are well preserved. Therefore, conversation at the bedside should be done with great caution (Box 8).

BIBLIOGRAPHY

Cairns H, Oldfield RC, Pennybacker JB, Whitteridge D. Akinetic mutism with an epidermod cyst of the 3rd ventricle. Brain 64:273–290, 1941.

Wieling W, Thijs RD, van Dijk N, Wilde AA, Benditt DG, van Dijk JG. Symptoms and signs of syncope: a review of the link between physiology and clinical clues. Brain 132:2630–2642, 2009. (review)

5.

BRAINSTEM AND CRANIAL NERVE TERRITORIES

1. BRAINSTEM

The brainstem is a cylindrical structure longitudinally situated in the posterior cranial fossa, and is formed of the **midbrain** (mesencephalon), **pons**, and **medulla oblongata** from rostral to caudal.

On transverse section of the midbrain at the level of the superior colliculus (Figure 5-1), a pair of large bulges is seen symmetrically at the anterior aspect (**cerebral peduncle** or crus cerebri), and on the posterior aspect there is a pair of small protrusions just lateral to the midline (**superior colliculus**) with another pair below them (**inferior colliculus**). These two pairs of protrusions together are called **quadrigeminal bodies**. This posterior region of the midbrain is called the **tectum**, and the region between the tectum and the cerebral peduncle is called the **mesencephalic tegmentum**, where the substantia nigra, red nucleus, periaqueductal gray substance, and other structures are located.

The anterior two-thirds of the pons (**pontine basis**) is formed by a large structure containing the descending fibers from the cerebral cortex through the cerebral peduncle and the transverse fibers originating from the pontine nucleus (Figure 5-2). The remaining part of pons is called the **pontine tegmentum**, which contains the medial lemniscus anteriorly and a number of nuclei and fiber tracts posteriorly.

The medulla oblongata is located at the caudal end of the brainstem, and anteriorly there is a pair of small protrusions just lateral to the midline (**pyramid**) (Figure 5-3). Through the pyramid, the descending fibers from the cerebral cortex project to the spinal anterior horn cells, and thus this fiber tract is called the **pyramidal tract**. Just lateral to each pyramid, there is another bulge formed by the **inferior olive**. Just posterior to the pyramid, the **medial lemniscus** is located. The posterior rim of the medulla oblongata forms the anterior wall of the fourth ventricle, and along the rim are situated the hypoglossal nucleus, dorsal motor nucleus of the vagus, and vestibular nuclei on each side away from the midline in this order.

2. COMMON STRUCTURES OF CRANIAL NERVES

There are 12 pairs of cranial nerves. Among these, the first, second, and eighth cranial nerves serve special sensory functions; olfaction, vision, and audiovestibular function, respectively. All of the remaining cranial nerves contain motor nerve fibers innervating the skeletal muscles, and the fifth, seventh, ninth, and tenth cranial nerves also contain somatosensory nerve fibers. Furthermore, the third, seventh, ninth, and tenth cranial nerves also contain autonomic nerve fibers.

Of the motor fibers contained in the cranial nerves, all of them originate from a corresponding motor nucleus, which is located within the brainstem tegmentum. In contrast, all of the primary somatosensory neurons are located in the somatosensory ganglia, which are located outside of the brainstem. Motor fibers of the cranial nerves do not cross between the sides, at least outside of the brainstem. Within the brainstem, the trochlear nerves cross at the anterior medullary velum (posterior rim of the midbrain at its caudal level), and some of the oculomotor nerve fibers are known to cross within the midbrain (see Chapter 9-1A).

Among the sensory fibers contained in the cranial nerves, only the optic nerves decussate partially (see Chapter 7-1B), but other sensory nerves do not cross. Therefore, if the sensory fibers are damaged, the symptoms will appear on the same side, corresponding to the innervated territory, with the exception of the optic nerve.

Cytoarchitecturally, the myelin sheath for the cranial nerves originates from the cell membrane of Schwann cells, except for the olfactory tract and the optic nerve.

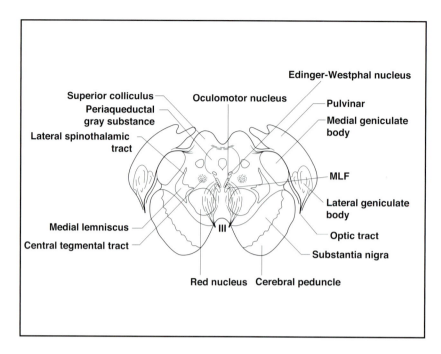

Figure 5-1 Schematic diagram showing a transverse section of midbrain at the level of the superior colliculus. III: oculomotor nerve, MLF: medial longitudinal fasciculus. (Modified from Haymaker, 1969)

Both the olfactory tract and the optic nerve are the secondary neuron of each sensory system, and thus their myelin sheath is formed of the cell membrane of oligodendroglia, in spite of the fact that those fibers are situated outside of the brain parenchyma. That is why the optic nerve is often affected in multiple sclerosis, which is a demyelinating disease affecting the central nervous system.

The autonomic nerve fibers contained in the cranial nerves generally innervate the ipsilateral side of the body except for the visceral organs, which are asymmetric in their location (see Chapter 14-5).

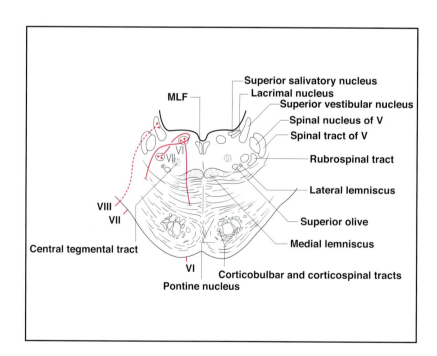

Figure 5-2 Schematic diagram showing a transverse section of pons at the level of the abducens nerve (VI) and the facial nerve (VII). V: trigeminal nerve, VIII: vestibulocochlear nerve, MLF: medial longitudinal fasciculus. (Modified from Haymaker, 1969)

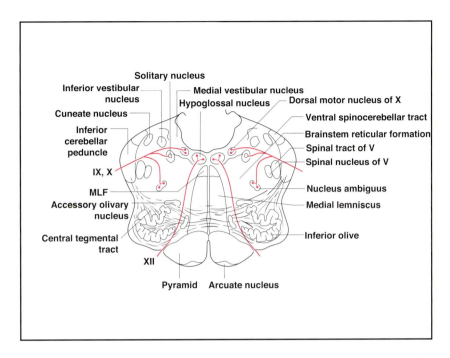

Figure 5-3 Schematic diagram showing a transverse section of medulla oblongata. V: trigeminal nerve, IX: glossopharyngeal nerve, X: vagus nerve, XII: hypoglossal nerve, MLF: medial longitudinal fasciculus. (Modified from Haymaker, 1969)

3. CRANIAL NERVES RELATED TO SOMATOSENSORY FUNCTION

Primary somatosensory neurons of the fifth, seventh, ninth, and tenth cranial nerves are all situated outside of the brainstem. Like the spinal nerve (see Figure 19-1), the primary sensory neuron is a bipolar cell located in a sensory ganglion. The impulses generated in the peripheral sensory receptors are conducted through the peripheral axon to the neuronal soma, and are further conducted through the central axon to reach the brainstem parenchyma. Cytoarchitecturally, therefore, the central axon belongs to the peripheral nervous system until it enters the brainstem parenchyma, and once it enters the brainstem, it belongs to the central nervous system. Thus, this single neuron is formed of two different components, peripheral and central, due to this difference in the histological origin of the myelin sheath.

Regarding axonal flow, which is important for the transport of neurotrophic factors from the neuronal soma to the distal axon, the nerve impulse in the motor fibers is conducted in the same direction as the axonal flow. In the peripheral axon of the sensory fibers, in contrast, the nerve impulse is conducted in the opposite direction to the axonal flow. Namely, in the peripheral axon of the sensory nerves, the electric impulse is conducted from the distal terminal to the sensory ganglion cell, whereas the neurotrophic factors are transported from the sensory cell to the distal terminal of the axon. In the central axon of the sensory nerves, the nerve impulse is conducted in the same direction as the axonal flow.

4. CRANIAL NERVES RELATED TO AUTONOMIC NERVOUS FUNCTION

The autonomic nervous system is described in detail later in this book (Chapter 20). The third, seventh, ninth, and tenth cranial nerves contain the parasympathetic efferent fibers. For the sympathetic nervous system, the preganglionic neuron is located in the intermediolateral nucleus, which is located at the lateral column of the spinal cord extending from the first thoracic segment to the first lumbar segment (see Figure 14-5). Then the preganglionic fibers leave the cord through the anterior spinal root to reach the sympathetic ganglion, from which the postganglionic fibers originate to innervate the whole body (see Figure 20-1). Regarding sympathetic innervation of the head, face, and cranial nerve territories, the preganglionic fibers originate from the intermediolateral nucleus at the first thoracic segment and run through the inferior and middle cervical sympathetic ganglia to reach the superior cervical sympathetic ganglion, where the postganglionic fibers originate (see Figure 8-4).

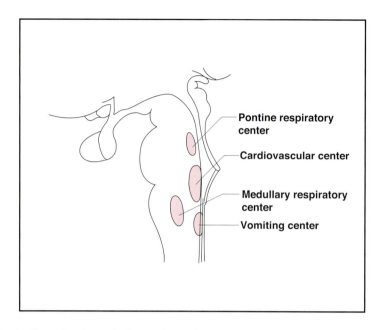

Figure 5-4 Schematic diagram showing the centers for respiration, cardiovascular system, and vomiting in the brainstem.

In the brainstem reticular formation, there are important centers for controlling the vital signs such as respiration, cardiovascular functions, and vomiting (Figure 5-4). In addition, the micturition centers also exist in the brainstem, and an isolated lesion involving some areas of pons or medulla oblongata can cause urinary retention.

5. LOCATION OF THE CRANIAL NERVE NUCLEI IN THE BRAINSTEM

With the exception of the first cranial nerve (olfactory nerve), the second cranial nerve (optic nerve) and the eleventh cranial nerve (accessory nerve), the nuclei of all cranial nerves are located in the tegmentum of the midbrain, pons,

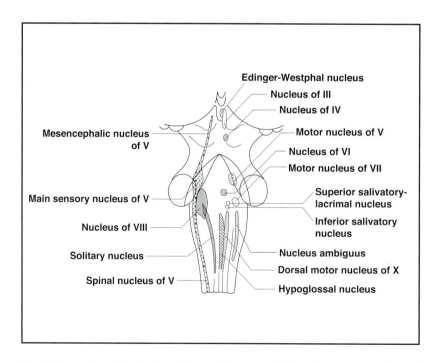

Figure 5-5 Schematic diagram showing the rostrocaudal extension of the cranial nerve nuclei. III: oculomotor nerve, IV: trochlear nerve, V: trigeminal nerve, VI: abducens nerve, VII: facial nerve, VIII: vestibulocochlear nerve, X: vagus nerve.

THE NEUROLOGIC EXAMINATION

or medulla oblongata. As the location of nuclei of these cranial nerves is often indicated on the transverse section of the brainstem at various levels, it tends to give a wrong impression as to the length of each nucleus. Since some nuclei, in fact, extend for a relatively long distance (Figure 5-5), the topographic interrelationship should be kept in mind when estimating the location of the lesion from the clinical symptoms and signs.

Neurologic Examination of the Cranial Nerve Territory

Functions of the cranial nerves can be tested in the order of their numbers, but the emphasis can be placed on certain cranial nerves depending on the information obtained from the history taking. In the following chapters, anatomical structures, functions, and the method of neurologic examination of each cranial nerve are described in the order of actual examination. However, the eleventh cranial nerve (accessory nerve) is dealt with in the chapter on the neck and trunk (Chapter 15), because its functions are related to the posture and movement of the neck.

BIBLIOGRAPHY

Haymaker W. Bing's Local Diagnosis in Neurological Diseases. 5th ed., Mosby, St Louis, 1969.

6.

OLFACTORY SENSATION

1. STRUCTURES AND NEUROTRANSMITTERS OF THE OLFACTORY SYSTEM

The primary neurons of the olfactory system are the bipolar cells located in the olfactory epithelium of the nasal mucous membrane (Figure 6-1). Their peripheral axonal endings serve as the olfactory receptors, and an electric impulse generated there is conducted to the cell body, from which the central axon originates as the olfactory nerve. The **olfactory nerve** is an unmyelinated fiber. After passing through the lamina cribrosa of the ethmoid bone, it projects to the **olfactory bulb** in the anterior cranial fossa. The secondary neurons originate from the mitral cells in the olfactory bulb, which then run posteriorly in the **olfactory tract** in the olfactory groove and enter the brain parenchyma from the anterior polar region of the temporal lobe. As described in Chapter 5-2, the olfactory tract belongs to the central nervous system, because its myelin sheath is derived from oligodendroglia. As the olfactory groove is a common site for a meningioma, unilateral anosmia is a representative sign of such a meningioma.

In the olfactory bulb, the neurotransmitter of the mitral cells is glutamate, while dopamine is considered to be involved in the interneurons. In relation to this, in Parkinson disease olfactory sensation is impaired from its early stage (Boesveldt et al, 2008). In fact, Lewy bodies appear in the olfactory bulb in the earliest stage of Parkinson disease (Braak & Del Tredici, 2008, for review).

Olfactory sensation is believed to be perceived in the limbic system of the brain, which includes, among others, the uncus, hippocampus, and amygdala (Figure 6-1). A patient with mesial temporal lobe epilepsy might complain of an unusual smell as an aura. This phenomenon is considered to be due to involvement of the olfactory centers by epileptic discharges, and this type of attack is called an **uncinate fit** according to its anatomical site.

2. EXAMINATION OF OLFACTORY SENSATION

The sense of smell is tested by using a nonpungent stimulus such as a mild perfume. It is important to test the left and right nose separately. Bilateral disturbance of olfactory sensation is commonly seen in inflammation of the nasal mucosa such as rhinitis or the common cold. **Bilateral anosmia** may be a manifestation of some

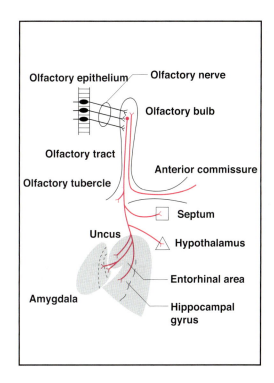

Figure 6-1 Schematic diagram showing the olfactory pathways. (Modified from Brodal, 2010, with permission)

hereditary neurodegenerative diseases. A typical example is an X-linked hereditary disease called **Kallmann syndrome**, which is characterized by anosmia, congenital mirror movements, and hypogonadotropic hypogonadism. Anosmia in this condition is believed to be due to developmental abnormality of the olfactory bulb. It is not difficult to distinguish congenital bilateral anosmia from upper respiratory infection by taking into account the accompanying symptoms. As described earlier, bilateral disturbance of olfactory sensation may be seen in patients with Parkinson disease, but total loss of this sense is rare in this disease.

Unilateral anosmia is a characteristic sign of **olfactory groove meningioma**, especially when the history of present illness suggests the presence of an intracranial space-occupying lesion, and, in fact, it may be the only neurological deficit seen in this slowly progressive tumor.

BIBLIOGRAPHY

Boesveldt S, Verbaan D, Knol DL, Visser M, van Rooden SM, van Hilfen JJ, et al. A comparative study of odor identification and odor discrimination deficits in Parkinson's disease. Mov Disord 23:1984–1990, 2008.

Braak H, Del Tredici K. Invited article: nervous system pathology in sporadic Parkinson disease. Neurology 70:1916–1925, 2008. (review)

Brodal P. The Central Nervous System: Structure and Function. 4th ed. Oxford University Press, New York, 2010.

7.

VISUAL FUNCTIONS

1. ANATOMY AND FUNCTION OF THE VISUAL SYSTEM

A. RETINA

Visual receptors are **photoreceptor cells** that are located in the outer layer of the retina (Figure 7-1). There are two kinds of photoreceptor cells: cones and rods. **Cones** are located mainly at the macular area and control photopic vision in the light condition, and **rods** are distributed more toward the periphery of the retina and control scotopic vision in the dimly lit condition. The primary neurons of the visual system are bipolar cells, which receive impulses through their peripheral axons and transmit them through their central axons to the retinal ganglion cells. The **retinal ganglion cells** serve as the secondary neurons of the visual system. Axons of ganglion cells from all parts of the retina project to the central part of the retina and form the **optic disc** (optic papilla) (Figure 7-2). From the optic disc, a bundle of axons runs posteriorly as the **optic nerve** and enters the cranial cavity through the **optic foramen**.

As described in Chapter 5-2, the optic nerve histologically belongs to the central nervous system, and it is often involved in multiple sclerosis and neuromyelitis optica. Isolated demyelination of the optic nerve is called **optic neuritis**, and it may also be called **retrobulbar neuritis** because the lesion commonly involves a part of the optic nerve behind the ocular bulb. It is usually unilateral, but it may be bilateral, as is often the case in neuromyelitis optica (Box 9).

In **Leber hereditary optic neuropathy (atrophy)**, vision is impaired relatively acutely in young adults. Usually it starts unilaterally, but in most cases the opposite eye is also involved within a year. As visual acuity may occasionally improve to some degree, it may have to be differentiated from bilateral optic neuritis. This condition belongs to the mitochondrial encephalomyopathies (see Box 57). It is due to a point mutation of mitochondrial DNA transmitted by maternal inheritance. Various treatments are being tried for this disease, including trials of antioxidant agents like idebenone (Newman, 2011, for review).

Fovea Centralis and Optic Disc

The **fovea centralis** (fovea) is in the center of the macula lutea (macula) and plays an important role in central vision. A bundle of nerve fibers arising from the fovea runs nasally to enter the optic disc from its temporal rim, the **maculopapillary bundle** (Figure 7-2). This bundle is considered to occupy the central portion of the optic nerve, which is commonly affected by demyelinating lesions in optic neuritis or retrobulbar neuritis. In this condition, therefore, it is common to find pale discoloration at the temporal part of the optic disc (**temporal pallor**). This phenomenon is due to retrograde degeneration of the optic nerve axons as a result of axonal involvement at the demyelinating site (Figure 7-2). For the same reason, a **central scotoma** is often seen in this condition. Thus, an ophthalmoscopic finding of temporal pallor in this condition suggests that the axons have also been involved secondary to the demyelination at least several days prior to the time of examination, and thus it suggests poor prognosis for visual acuity. By contrast, in conditions associated with primary degeneration of the macula, temporal pallor is seen as a result of orthograde degeneration of the axons (Figure 7-3).

Blood Supply to the Retina

The retina receives its blood supply from the **ophthalmic artery**, which bifurcates from the internal carotid artery soon

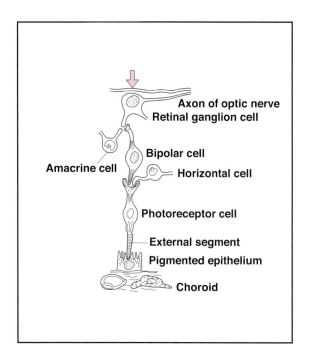

Figure 7-1 Cytoarchitecture of retina. The outer layer is shown below and the inner layer is shown upward of the figure. Arrow on top indicates direction of the incoming light. (Modified from Brodal, 2010, with permission)

after it enters the cranial cavity through the carotid canal. The ophthalmic artery enters the orbit along with the optic nerve through the optic foramen, and it supplies blood to the retina as the **central retinal artery** (Figure 7-4). Occlusion of this artery, for example by embolism, causes ipsilateral **blindness**.

Temporal arteritis is an arteritis of the temporal artery affecting elderly people. This special arteritis might cause ipsilateral blindness and optic atrophy due to secondary thrombosis in the ophthalmic artery. It has been reported that varicella-zoster virus might trigger the immunopathology of this giant cell arteritis (Gilden et al, 2015). Temporal arteritis is often combined with **polymyalgia rheumatica**, and it shows marked elevation of the erythrocyte sedimentation rate and responds to corticosteroid therapy (see Chapter 16-3C). If the central retinal artery is transiently occluded by an embolus originating from atherothrombotic plaque of the internal carotid artery, it causes transient blindness as a result of transient ischemic attack (**amaurosis fugax**). If this attack is accompanied by contralateral hemiparesis, it suggests the presence of atherothrombosis in the internal carotid artery on the side of blindness.

Transient blindness may be also seen as a prodromal symptom of migraine. In **retinal migraine**, spasm in the ophthalmic artery or in the central retinal artery may cause visual disturbance as a result of ischemia, followed by pulsating pain in the orbit or in the surrounding region. Acute visual loss in optic neuritis or retrobulbar neuritis is characterized by a central scotoma. In this case, ocular pain is induced by upward gaze, because the optic nerve is mechanically stretched by this maneuver, which in turn provokes the inflammatory pain.

B. OPTIC NERVE AND OPTIC CHIASM

The optic nerve runs posteromedially after leaving the orbit and about half of the nerve fibers cross at the **optic**

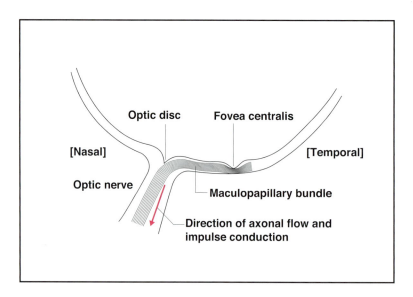

Figure 7-2 Schematic diagram showing the interrelationship of optic disc and fovea. View from top of the right eye. The maculopapillary bundle originating from the fovea centralis enters the optic disc from its temporal margin.

It is known that in patients with multiple sclerosis (MS) symptoms such as motor paresis worsen while taking a bath. In 1890, a German ophthalmologist named Uhthoff reported that, in four among 105 patients with MS, visual loss and abnormality of color vision and visual field were induced by physical exercise. In one of the four patients, in addition to visual loss of the left eye, motor paresis of the right leg and sensory disturbance of the left arm were also induced when standing by the stove (Guthrie & Nelson, 1995). In fact, this phenomenon is considered to be common in patients with MS. Uhthoff initially thought that this phenomenon was due to physical exercise rather than an increase in the body temperature. Based on subsequent observation by many neurologists, it is currently believed that this phenomenon is caused by an increase in the body temperature rather than by physical exercise. By using the technique of transcranial magnetic stimulation in MS patients, it was shown that a change in body temperature worsens the conduction block (Humm et al, 2004). Physiologically, it is known that, at the site of incomplete demyelination where the conduction block takes place, the conduction rate is decreased by the temperature increase, whereas, in intact nerve fibers, the temperature elevation increases the conduction velocity. However, it is also known that, in some cases, symptoms worsen with a decrease in the body temperature. Nerve conduction in demyelinated nerve can be described as an inverted U-shaped function, slowing with both increasing and decreasing temperature. A similar phenomenon can be seen in multifocal motor neuropathy, which is characterized by conduction block in the peripheral motor nerve fibers (see Chapter 16-3C). In this condition, fatigue is caused as a result of increased conduction block after strong contraction of the corresponding muscle (activity-dependent conduction block) (Kaji et al, 2000).

chiasm. Namely, those fibers coming from the nasal half of the retina, which corresponds to the temporal visual field of that eye, run through the medial half of the optic nerve and cross at the chiasm to form the contralateral optic tract together with the uncrossed fibers coming from the temporal half of the contralateral retina, which corresponds to the nasal visual field of that eye (Figure 7-5). Thus, the optic tract transmits the visual input arising from the contralateral hemifield of both eyes.

If the optic chiasm is compressed by a pituitary adenoma from below, only the crossed fibers of optic nerves are affected, resulting in **bitemporal hemianopsia** (2 of Figure 7-5). It is known that the crossing fibers originating from the inferior nasal aspect of the retina first enter the contralateral optic nerve forming an arc for a short distance before crossing at the chiasm. Thus, if the optic nerve is compressed from below just before entering the chiasm, it causes a defect of the superior temporal visual field of the contralateral eye in addition to visual loss of the ipsilateral eye. This phenomenon is, however, extremely rare. Theoretically, compression of the optic chiasm from below on both sides may damage those nerve fibers arising from the temporal half of both retinas and cause binasal hemianopsia, but this phenomenon is also extremely rare.

The **optic tract** is formed from the nerve fibers arising from the temporal half of the ipsilateral retina and the nasal half of the contralateral retina, and it runs posterolaterally and projects to the **lateral geniculate body (LGB)**. Thus, if the optic tract is damaged, it causes **homonymous hemianopsia** contralateral to the lesion (3 of Figure 7-5). Since the optic tract is located just below the globus pallidus and internal capsule, deep brain surgery targeting the globus pallidus should be carried out with caution (see Figure 16-8).

Nerve Fibers of the Optic Tract Related to Nonvisual Functions

While most nerve fibers of the optic tract project to LGB, some fibers turn medially just before reaching the LGB and enter the mesencephalic tectum to project to the superior colliculus and pretectal nucleus (Figure 7-6). The **superior colliculus** plays an important role in eye–head coordination (see Chapter 9-4), and the **pretectal nucleus** serves as the afferent arc of the light reflex (see Chapter 8-1). Furthermore, some nerve fibers of the optic tract project to the suprachiasmatic nucleus of hypothalamus, which is located just above the optic chiasm. Neurons in the **suprachiasmatic nucleus** are activated by bright light and activate the pineal body to produce melatonin, which then activates a part of the hypothalamus involved in the control of the **circadian rhythm** (see Chapter 28-3). This is why it is believed that exposure to sunlight and the use of melatonin improve jet lag during an overseas trip and changing time zones.

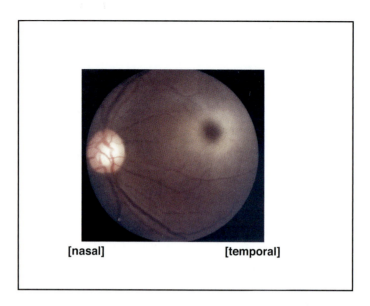

[nasal]   [temporal]

Figure 7-3 Ophthalmoscopic view of the left eye in a case of sialidosis type 2. The fovea centralis appears "cherry-red" in color (cherry-red spot), and is surrounded by white color due to the lipid deposit. The optic disc shows "temporal pallor" due to orthograde degeneration of the maculopapillary bundle as a result of macular degeneration. A white spot in the center of the optic disc is due to physiological cupping.

C. LATERAL GENICULATE BODY AND OPTIC RADIATION

The tertiary neurons of the visual system send projections from the LGB to the visual cortex (**geniculocalcarine tract**). The tract runs laterally through the posterior limb of the internal capsule and spreads as **optic radiation**. Therefore, a vascular lesion of that part of the internal capsule causes contralateral hemiplegia and homonymous hemianopsia. The dorsolateral portion of optic radiation runs posteriorly along the posterior horn of the lateral ventricle and reaches the upper half of the visual cortex through the parietal lobe. The ventral portion of optic radiation runs laterally just above the inferior horn of the lateral ventricle forming **Meyer's loop**. Then it reaches

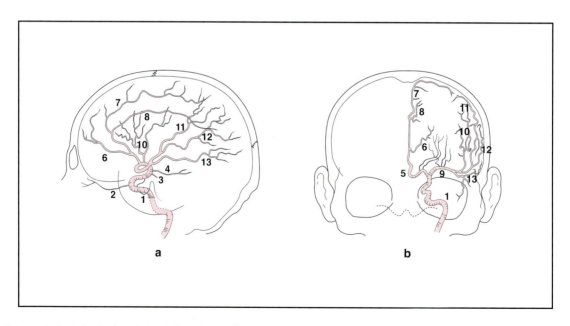

a   b

Figure 7-4 Main cerebral arteries (a: lateral view, b: frontal view). 1: internal carotid artery, 2: ophthalmic artery, 3: posterior communicating artery, 4: anterior choroidal artery, 5: anterior cerebral artery, 6: orbitofrontal artery, 7: callosomarginal artery, 8: pericallosal artery, 9: middle cerebral artery, 10: arteries of precentral and central sulci, 11: parietal artery, 12: angular artery, 13: temporal artery. See Figure 9-3 for the vertebrobasilar artery territory. (Reproduced from List et al, 1945, with permission)

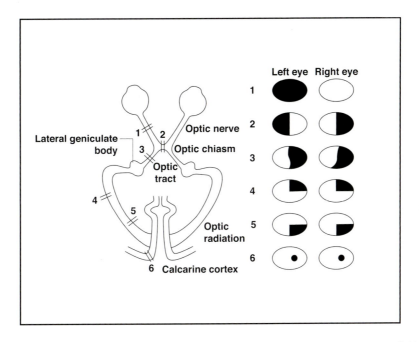

Figure 7-5 Schematic diagram of the visual pathway and defect of visual field caused by lesion of each site. 1: blindness, 2: bitemporal hemianopsia, 3: homonymous hemianopsia, 4: homonymous superior quadrantanopsia, 5: homonymous inferior quadrantanopsia, 6: homonymous visual field defect (homonymous scotoma). Note that hemianopsia due to lesion of optic tract (3) is incongruous in shape between the two eyes.

the lower half of the visual cortex through the temporal lobe. If Meyer's loop is damaged by surgical resection of the anterior portion of the temporal lobe for treatment of medically intractable mesial temporal lobe epilepsy, contralateral homonymous superior quadrantanopsia may appear.

A lesion of the retrochiasmatic portion of the visual system causes contralateral homonymous hemianopsia, but the shape of the visual field defect differs depending on which part of the visual pathway is damaged. In a lesion of the optic tract, the visual field defect is incongruous in its shape between the two hemifields (3 of Figure 7-5). By

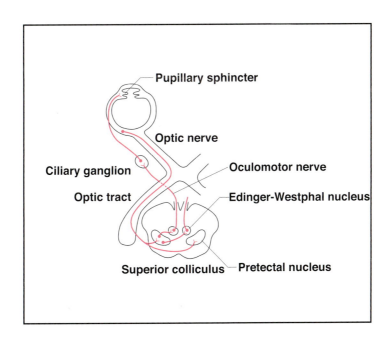

Figure 7-6 Schematic diagram showing the afferent and efferent pathways related to the light reflex. (Modified from Brodal, 2010, with permission)

contrast, the visual field defect caused by a lesion of the optic radiation near the visual cortex is more congruous between the left and right eyes. As the optic radiation is separated into the temporal pathway and the parietal pathway as described above, a lesion of the temporal lobe causes **homonymous superior quadrantanopsia** (4 of Figure 7-5) while a lesion of the parietal lobe causes **homonymous inferior quadrantanopsia** (5 of Figure 7-5), both contralaterally.

In hemianopsia caused by a vascular lesion of the visual cortex, the central visual field is often spared (**macular sparing**). The mechanism underlying this phenomenon has not been precisely elucidated, but it has been postulated that a part of the occipital cortex receiving input from the macular portion of retina might receive blood supply from bilateral posterior cerebral arteries. However, in view of the fact that this phenomenon is seen not only in ischemic stroke of the posterior cerebral artery territory but also in hemorrhage of the occipital lobe, the above hypothesis is unlikely.

D. VISUAL CORTEX

On a histological section of cortex around the calcarine fissure, a white line called **the line of Gennari** is seen, which is due to abundant myelinated fibers in the fourth layer of the calcarine cortex. This cortex is also called the **striate area** based on this appearance. There is precise topographical organization throughout the whole visual system starting from the retina and terminating at the calcarine cortex. Namely, visual input coming from a certain part of the visual field activates retinal ganglion cells localized to the corresponding part of each retina, and their impulses activate a group of neurons in the corresponding part of LGB contralateral to the visual field, which then activates neurons in the corresponding part of the striate area (**retinotopic organization**). Thus, if there are blind spots of congruous shape in the visual fields of the two eyes, it may be due to a localized lesion involving a small part of the contralateral striate area (**homonymous scotoma**) (6 of Figure 7-5).

E. BLOOD SUPPLY TO THE VISUAL PATHWAY

As the visual system extends from eyes to the occipital cortex, it receives blood supply from multiple arteries. The retina and its ganglion cells receive blood supply from the ophthalmic artery. The optic chiasm is supplied by a branch of the anterior cerebral artery. The optic tract and LGB are supplied by the anterior choroidal artery, which bifurcates from the internal carotid artery, and the optic radiation is supplied by branches of the internal carotid artery. Finally the occipital cortex receives blood supply from the posterior cerebral artery (Figures 7-4 and 7-7). Therefore, visual field defects caused by ischemic vascular diseases differ depending on which artery is involved. The responsible artery can be estimated from the mode of visual field defect and other accompanying neurologic deficits.

F. CYTOARCHITECTURE OF THE VISUAL SYSTEM AND HIGHER CORTICAL FUNCTIONS

The LGB is divided into six layers, the ventral two layers mainly formed of large neurons (**magnocellular layer**) and the dorsal four layers mainly formed of small neurons (**parvocellular layer**) (Figure 7-8). The magnocellular layer receives projections from large retinal ganglion cells, and the parvocellular layer receives axons originating from small retinal ganglion cells.

The **primary visual cortex** is in the striate area of the occipital cortex (**Brodmann area 17**), and it is connected to the extrastriate area including Brodmann areas 18 and 19 (Figure 7-9) (Brodmann, 1910). The primary visual area is engaged in the processing of basic visual information, and more advanced visual information is processed in the extrastriate area. In general, it is believed that recognition of visual objects is processed in the **ventral pathway** projecting from the occipital cortex to the temporal cortex ("what" pathway) while spatial information and recognition of movement are processed in the **dorsal pathway** projecting from the occipital cortex to the parietal cortex ("where" pathway). It is also believed that the projection fibers originating from the magnocellular layer of LGB are engaged in the processing of movement and depth while those originating from the parvocellular layer of LGB are related to the processing of shape, pattern, and color of objects.

Special Visual Functions

Several cortical areas are known to be involved in special visual functions. Area V4 (the posterior part of the lingual gyrus and the posterior part of the fusiform gyrus) is important for **color vision**. Area V5 (the posterior part of the middle temporal gyrus, corresponding to middle temporal [MT] of monkey) plays a special role in visual recognition of movement (**motor vision**). The fusiform gyrus in the inferior temporal lobe is known to be important

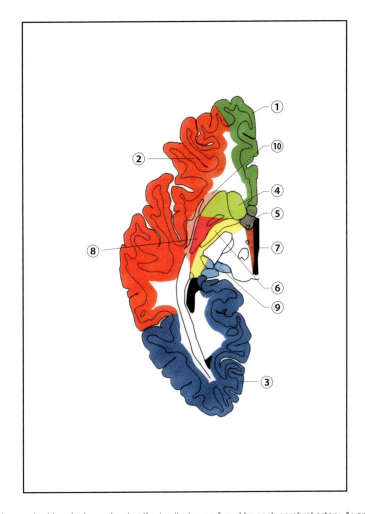

Figure 7-7 A horizontal section of the cerebral hemisphere showing the territories perfused by each cerebral artery. 1: anterior cerebral artery, 2: middle cerebral artery, 3: posterior cerebral artery, 4: perforating branches of the anterior cerebral artery, 5: anterior communicating artery, 6: anterior choroidal artery, 7: perforating branches of the posterior communicating artery, 8: perforating branches of the middle cerebral artery, 9: posterior choroidal artery. (Reproduced from Duvernoy, 1999, with permission)

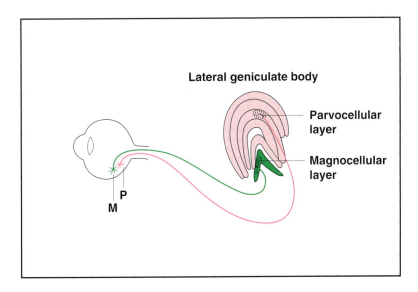

Figure 7-8 Structure of the lateral geniculate body and the projection it receives from the retina. M: large ganglion cells of the retina, P: small ganglion cells of the retina. (Modified from Brodal, 2010, with permission)

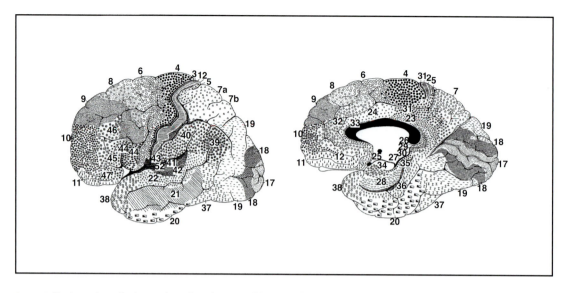

Figure 7-9 Brodmann's cortical areas based on the cytoarchitecture. (Reproduced from Brodmann, 1910)

for **recognition of faces**, and a bilateral lesion of this area causes **prosopagnosia**. In this condition, the patient cannot recognize a familiar face visually, but once the voice is heard, the person can be easily identified. Information about these higher visual functions has been obtained by observation of the patients with localized cortical lesions and by recently developed, noninvasive techniques such as magnetoencephalography and functional neuroimaging (Shibasaki, 2008, for review).

2. EXAMINATION OF VISUAL FUNCTIONS

A. VISUAL ACUITY

Before examining visual acuity from a neurologic point of view, it is better to pay attention to the presence or absence of any abnormality in the cornea, lens, and vitreous body. Presence of these ophthalmological abnormalities can be estimated from the past medical history, but if there is any question, ophthalmological evaluation will be needed. If a patient usually wears glasses for accommodation failure or astigmatism, it is advisable to examine visual acuity with the glasses on for the neurologic examination.

How much detail of visual acuity should be measured depends on the tentative diagnosis based on the history taking and on the clinical set-up in the hospital. At any rate, it is important to examine the visual acuity of each eye independently. For quantitative measurement of visual acuity, various charts are available. Visual acuity can be measured for both near and far, relevant for reading and seeing at a

distance, respectively. Differences in acuity for near and far are indicative of ophthalmological causes.

If abnormality of visual acuity is found in one eye, or in both eyes but with significant asymmetry between the two eyes, it may suggest either ophthalmological abnormalities including the retina or an optic nerve lesion in that eye. In that case, it is important to check whether it is a defect of the central visual field (**central scotoma**) or it involves the whole visual field. The presence of a central scotoma suggests a lesion either in the macula of the retina or in the optic nerve.

B. VISUAL FIELD

Examination of the visual field may be initiated by a **confrontation test**, in which the visual field of two eyes is simultaneously tested by using examiner's hands. For example, the examiner sits about 50 cm in front of and facing the patient, and holds the examiner's hands about 30 degrees apart. Then the examiner wiggles fingers of the left or right hand and asks the patient to tell which hand was moved.

When doing the confrontation test, it is important to test also simultaneous presentation of visual targets in the left and right visual fields. If the patient constantly neglects one side, it suggests either homonymous hemianopsia or hemispatial neglect (see Chapter 23-2C), and in this case the visual field of each eye should be examined in more detail. For testing the visual field of one eye on the confrontation test, for example, the examiner's left eye serves as a control for the patient's right eye by keeping the other eye closed or masked. Then the patient is asked to fix his/her gaze on the examiner's hand held just halfway between the patient and the examiner, while the examiner moves a visual target with the other hand in the central and peripheral visual field.

If there is any difficulty in testing the upper visual field, it is useful to test it again with the upper eyelid lifted. Furthermore, in subjects who have a very high nose, the confrontation test might show an apparent defect in the inferior nasal field for both eyes.

As expected, sensitivity of the confrontation test is not very high (Kerr et al, 2010), but gross abnormality of the visual field can be detected if carefully tested. Needless to say, however, if any abnormality of visual system is suggested from the history taking or from the confrontation test, the visual field should be measured precisely by using the perimetry.

Central Scotoma

The presence of a central scotoma in one eye suggests that either the macular region of the retina or the optic nerve is damaged. When doing the confrontation test, one may find a blind spot just lateral (temporal) to the central field. This field defect is called the **Mariotte blind spot**, which corresponds to the optic disc, where there are no photoreceptor cells (Figure 7-2). Therefore, this blind spot is enlarged in case of papilledema. Furthermore, in case of central retinitis, a blind spot of racket shape may be formed as a result of fusion of the central scotoma and the Mariotte blind spot.

Other Visual Field Defects

A defect of temporal fields of both eyes (**bitemporal hemianopsia**) is caused by a lesion of the optic chiasm, in particular its compression by a pituitary adenoma from below (2 of Figure 7-5). A hemifield defect of the same side in both eyes (for example, nasal of one eye and temporal of the other eye) is called **homonymous hemianopsia** and is caused by a lesion involving the contralateral visual pathway central to the optic chiasm, namely the optic tract (3 of Figure 7-5), LGB, optic radiation, or occipital cortex. Likewise, a defect of either the upper half or the lower half of hemifield of the same side in both eyes is called **homonymous superior quadrantanopsia** (4 of Figure 7-5) or **homonymous inferior quadrantanopsia**, respectively (5 of Figure 7-5). The former is caused by a lesion of the

contralateral temporal lobe, and the latter is caused by a lesion of the contralateral parietal lobe. Unilateral lesion of the calcarine cortex causes a congruous defect of the contralateral hemifield, often associated with macular sparing, in both eyes.

If the occipital pole is unilaterally affected, by head trauma for example, a localized field defect (scotoma) may be seen in the contralateral half of the central visual field of both eyes (6 of Figure 7-5). This homonymous scotoma may resemble bilateral central scotoma due to bilateral optic neuritis. These two cases, however, can be differentiated from the history of present illness, a precise pattern of the field defect, and results of light reflex. In bilateral optic neuritis, the shape of the scotoma may not be exactly the same in the two eyes and the light reflex may be absent or decreased if a light stimulus is projected from the defective visual field, whereas the light reflex is always intact in an occipital lesion (see Chapter 8-2).

Constriction of Peripheral Visual Field

Constriction of the peripheral visual field is encountered in lesions primarily involving the periphery of the retina. A typical example is **retinal pigment degeneration**, which is also called retinitis pigmentosa although it is not an inflammatory disease. This condition is usually seen for both eyes. In this case, the patient complains of **night blindness (nyctalopia)**. The diagnosis is confirmed by ophthalmoscopic observation of pigments in the periphery of the retina.

Constriction of the visual field may be also seen in diffuse lesions of the occipital cortex. A typical example is **Minamata disease**, which is due to organic mercury poisoning. Other neurologic symptoms seen in this condition include cerebellar ataxia, dysarthria, and sensorineural hearing deficit (**Hunter-Russell syndrome**) (see Chapter 1-1). Pathologically there is marked atrophy in the cerebellar cortex and the calcarine cortex.

In a patient showing constriction of the peripheral visual field due to an organic lesion of the calcarine cortex, the visual field is expected to become increasingly wider as the patient moves away from the visual target. In a patient with a psychogenic visual field defect, however, the field defect does not change in its angle even if the patient moves away from the target. This phenomenon is called **tunnel vision** or **tubular vision** and is considered to be characteristic of psychogenic field constriction.

C. OPHTHALMOSCOPIC EXAMINATION OF OCULAR FUNDUS

For the purpose of neurologic examination, it is usually sufficient to examine the ocular fundus by an ophthalmoscope without using eye drops for dilating the pupils, but turning out the lights in the examining room is often valuable. In case the precise ophthalmoscopic findings are important, eye drops can be used after completing all other neurologic examinations, or at least after examining the pupils (see Chapter 8-2).

Optic Disc

In the ophthalmoscopic examination as a part of the neurologic examination, it is practical to identify the optic disc (optic papilla) first. At the initial stage of **papilledema**, color of the optic disc becomes more red than usual and the surrounding veins look enlarged. At a little more advanced stage of papilledema, the optic disc appears poorly demarcated, and the ophthalmoscope can be focused differently between the disc and the nearby blood vessels, which suggests the presence of swelling in the optic disc. Papilledema is caused by either intracranial hypertension or a pathological process directly occluding the central retinal vein.

Pale discoloration of the optic disc is characteristic of **optic atrophy**. It is caused by either orthograde axonal degeneration from a primary pathology of the retina or retrograde axonal degeneration following a pathological process of the optic nerve. Optic atrophy is commonly found in patients with **multiple sclerosis** or **optic neuritis (retrobulbar neuritis)**, and this finding suggests that axons of the optic nerve have been involved as the result of retrograde degeneration. The nerve fibers originating from the macular region of the retina enter the optic disc from its temporal rim and pass through the central section of the optic nerve. Consequently, a demyelinating lesion involving the central section of the optic nerve causes atrophy in the temporal portion of the optic disc as a result of retrograde degeneration (**temporal pallor**) (Figure 7-2).

Physiological Cup of Optic Disc

The central part of optic disc looks pale due to a physiological cup even in healthy subjects. If the optic disc is tilted laterally due to, for example, myopia, the physiological cup is seen at the temporal portion of the disc, resembling temporal pallor. Distinction from real temporal pallor is possible based on the history of myopia and correction of visual acuity by the use of glasses.

Fovea Centralis

The fovea can be identified by shifting the ophthalmoscope light laterally away from the optic disc or by asking the subject to look at the ophthalmoscope light. In patients with lipidosis, the surrounding area of the fovea looks white due to deposit of lipid, and the fovea looks purple-red. As this color resembles that of a cherry, it is called a **cherry-red spot** (Figure 7-3). In this condition, examination of the visual field discloses a central scotoma, and temporal pallor is seen in the optic disc due to orthograde axonal degeneration of the maculopapillary bundle.

Retinal Pigment Degeneration

In this condition, star-shaped black spots are observed mainly in the equatorial (peripheral) region of retina. The patient complains of night blindness, and the visual field is constricted on the perimetric examination. Retinal pigment degeneration is associated with various kinds of neurodegenerative diseases; among others Kearns-Sayre syndrome (a form of mitochondrial encephalomyopathy) (see Box 57), Bassen-Kornzweig disease (see Box 30), Refsum disease (see Chapter 3-1), and Cockayne disease (see Chapter 3-1).

Observation of Retinal Blood Vessels

In patients with hypertension, narrowed vessel diameter and compression of veins at arteriovenous crossings might be seen. In patients with diabetes mellitus, red spots might be seen in the arterial wall. This had been thought to be due to microaneurysms, but histologically these are small hemorrhages. In addition, attention should be paid to homogeneity of the retinal color and the presence or absence of hemorrhage.

BIBLIOGRAPHY

Brodal P. The Central Nervous System: Structure and Function. 4th ed. Oxford University Press, New York, 2010.

Brodmann K. Feinere Anatomie des Grosshirns. In Lewandowsky M (ed.). Handbuch der Neurologie. Erster Band: Allgmeine Neurologie. Verlag von Julius Springer, Berlin, 1910. pp. 206–307.

Duvernoy HM. The Human Brain: Surface, Blood Supply, and Three-Dimensional Sectional Anatomy. 2nd ed. Springer-Verlag, Wien, 1999.

Gilden D, White T, Khmeleva N, Heintzman A, Choe A, Boyer PJ, et al. Prevalence and distribution of HZV in temporal arteries of patients with giant cell arteritis. Neurology 84:1948–1955, 2015.

Guthrie TC, Nelson DA. Influence of temperature changes on multiple sclerosis: critical review of mechanisms and research potential. J Neurol Sci 129:1–8, 1995.

Humm AM, Beer S, Kool J, Magistris MR, Kesselring J, Rösler KM. Quantification of Uhthoff's phenomenon in multiple sclerosis: a magnetic stimulation study. Clin Neurophysiol 115:2493–2501, 2004.

Kaji R, Bostock H, Kohara N, Murase N, Kimura J, Shibasaki H. Activity-dependent conduction block in multifocal motor neuropathy. Brain 123:1602–1611, 2000.

Kerr NM, Chew SSL, Eady EK, Gamble GD, Danesh-Meyer HV. Diagnostic accuracy of confrontation visual field tests. Neurology 74:1184–1190, 2010.

List CF, Burge CH, Hodges FJ. Intracranial angiography. Radiology 45:1–14, 1945.

Newman NJ. Treatment of Leber hereditary optic neuropathy. Brain 134:2447–2450, 2011. (review)

Shibasaki H. Human brain mapping: hemodynamic response and electrophysiology. Clin Neurophysiol 119:731–743, 2008. (review)

8.

PUPILS AND ACCOMMODATION

There are two kinds of muscles in the eyes: extraocular muscles, which move the ocular bulb, and intraocular muscles, which are innervated by the autonomic nervous system. The intraocular muscles have two functions: one controls the diameter of pupils, and the other controls thickness of the lens (**accommodation**). For examining the ocular muscles, we can start from either muscle, but it is practical to examine the intraocular muscles first in order to avoid overlooking them by examining the extraocular muscles first.

1. NERVE INNERVATION OF INTRAOCULAR MUSCLES

The preganglionic fibers of the parasympathetic nerves innervating pupils originate from the Edinger-Westphal nucleus, which is situated in the midbrain tegmentum (see Figures 5-1 and 7-6). They run anteriorly in the oculomotor nerve and exit the midbrain just medial to the cerebral peduncle (see Figure 5-1). Then they run through the cavernous sinus (Figure 8-1) and enter the orbit through the superior orbital fissure (Figure 8-2) to reach the ciliary ganglion. The postganglionic fibers originate from the ciliary ganglion and innervate the pupillary sphincter (see Figure 7-6). As the pupillary sphincter encircles the pupil in the iris, its contraction decreases the pupillary diameter (Figure 8-3).

Acetylcholine is the neurotransmitter for both the pre- and postganglionic fibers, but the mode of transmission is nicotinic for the preganglionic fibers and muscarinic for the postganglionic fibers. When these nerve fibers are involved in a lesion, the pupillary diameter of the affected eye becomes larger compared with the contralateral pupil (**mydriasis**).

A. LIGHT REFLEX AND CONVERGENCE REFLEX

There are two reflexes related to the pupil: the light reflex and the convergence reflex. The **light reflex** is manifested as shrinkage of the pupillary diameter in response to a light stimulus. Its reflex center is in the midbrain tegmentum with the afferent arc served by the optic nerve and the efferent arc served by the autonomic fibers of the oculomotor nerve (see Figure 7-6). The afferent fibers separate from the optic tract just before they reach the lateral geniculate body, and project to the pretectal nucleus of the midbrain bilaterally. The fibers originating from the pretectal nucleus project to the Edinger-Westphal nucleus, which is located just anteriorly. The efferent fibers originating from the Edinger-Westphal nucleus run anteriorly as a part of the oculomotor nerve and project to the ipsilateral ciliary ganglion, which then innervates the **pupillary sphincter.**

A light stimulus presented to one eye elicits the light reflex in both eyes because of partial crossing of the optic nerve fibers at the optic chiasm and because of projection of the afferent fibers from the optic tract to the pretectal nucleus on both sides. The light reflex elicited in the stimulated eye is called the direct pupillary reaction, and the reflex elicited in the opposite (nonstimulated) eye is called the indirect or consensual pupillary reaction.

The **convergence reflex** is manifested as shrinkage of the pupillary diameter when one looks at a near object placed just in front of the eyes. The efferent pathway of this reflex is the same as that of the light reflex, but the afferent pathway is not precisely known. It used to be thought that the proprioceptive afferent impulse originating from the medial rectus muscle might serve as its afferent pathway, but another theory is the near vision itself acts as the afferent because unilateral near vision can elicit this reflex. If the latter theory is correct, this reflex might more properly

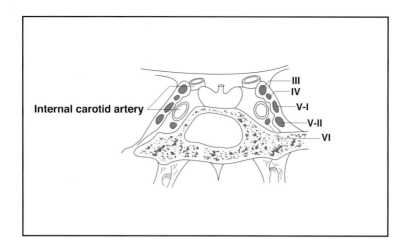

Figure 8-1 Frontal section of the cavernous sinus and the position of cranial nerves that pass through the sinus. III: the third cranial nerve (oculomotor nerve), IV: the fourth cranial nerve (trochlear nerve), V-I: the first branch of the fifth (trigeminal) nerve, V-II: the second branch of the trigeminal nerve, VI: the sixth cranial nerve (abducens nerve). (Reproduced from from Haymaker, 1969, with permission)

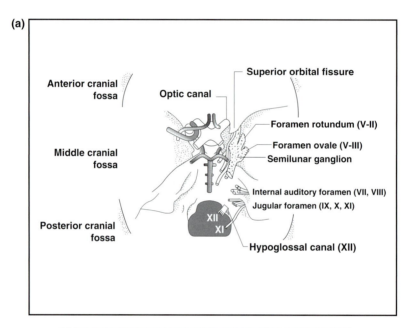

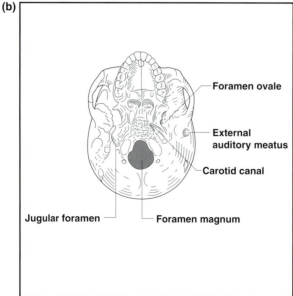

Figure 8-2 Foramina and canals through which the cranial nerves pass. (a) view from inside of the cranial fossa, (b) view from the skull basis. [Figure (a) reproduced from Haymaker, 1969, with permission, (b) modified from Chusid & McDonald, 1964]

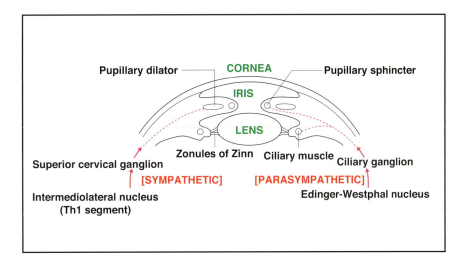

Figure 8-3 Schematic illustration of the nerve tracts controlling the pupil and accommodation. The iris is shown in relative large size in order to show the pupillary sphincter and dilator.

be called the accommodation reflex rather than the convergence reflex.

B. SYMPATHETIC NERVOUS SYSTEM AND HORNER SYNDROME

The pupils are dilated by a function of the sympathetic nerve fibers (Figure 8-4). The preganglionic fibers originate from the **intermediolateral nucleus** at the level of the first thoracic segment, which is called the **ciliospinal center of Budge**. The fibers exit the spinal cord through the anterior root of the first thoracic nerve and enter the sympathetic trunk. After passing through the inferior cervical ganglion (**stellate ganglion**) and the middle cervical ganglion, they make synaptic connection with the postganglionic fibers of the superior cervical ganglion. Then the postganglionic fibers ascend along with the internal carotid artery and the ophthalmic artery and innervate the **pupillary dilator** in the orbit (Figure 8-3).

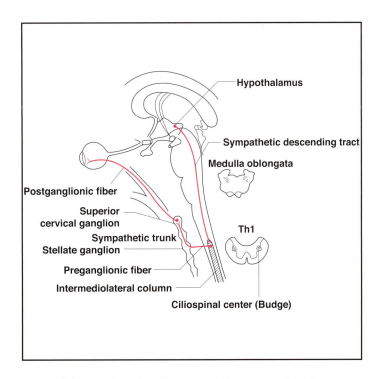

Figure 8-4 Schematic illustration of the sympathetic nervous pathway for controlling the pupils. Th1: the first thoracic cord.

The neurotransmitter for the preganglionic fibers is acetylcholine, which acts in a nicotinic way, and that for the postganglionic fibers is noradrenaline. As the pupillary dilator surrounds the pupil radially, its contraction dilates the pupil. Therefore, impairment of unilateral sympathetic pathway results in the smaller pupillary diameter as compared to the intact side (**miosis**). In a stellate ganglion block with an anesthetic agent that is applied for the treatment of pain, miosis is seen on the side of the block because the preganglionic fibers are blocked in the ganglion.

The sympathetic nerve fibers also innervate the superior tarsal muscle (Müller muscle). This muscle does not function in voluntary eyelid opening, but it acts to spontaneously maintain the elevated position of the upper eyelid. Therefore, impairment of those sympathetic nerve fibers causes drop of the upper eyelid (**ptosis**). In addition, the sympathetic nerve fibers are distributed to the mucous membrane of the eyes, nasal cavity, and oral cavity to inhibit secretion, to the facial skin to increase sweating, and to the arteries inside as well as outside of the cranial cavity to contract them.

A combination of miosis, ptosis and retraction of the ocular bulb (enophthalmos) constitutes **Horner syndrome**. This condition is caused by involvement of the sympathetic nervous system innervating that eye. In most cases of Horner syndrome, in addition to the above triad, hyperemia of the palpebral and bulbar conjunctiva and decreased sweating and increased temperature of the facial skin are seen on the affected side. In clinical practice, these additional symptoms/signs often serve to confirm the presence of Horner syndrome. Hyperemia and skin temperature elevation result from dilation of arterioles and capillaries. The mechanism as to how the enophthalmos occurs has not been elucidated. Decreased sweating and skin temperature elevation are limited to the face if the sympathetic nervous system is involved peripheral to the ciliospinal center of Budge, but when the descending sympathetic tract is involved in the brainstem or cervical cord, the above symptoms/signs are seen not just on the face but also on the affected side of the whole body (Figure 8-4).

The center of the sympathetic nervous system is in the hypothalamus. The central sympathetic fiber tracts originating from the hypothalamus descend through the medial part of the brainstem tegmentum and cervical cord and project to the intermediolateral nucleus of the spinal cord, which extends from the first thoracic to the first lumbar segment. As described earlier, those descending fibers related to the pupillary control make synaptic connection at the first thoracic segment of the intermediolateral nucleus (ciliospinal center of Budge). As the central sympathetic fibers run relatively deep in the brainstem and cervical cord, the presence of Horner syndrome in patients with brainstem or cervical cord lesion suggests the presence of an intramedullary lesion. In cervical spondylosis, for example, the extramedullary compression does not cause Horner syndrome unless the anterior root is compressed at the first thoracic segment.

In the lateral medullary syndrome of Wallenberg, which is caused by infarction of the posterior inferior cerebellar artery, Horner syndrome is a cardinal feature because the descending sympathetic fibers are involved in the medulla oblongata (Table 8-1, see Figures 14-1, 14-2 and 14-3, Box 21).

Contrary to the above, if the sympathetic pathway becomes hyperactive for some reason, it is expected to cause mydriasis, elevation of the upper eyelid, protrusion of the ocular bulb (exophthalmos), anemia of the palpebral conjunctiva, and increased sweating and decreased skin temperature of the ipsilateral face. This condition is called **Pourfour du Petit syndrome**, but it is rare. In view of the fact that exophthalmos is also seen in patients with hyperthyroidism along with tachycardia and hyperhidrosis, the sympathetic nervous system is considered to be hyperactive in hyperthyroidism.

C. ACCOMMODATION AND ITS ABNORMALITY

Accommodation is a function of the ciliary muscle, which is innervated by the parasympathetic fibers of the oculomotor nerve. Its action is to focus the visual image on the fovea by controlling the thickness of the lens. As the ciliary muscle surrounds the lens in a ring-like fashion, its contraction loosens the zonules of Zinn, which radially support the lens, and it allows the lens to increase its thickness due to its own elasticity (Figure 8-3). Owing to this special function of the ciliary muscle, it becomes possible to clearly see a visual target placed as near as 15 cm in front of eyes (**near point**). If accommodation becomes hyperactive, a far object is focused in front of the fovea causing the nearsightedness (myopia). On the contrary, if the refraction becomes hypoactive, a near object is focused behind the fovea, causing hyperopia. Thus, involvement of the parasympathetic nerve fibers of the oculomotor nerve causes accommodation failure, and the near point is extended to longer than 15 cm. Thus, if a patient with oculomotor nerve palsy complains of visual disturbance, accommodation failure should also be considered as its possible cause.

TABLE 8-1 SYNDROME CAUSED BY LOCALIZED LESION OF THE BRAINSTEM

| Syndrome | Symptoms/Signs | | Sites of Lesion |
	Ipsilateral	Contralateral	
[CROSSED]			
Weber*	III nerve palsy	Hemiplegia	Cerebral peduncle
Claude*	III nerve palsy	Motor ataxia	Midbrain medial tegmentum, red nucleus
Benedikt	III nerve palsy	Hemiplegia, tremor, involuntary movement	Midbrain medial basis, red nucleus, substantia nigra
Millard-Gubler*	Facial nerve palsy	Hemiplegia	Caudal pons lateral basis
Foville*	Facial nerve palsy Conjugate gaze palsy	Hemiplegia	Caudal pons basis, paramedian tegmentum
Raymond-Cestan	INO	Dysesthesia, motor ataxia, hemiplegia	Rostral pons tegmentum
Wallenberg	Horner, facial nociceptive sensory loss, vertigo, dysphagia, motor ataxia	Nociceptive sensory loss below neck	Lateral medullary tegmentum
Cestan-Chenais	Horner, facial nociceptive sensory loss, dysphagia	Nociceptive sensory loss below neck, hemiplegia	Lateral medulla
Babinski-Nageotte*	Horner, facial nociceptive sensory loss, vertigo, dysphagia, motor ataxia	Nociceptive sensory loss below neck, hemiplegia	Unilateral medulla except for medial lemniscus and hypoglossal nucleus
[UNCROSSED]			
Parinaud*	Vertical gaze palsy, convergence palsy		Rostral midbrain-thalamus

III nerve: oculomotor nerve, INO: internuclear ophthalmoplegia

* Original reports are listed in the bibliography at the end of this chapter.

2. EXAMINATION OF INTRAOCULAR MUSCLES

First, the shape and diameter of pupils should be observed, paying special attention to possible asymmetry between the two eyes. Asymmetry of pupillary diameter is called **aniso-coria**. A pathologically large pupil is called **mydriasis**, and a pathologically small pupil is called **miosis**. Of course, judgment of this asymmetry is impossible in a condition in which any eye-drop such as pupillary dilator has been applied. Furthermore, if the patient underwent any ophthalmological surgery in the past, the pupil might look irregular in shape.

In general, pupils tend to be small in the aged population. In that case, it is useful to examine the pupils in a dark room in order to dilate the pupils as much as possible. Normal pupils are usually **round and isocoric**, meaning the same diameter. When the iris looks dark as in some races, the pupils can be better observed by lighting the eyes from

either side. Projection of the light from the front should be avoided, because it changes the pupillary diameter as the result of light reflex.

A. OCULOMOTOR NERVE PALSY AND HORNER SYNDROME

If a pupil is extremely large or extremely small as compared with the other side, the pupil of that side is likely abnormal. Sometimes, however, it might be difficult to judge which side is abnormal. If there is any asymmetry in the level of the upper eyelid, then it helps determining the abnormal side. If there is ptosis in one eye, that side is often abnormal. If the pupil is larger in the eye with ptosis, it is likely to be oculomotor nerve palsy. In this case, the light reflex and convergence reflex are often lost, insufficient, or sluggish on the affected side.

By contrast, if the pupil is smaller in the eye with ptosis, it is most likely to be Horner syndrome and suggests involvement of the sympathetic nerve fibers on that side. As the tarsal levator muscle is not a skeletal muscle, ptosis due to impairment of the sympathetic nerve fibers is milder in its degree as compared with paralysis of the levator muscle of the upper eyelids due to impairment of the oculomotor nerve fibers. As described above, the accompanying symptoms/signs such as enophthalmos, conjunctival hyperemia, and decreased sweating and elevated temperature of the facial skin support the diagnosis of Horner syndrome. Among these signs, enophthalmos, though it is one of the triad of Horner syndrome, is sometimes difficult to confirm. In that case, other accompanying signs might help making the diagnosis.

Horner syndrome is often congenital due to a traumatic injury of the sympathetic tract in the neck. Anisocoria due to unilateral miosis is sometimes difficult to detect in a bright room, because both pupils react to the light stimulus. In that case, it is useful to examine the patient in a dark room, where the intact pupil dilates more than the affected pupil, making the anisocoria more easily detectable.

B. EXAMINATION OF THE LIGHT REFLEX AND ITS ABNORMALITY

With the eyes kept open, the examiner projects a penlight to either eye and observes the reaction of both pupils simultaneously. In order to avoid overlap of the convergence reflex, the light should be projected to the eye obliquely from the temporal side instead of projecting straight from the front.

If the light reflex is absent or decreased in the stimulated eye (direct reaction absent) while it is present in the opposite (nonstimulated) eye (indirect reaction present), it suggests impairment of the efferent pathway, namely the midbrain or oculomotor nerve, of the stimulated eye (Figure 8-5, see also Figure 7-6). By contrast, if the light reflex is absent or decreased in the nonstimulated eye (indirect reaction absent) while it is present in the stimulated eye (direct reaction present), it suggests impairment of the efferent pathway of the nonstimulated eye. In other words, if the light reflex is absent in one eye regardless of the side of stimulation, it suggests impairment of the efferent pathway of that eye. By contrast, if the light reflex is absent in both eyes (both direct and indirect reactions absent), it suggests either the visual impairment (afferent pathway) of the stimulated eye or bilateral impairment of the efferent pathway. For example, if the light reflex in response to the

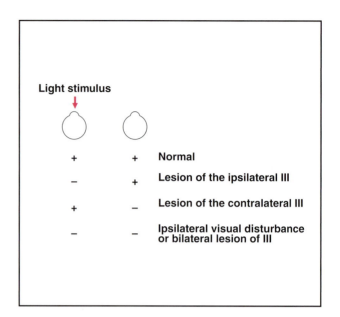

Figure 8-5 Presence (+) or absence (−) of the light reflex and its interpretation. Ipsilateral: ipsilateral to the light stimulus, contralateral: contralateral to the light stimulus, III: oculomotor nerve.

right eye stimulation is absent in both eyes, it suggests either the visual loss of the right eye or bilateral impairment of the autonomic fibers of the oculomotor nerves.

If visual loss is limited to one eye, the light stimulation of the other (intact) eye will elicit the light reflex in both eyes. In this case, if the light stimulus is shifted from the normal eye to the blind eye, it is expected to lead to pupillary dilation in both eyes, and this phenomenon can be repeated by shifting the light stimulus between the two eyes. As this phenomenon is paradoxical to the ordinary reaction, it is called **paradoxical pupillary reaction**. This paradoxical reaction is often encountered in patients with multiple sclerosis or optic (retrobulbar) neuritis. This phenomenon is called Marcus Gunn pupil, while Marcus Gunn is also attached to jaw-winking as a Marcus Gunn phenomenon (see Box 14).

Bilateral loss of the light reflex is an important finding for the diagnosis of brain death (see Chapter 29-5C). In relation to this, in a patient lying supine in a bright room such as an intensive care unit (ICU), the pupils might already be constricted to the room light before testing. In that case, a very bright light stimulus might be needed to elicit the remaining reflex. An alternative practical way would to test the light reflex immediately after opening the eyelids or to test the reflex after darkening the room. As a comatose patient usually lies supine in a bright room, the above caution is important in order to avoid misjudgment.

C. SPECIAL ABNORMAL FINDINGS OF PUPILS

A condition in which the light reflex is lost or decreased in spite of normal vision while the convergence reflex is preserved is called **Argyll Robertson pupil**. In this condition, the pupillary diameter is relatively small. This pupil is seen in patients with neurosyphilis, especially with tabes dorsalis, but it is also seen in diabetic impairment of the autonomic nervous system.

Pupillotonia is characterized by marked mydriasis in which the light reflex is extremely slow, and continuous exposure to the light stimulus in a dark room will shrink the pupil extremely slowly. Then, if the patient is placed in a very dark room immediately afterward, the pupil will dilate again very slowly. It is, therefore, believed that, in this condition, both the pupillary sphincter and dilator muscles are in a tonic state so that they contract only with extreme slowness. In this condition, the convergence reflex is relatively better preserved than the light reflex.

A typical example of pupillotonia is seen in **Adie syndrome**, which is usually accompanied by loss of the Achilles tendon reflex. Pupillotonia associated with segmental anhidrosis and loss of tendon reflexes is called **Ross syndrome**. In most cases of pupillotonia, the affected pupil overreacts to eye drops of a cholinesterase inhibitor causing extreme miosis, which is supposed to be due to hypersensitivity of synaptic receptors of the postganglionic fibers. A similar condition is seen following a lesion of the postganglionic fibers and is explained as **denervation supersensitivity**. Pupils may display small amplitude fluctuations in size under constant illumination. This phenomenon is called **hippus,** but its clinical significance has not been clarified.

D. EXAMINATION OF THE CONVERGENCE REFLEX

Convergence reflex is tested by moving a visual target toward the nasion with both eyes kept open or by asking the subject to look at a near object. The reaction is judged in the same way as for the light reflex. If the reaction is absent or decreased in one eye, it suggests impairment of the autonomic fibers of the oculomotor nerve. As the light reflex can be tested and judged more easily than the convergence reflex, the latter is often used as supplementary to the light reflex.

E. EXAMINATION OF ACCOMMODATION

As described earlier, accommodation is a function of the ciliary muscle to control refraction by changing the thickness of the lens. It is tested by measuring the near point while moving a visual target toward each eye. The near point in healthy subjects is usually 15 cm. In accommodation failure, the near point becomes longer. In other words, the subject cannot see clearly an object placed 15 cm or further in front of eye. This may be one of the reasons for complaints of visual disturbance by patients with disorders of the autonomic nervous system.

BIBLIOGRAPHY

Babinski J, Nageotte J. Hémiasynergie, latéropulsion et myosis bulbaires avec hémianesthésie et hémiplégie croisées. Rev Neurol (Paris) 10: 358–365, 1902.

Chusid JG, McDonald JJ. Correlative Neuroanatomy and Functional Neurology. 12th ed. Lange, Maruzen Asian Edition, Tokyo, 1964.

Claude H. Syndrome pédonculaire de la région du noyau rouge. Rev Neurol (Paris) 23:311–313, 1912.

Claude H, Loyez M. Ramollissement du noyau rouge. Rev Neurol (Paris) 24: 49–51, 1912.

Foville A. Note sur une paralysie peu connue de certains muscles de l'oeil, et sa liaison avec quelques points de l'anatomie et la physiologie de la protubérance annulaire. Bull Soc Anat Paris 33:393–414, 1858.

Haymaker W. Bing's Local Diagnosis in Neurological Diseases. 5th ed., Mosby, St Louis, 1969.

Millard M. Extrait du rapport de M. Millard sur les observations précédentes. Bull Soc Anat Paris 31:217–221, 1856.

Parinaud H. Paralysis of the movement of convergence of the eyes. Brain 9:330–341, 1886.

Weber H. A contribution to the pathology of the crura cerebri. Medico Chirurg Trans 46:121–139, 1863.

EXTRAOCULAR MUSCLES, GAZE, AND EYE MOVEMENTS

1. NERVE INNERVATION OF EXTRAOCULAR MUSCLES

There are six extraocular muscles attached to each eyeball: medial rectus, lateral rectus, superior rectus, inferior rectus, superior oblique, and inferior oblique (Figure 9-1a). Contraction of the medial rectus and lateral rectus muscles rotates the eyeball medially and laterally, respectively. The exact action of the other four muscles depends on the position of eye (Figure 9-1b). The superior and inferior rectus muscles are attached to the top and the bottom, respectively, of the anterior hemisphere of the eyeball, and act most efficiently when the eye is slightly abducted. Therefore, contraction of the superior rectus muscle rotates the eyeball upward diagonally in the lateral direction, and contraction of the inferior rectus muscle rotates the eyeball downward diagonally in the lateral direction. The superior and inferior oblique muscles are attached to the top and the bottom, respectively, of the posterior hemisphere of the eyeball, and act most efficiently when the eye is slightly adducted. Furthermore, the direction of muscle power for these two muscles is reversed by a hook (trochlea), which is attached to the upper and lower medial wall, respectively, of the orbit. Therefore, contraction of the superior and inferior oblique muscles rotates the eyeball downward and upward, respectively, diagonally in the medial direction (Figure 9-1b).

Thus, simultaneous contraction of the superior rectus and inferior oblique muscle rotates the eyeball upward, and simultaneous contraction of the inferior rectus and superior oblique muscle rotates the eyeball downward. Among these six extraocular muscles, the medial rectus, superior rectus, inferior rectus, and inferior oblique muscles are innervated by the oculomotor nerve. The superior oblique muscle is innervated by the trochlear nerve, and the lateral rectus muscle is innervated by the abducens nerve.

A. THIRD CRANIAL NERVE (OCULOMOTOR NERVE)

As just described, the oculomotor nerve innervates four extraocular muscles: medial rectus, superior rectus, inferior rectus, and inferior oblique. Therefore, when the oculomotor nerve is involved by a lesion, medial rotation and upward rotation of the eyeball are paralyzed, but its lateral rotation is preserved. Downward rotation is partially possible because the superior oblique muscle is spared. The oculomotor nucleus is located in the midbrain at the level of superior colliculus, in front of the periaqueductal gray substance and just medial to the **medial longitudinal fasciculus (MLF)** (see Figure 5-1). The oculomotor nucleus is formed from four groups of neurons, one innervating each extraocular muscle, and a fifth group innervating the levator muscle of the upper eyelid. Within the oculomotor nucleus, there is some topographic arrangement of those neuronal groups in terms of functions. For example, the neuronal groups related to the upward rotation of the eyeball (superior rectus, inferior oblique, and levator muscle of the upper eyelid) are located close to each other.

Motor fibers originating from the oculomotor nucleus, together with the autonomic fibers originating from the Edinger-Westphal nucleus, run anteriorly through the medial part of the red nucleus, and exit from the midbrain just medial to the cerebral peduncle (see Figure 5-1). As the fibers of the oculomotor nerve are relatively spread apart within the midbrain parenchyma, an intramedullary lesion may affect some fiber groups selectively. In this case, therefore, weakness of the extraocular muscles might be different in its degree among muscles. As the fiber groups assemble to form a small bundle at the exit from the midbrain, the closer the lesion is to the anterior rim of the midbrain, the more muscles are equally paralyzed to produce complete oculomotor nerve palsy, as seen in Weber syndrome (Figure 9-2).

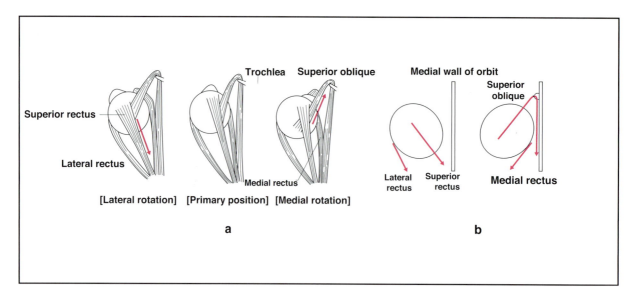

Figure 9-1 Structure of extraocular muscles (a) and direction of action of each muscle shown by arrows (b). View of the left eye from above. The superior rectus muscle rotates the ocular bulb upward in its laterally rotated position, and the superior oblique muscle rotates the ocular bulb downward in its medially rotated position. At the base of the ocular bulb, the inferior rectus muscle and the inferior oblique muscle function according to the same principle.

Intramedullary Lesion of the Oculomotor Nerve and Crossed Hemiplegia

As the oculomotor nerve passes just medial to the red nucleus, its lesion there might have an associated ataxia of the contralateral extremities in addition to the ipsilateral oculomotor nerve palsy (**Claude syndrome**) (Figure 9-2, see Table 8-1). In this case, the ataxia is caused by a lesion of the superior cerebellar peduncle, which originates from the contralateral dentate nucleus of cerebellum and crosses before reaching the red nucleus (see Chapter 16-2C). Claude in 1912 reported a 56-year-old man who presented

with complete paralysis of the right oculomotor nerve and probably also paralysis of the trochlear nerve associated with ataxia of the left extremities (Claude, 1912). Later the autopsy findings of that case were reported, which showed a small infarction at the right midbrain involving the oculomotor nerve, the rostral part of the superior cerebellar peduncle, the medial part of the red nucleus, and the MLF (Claude & Loyez, 1912). Following this case report, a combination of oculomotor nerve palsy and the contralateral cerebellar ataxia was called Claude syndrome, but it is estimated from the original report that there might have also

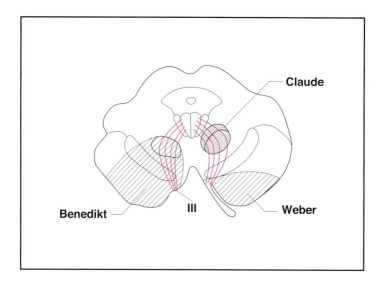

Figure 9-2 Crossed syndrome due to localized lesion of the midbrain. III: oculomotor nerve.

THE NEUROLOGIC EXAMINATION

been **internuclear ophthalmoplegia (INO)** due to involvement of the MLF, although it must have been impossible to clinically confirm INO because of the presence of complete oculomotor nerve palsy.

It is noteworthy that Guillain commented to Claude's report based on his own research that, following a lesion of the red nucleus, retrograde degeneration could occur in the superior cerebellar peduncle down to the dentate nucleus of cerebellum (Claude & Loyez, 1912).

A condition in which oculomotor nerve palsy is associated with contralateral tremulous involuntary movements and hemiplegia or pyramidal signs is called **Benedikt syndrome**. In this condition, the lesion also involves the substantia nigra and cerebral peduncle (Figure 9-2, see Table 8-1) (Liu et al, 1992). A lesion at the site of exit of the oculomotor nerve from the midbrain causes ipsilateral oculomotor nerve palsy and contralateral hemiplegia or pyramidal signs (**Weber syndrome**) (Figure 9-2, Box 10). Weber syndrome is caused by a vascular lesion of the midbrain basis, but it is also seen in an extramedullary lesion compressing the midbrain from anteriorly.

The above-described conditions manifesting a cranial nerve lesion associated with contralateral hemiplegia used to be called alternate hemiplegia or alternating hemiplegia. However, as "alternate" and "alternating" is more commonly used in a temporal meaning than in a spatial meaning, "**crossed hemiplegia**" might be a more appropriate terminology for these conditions (Liu et al, 1992, for review). Hemiplegia encountered in crossed hemiplegia is not necessarily severe in its degree, and it may be just a positive Babinski sign due to mild impairment of the corticospinal tract.

It is known in animals that the nerve fibers innervating the superior rectus muscle cross at the level of the oculomotor nucleus and join the contralateral oculomotor nerve, and that the levator muscle of the upper eyelid is bilaterally innervated (Bienfang, 1975). In relation to this, some human cases with small infarctions in the midbrain tegmentum have been reported to manifest the isolated paralysis of the contralateral superior rectus muscle (Kwon et al, 2003; Tsukamoto et al, 2005).

Extramedullary Lesion of the Oculomotor Nerve

After exiting from the midbrain, the oculomotor nerve passes between the posterior cerebral artery and the superior cerebellar artery (Figure 9-3), then passes through the upper part of the cavernous sinus (see Figure 8-1), enters the orbit through the superior orbital fissure (see Figure 8-2a), and sends its branches to the four extraocular muscles and

the levator muscle of the upper eyelid. Impairment of the oculomotor nerve is an important sign in tentorial herniation (see Chapter 29-5C). In this case, the oculomotor nerve is believed to be entrapped between the posterior cerebral artery and the superior cerebellar artery as a result of supratentorial compression rather than being involved intramedullary in the midbrain.

Cavernous Sinus Syndrome

As the oculomotor nerve passes through the cavernous sinus, it is easily impaired by inflammation of the

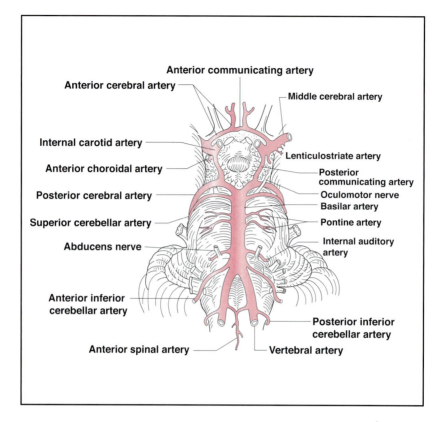

Figure 9-3 Spatial relationship between arteries at the base of the brainstem and cranial nerves. (Modified from Chusid & McDonald, 1964)

cavernous sinus, either by an autoimmune mechanism or as a result of infectious diseases. As it is often associated with severe ocular pain, this condition is called **painful ophthalmoplegia (Tolosa-Hunt syndrome)**. Similar symptoms/signs can be seen in the **orbital apex syndrome**, which is due to inflammation or tumor of the orbital apex and is characterized by exophthalmos and palpebral swelling in addition to painful ophthalmoplegia.

B. FOURTH CRANIAL NERVE (TROCHLEAR NERVE)

The nucleus of the trochlear nerve is located in the caudal midbrain at the level of the inferior colliculus just posterior to the MLF. From there the fibers run medioposteriorly, cross at the anterior medullary velum, and exit from the contralateral midbrain through its posterior rim. Then the fibers run anteriorly, pass through the cavernous sinus, and enter the orbit through the superior orbital fissure (see Figures 8-1 and 8-2a). This is the only cranial nerve that crosses in the brainstem, except for the fibers of the oculomotor nerve innervating the superior rectus muscle, but it is extremely rare for this nerve to be solely affected by an intramedullary lesion.

C. SIXTH CRANIAL NERVE (ABDUCENS NERVE)

The nucleus of the abducens nerve is located near the anterior wall of the fourth ventricle. Its nerve fibers run anteriorly through the medial pons and exit from the pons

BOX 11 TOP OF THE BASILAR ARTERY SYNDROME

A number of branches originate from the distal part of the basilar artery (Figure 9-3). Therefore, infarction or embolism involving the top of the basilar artery causes ischemic lesions in multiple structures such as the thalamus, the midbrain, the cerebellum, and the mesial part of the temporal and occipital lobes, and, depending on the anatomy, there can be a variety of clinical symptomatology. These symptoms/signs include bilateral ptosis, extraocular muscle palsy, internuclear ophthalmoplegia, pupillary abnormalities, motor disturbance, impairment of consciousness, confusion, visual field defect, and cerebellar ataxia. The symptom complex is sometimes called "top of the basilar artery syndrome," but there are no strict criteria for this diagnosis. In some cases of this syndrome, generalized convulsion as the initial symptom or locked-in syndrome has been reported. The diagnosis can be confirmed by magnetic resonance angiography.

through the corticospinal tract (see Figure 5-2). Then the nerve fibers pass between the internal auditory artery and the anterior inferior cerebellar artery (Figure 9-3) and through the cavernous sinus, and enter the orbit through the superior orbital fissure to innervate the lateral rectus muscle (see Figures 8-1 and 8-2a). If the abducens nerve is involved together with the corticospinal tract by either an intramedullary lesion or extramedullary compression, an abducens palsy and spastic paralysis of the contralateral extremities are simultaneously seen (**abducens crossed hemiplegia**). This condition, like Weber syndrome, is a representative case of crossed hemiplegia.

The abducens nerve runs in the cranial cavity a longer distance than any other cranial nerve, extending from the posterior cranial fossa along the clivus to the orbit. Therefore, in a state of intracranial hypertension, this nerve tends to be impaired either unilaterally or bilaterally, though to a relatively mild degree. As this is not due to direct compression of the nerve by a mass lesion, this circumstance belongs to the **false localizing signs**.

As is described later (see Chapter 11-1A), the facial nerve first runs posteriorly from its nucleus, turns around the abducens nucleus, and exits from the lateral rim of the pons. Thus, the abducens nerve and the facial nerve are very close together at the pontine tegmentum, but once they exit from the pons, they do not meet again (see Figure 5-2). Therefore, when these two nerves are simultaneously affected, it suggests the presence of an intramedullary lesion in the pontine tegmentum. However, it has to be kept in mind that the above two nerves may still be affected simultaneously by an inflammatory process outside of the brainstem, as seen in multiple cranial neuritis.

2. NEURAL CONTROL MECHANISM OF GAZE

Voluntary movement of both eyes either horizontally or vertically is called **gaze**. This important mechanism is controlled by elaborate central networks.

A. CENTRAL CONTROL MECHANISM OF GAZE

The main cortical gaze centers are located in the frontal lobe. The **frontal eye field (FEF)** is located at the lateral frontal convexity just anterior to the face/hand area of the primary motor cortex, and the **supplementary eye field (SEF)** is located in the mesial frontal cortex just anterior and superior to the supplementary motor area proper (SMA proper) (see Figure 11-3). Visual information is transferred from the posterior parietal cortex (area 7) to the FEF. The nerve fibers originating from FEF and SEF pass through the corona radiata and the centrum semiovale of the cerebral hemisphere, cross at the upper brainstem, and project to the **paramedian pontine reticular formation (PPRF)**, which serves as the lateral gaze center (Figure 9-4). Physiologically, there are saccadic burst neurons in the PPRF. The nerve fibers originating from the PPRF project to the ipsilateral abducens nucleus, in which two different groups of neurons are present. The nerve fibers originating from one group form the abducens nerve and pass through the medial part of pons anteriorly, and those originating from another group of neurons (internuclear neurons) cross at the same level to form the MLF. The MLF ascends through the medial part of the pontine tegmentum and projects to the ventral nucleus of the oculomotor nucleus, which innervates the medial rectus muscle. Thus, activation of PPRF causes contraction of the ipsilateral lateral rectus muscle and the contralateral medial rectus muscle simultaneously, resulting in the lateral gaze to the side ipsilateral to the PPRF or contralateral to the cortical gaze center (Figure 9-4).

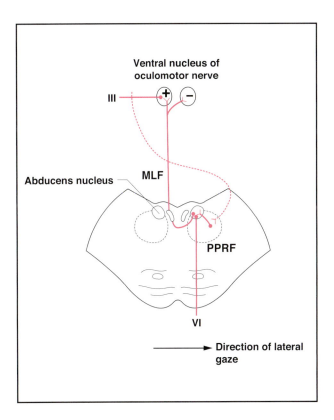

Figure 9-4 Schematic illustration of the nerve pathway to explain the lateral gaze and internuclear ophthalmoplegia. III: oculomotor nerve, VI: abducens nerve, MLF: medial longitudinal fasciculus, PPRF: paramedian pontine reticular formation.

B. LATERAL GAZE AND LATERAL GAZE PALSY

A unilateral lesion of the frontal lobe may cause disturbance of lateral gaze to the other side. This condition may not necessarily present with gaze palsy, but it may just slow down the saccadic movement to the contralateral side. If consciousness of the patient is disturbed in this condition, the eyes are often deviated toward the side of the lesion due to the preserved activity of the contralateral eye fields (**conjugate deviation of eyes**).

A similar phenomenon can also be seen in a parieto-occipital lesion, but in this case the head may be also rotated toward the side of the lesion. This condition is also seen in patients with some disturbance of consciousness, most likely because visual attention is intact toward the side of the lesion and impaired toward the side contralateral to the lesion. It is not completely clear why the conjugate deviation of eyes is more common in a state of impaired consciousness, but it is conceivable that, in conscious patients, visual attention can compensate for the tendency to deviate by intact visual attention.

In the acute phase of thalamic hemorrhage, eyes are often deviated toward the contralateral side. This is considered to be a positive symptom (see Chapter 1-1), and the direction of deviation may be reversed later during the clinical course.

As expected from Figure 9-4, a unilateral lesion of the pontine tegmentum causes lateral gaze palsy to the side of the lesion, and the eyes tend to be deviated to the contralateral side. Contrary to the conjugate deviation due to a hemispheric lesion, conjugate deviation due to a pontine lesion can be also seen in patients with intact consciousness.

When the lateral gaze center of the pons (PPRF) is involved by a lesion, the lesion commonly involves the ipsilateral MLF as well. In this condition, lateral gaze may not be conjugate (meaning that the two eyes are not paralyzed to the same degree). In a lesion of the right pontine tegmentum, for example, the left eye is deviated to the left whereas the right eye is not deviated at all or is deviated just a little to the left because of the associated lesion of the right MLF.

Lateral gaze palsy due to a PPRF lesion varies in its severity depending on the nature and degree of the lesion. It could be complete lateral gaze palsy, but in case of relatively mild impairment or during recovery from an acute phase, it may just show incomplete lateral gaze palsy or it may just decrease the speed of the lateral gaze.

C. VERTICAL GAZE AND VERTICAL GAZE PALSY

In contrast with the lateral gaze center, which is in the pons, the vertical gaze center is located in the midbrain. The **rostral interstitial nucleus of MLF** plays a main role in the control of vertical gaze, but the interstitial nucleus of Cajal is also known to participate. Like the lateral gaze center, saccadic burst neurons exist in these gaze centers. These structures are believed to receive input from the frontal eye field, vestibular nucleus, and superior colliculus, but the distinction of upward and downward gaze is not clearly known.

Compression of the quadrigeminal body by a pineal tumor, for example, causes **vertical gaze palsy** and convergence palsy. A combination of vertical gaze palsy and convergence palsy is called **Parinaud syndrome**. This condition is often associated with pupillary abnormalities and up-beat nystagmus. The gaze palsy seen in Parinaud syndrome may be solely upward or solely downward, or may be in both directions (Parinaud, 1886). In four autopsied cases with Parinaud syndrome studied by Pierrot-Deseilligny, infarction was commonly found in the border zone area between the midbrain and the thalamus, involving the rostral interstitial nucleus of the MLF and its efferent fibers (Pierrot-Deseilligny et al, 1982). In this case, the oculocephalic reflex or doll's eye sign (see 5-C of this chapter) is usually preserved.

Progressive supranuclear palsy (PSP, Steele-Richardson-Olszewski syndrome) is characterized by vertical gaze palsy, especially downward gaze palsy, in which the oculocephalic reflex is preserved. In this condition, the superior colliculus is pathologically affected, and demonstration of its atrophy on MRI serves as one of its diagnostic criteria.

Vertical supranuclear palsy is seen in children with neurolipidosis, especially Niemann-Pick disease type C (**ophthalmoplegic lipidosis**).

D. CONVERGENCE AND CONVERGENCE PALSY

In order to see a near object, convergence is produced by bilateral contraction of the medial rectus muscles. The convergence center is called the Perlia nucleus, which is located in the midbrain. Diagnosis of **convergence palsy** is only possible when the medial rectus muscles are not paralyzed. However, as the Perlia nucleus is located near the oculomotor nucleus, the two nuclei are commonly affected by the same lesion. In this case, it is difficult to confirm the presence of convergence palsy. When examining the aged population, it should be kept in mind that convergence and vertical gaze tend to be incomplete even in healthy subjects.

In order to see a far object, the lateral rectus muscles contract bilaterally. This is called **divergence**. If double vision is a complaint when looking at a far object, it may be due to bilateral paralysis of lateral rectus muscles or divergence palsy, and the distinction between the two conditions is sometimes difficult. If the lateral rectus muscle is paralyzed, it is expected to worsen double vision when looking laterally toward the impaired side whereas, in divergence palsy, double vision is expected to disappear or decrease when looking toward either side.

3. MEDIAL LONGITUDINAL FASCICULUS AND INTERNUCLEAR OPHTHALMOPLEGIA

As the MLF connects the abducens nucleus with the contralateral oculomotor nucleus (Figure 9-4), its interruption causes disconjugate lateral gaze palsy to the contralateral side. Namely, the contralateral eye can be abducted but the ipsilateral eye cannot be adducted (**internuclear ophthalmoplegia, INO**). In this case, horizontal nystagmus is seen on lateral gaze to the side contralateral to the lesion with the rapid phase directed toward the side of gaze. Characteristically, this nystagmus is seen solely or predominantly in the abducting eye (**dissociated nystagmus**). As the same phenomena can be seen in patients with horizontal nystagmus associated with oculomotor nerve palsy, it has to be proved that the medial rectus muscle is intact before making the diagnosis of INO. In this case, the presence of convergence is used for proving that it is intact. Thus, the diagnostic criteria for INO is composed of (1) impairment of adduction of the eye ipsilateral to the lesion, (2) dissociated nystagmus, and (3) relative preservation of convergence.

Since the MLF lies close to the midline in the brainstem, demonstration of an INO always suggests the presence of an intramedullary lesion. When the MLF is only mildly affected or during the recovery phase from an acute phase, the adduction of the ipsilateral eye may appear normal, and instead only the dissociated nystagmus might be seen. In that case, careful observation of the lateral saccade toward the side contralateral to the lesion might disclose slower speed of the adducting eye as compared with the speed of the abducting eye. INO is commonly seen in ischemic vascular disease or multiple sclerosis. The most common cause of bilateral INO in young subjects is multiple sclerosis.

In a unilateral lesion of the pontine tegmentum involving both the PPRF and the MLF, the lateral gaze to the side ipsilateral to the lesion is impaired while the lateral gaze to the contralateral side shows INO. In this condition, therefore, the eye ipsilateral to the lesion does not move to either side while the contralateral eye moves only laterally but not medially. Thus, this condition is called the **one-and-a-half syndrome** (Figure 9-5).

4. CENTRAL CONTROL MECHANISM OF EYE MOVEMENTS

Eye movements are categorized into two kinds: **saccadic eye movement (saccades)** and **smooth pursuit eye movement (smooth pursuit)**. Saccades occur when the eyes rapidly shift their fixation from one visual target to the other, and smooth pursuit occurs when the eyes pursue a smoothly moving visual target. For these two, the final

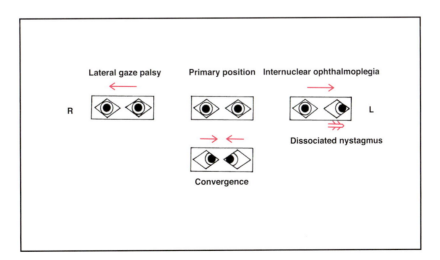

Figure 9-5 Schematic illustration to show the one-and-a-half syndrome. In this case, the lesion is in the right pontine tegmentum. Right lateral gaze is paralyzed due to the lesion of the right PPRF, and internuclear palsy is seen on the left lateral gaze due to the lesion of the right MLF. Convergence is normal. R: right, L: left. Single arrows indicate the direction of gaze.

common pathway from the brainstem nuclei to the extraocular muscles is the same, but the central control mechanism is different.

A. CENTRAL CONTROL MECHANISM OF SACCADES

Physiologically, saccades are grouped into two kinds, memory guided and visually guided. **Memory-guided saccades** (MGS) are generated when a subject is requested to look at a visual target after it has been removed. **Visually guided saccades** (VGS) are generated by asking a subject to look at a visual target. Thus the MGS is more voluntary while the VGS is more reflexive if done immediately upon presentation of the visual stimulus. Results of experimental studies in monkeys, clinical observations in patients, and neuroimaging studies in healthy subjects all indicate that MGS is mainly controlled by the frontal cortex including the SEF, FEF, dorsolateral prefrontal cortex, and anterior cingulate, and that VGS is mainly controlled by the posterior parietal cortex (Girard & Berthoz, 2005, for review; Ramat et al, 2007) (Figure 9-6).

It is believed that the nerve fibers originating from the frontal cortex project directly to the saccadic burst neurons in the gaze centers of midbrain and pons, but there is also a role of the superior colliculus in the control of saccades (Figure 9-6) (Girard & Berthoz, 2005, for review; Ramat et al, 2007; Terao et al, 2011). In the superior colliculus, a group of neurons is retinotopically organized and related to visual function, and another group of neurons is engaged in motor control. The superior colliculus receives input directly from the frontal and parietal cortices and the striatum, and its output projects to the saccadic burst neurons in the gaze centers and to the cerebellum. However, as an experimental lesion of the superior colliculus in animals does not alter the amplitude of saccades or smooth pursuit, it is believed that the superior colliculus is not a direct relay center from the cortex to the burst neurons but it controls selection of visual target and initiation and speed of eye movements (Ramat et al, 2007).

B. CENTRAL CONTROL MECHANISM OF SMOOTH PURSUIT

There is some overlap of the central control system of smooth pursuit with that of the above described VGS, but area V5, which corresponds to the middle temporal visual area (MT) and the medial superior temporal visual

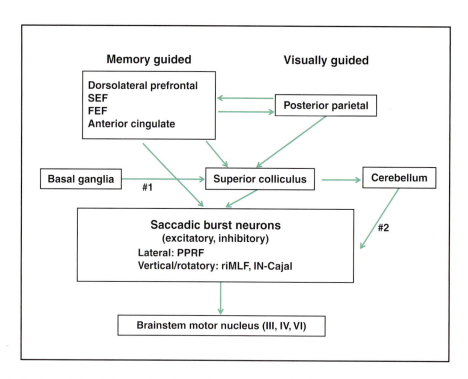

Figure 9-6 Diagram illustrating the central control mechanism of saccadic eye movement. The difference between a memory-guided saccade and a visually guided saccade is not absolute but relative. The arrows show the main flow of information between different structures, and in fact most connections are believed to be bidirectional. Furthermore, the ascending pathway from the subcortical structures to the cerebral cortex through the thalamic relay nuclei is not shown here. #1 is inhibitory and mainly related to motor selection. #2 controls accurate performance of the saccades. SEF: supplementary eye field, FEF: frontal eye field, PPRF: paramedian pontine reticular formation, riMLF: rostral interstitial nucleus of the medial longitudinal fasciculus, IN-Cajal: interstitial nucleus of Cajal. (Prepared by the authors based on Girard & Berthoz, 2005, and Ramat et al, 2007)

area (MST) of monkeys plays an important role in motion vision and thus in smooth pursuit (Figure 9-7) (Lencer & Trillenberg, 2008, for review). Area V5 in humans is located in the posterior part of the superior temporal sulcus at the site where its ascending branch bifurcates (Matsumoto et al, 2004) (see Chapter 23-1C). Area V5 receives input from the primary visual cortex directly or indirectly, and also from the vestibular nuclei, and it projects to the FEF and the parietal eye field. Furthermore, the FEF receives input from the SEF, dorsolateral prefrontal cortex, and parietal cortex, each of which controls the function of the FEF. The smooth pursuit-related neurons in the brainstem are considered to be in the reticular formation, which corresponds to the dorsolateral pontine nucleus and the nucleus reticularis tegmenti pontis in monkeys. The neuronal group receives input from area V5 and the FEF and projects indirectly via cerebellum and vestibular nuclei to the motor nuclei innervating the extraocular muscles (Figure 9-7, Box 12) (Mustari et al, 2009).

C. ROLES OF CEREBELLUM AND BASAL GANGLIA IN EYE MOVEMENTS

The cerebellum and basal ganglia play an important role in the control of eye movements. The cerebellum receives input from the superior colliculus and projects output

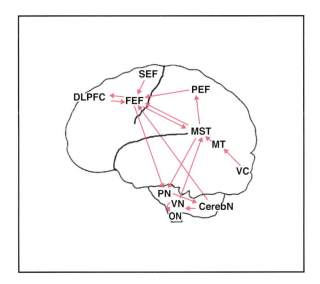

Figure 9-7 Schematic diagram showing the central pathway related to the control of smooth pursuit eye movement. CerebN: cerebellar nucleus, DLPFC: dorsolateral prefrontal cortex, FEF: frontal eye field, MST: medial superior temporal visual area, MT: middle temporal visual area, ON: motor nuclei innervating extraocular muscles, PEF: parietal eye field, PN: smooth pursuit-related nucleus in the pontine reticular formation, SEF: supplementary eye field, VC: primary visual cortex, VN: vestibular nuclei. (Reproduced from Lencer & Trillenberg, 2008 with permission).

BOX 12 SACCADIC EYE MOVEMENT AND SMOOTH PURSUIT EYE MOVEMENT

It is generally believed that a saccadic eye movement (saccade) is a rapid eye movement whereas a smooth pursuit eye movement (smooth pursuit) is a slow movement, but from the clinical point of view, the distinction between the two should be made not just based on the speed of ocular movements but rather on the way the eye movement was induced in the examination. A saccade is induced by shifting the visual fixation from one visual target rapidly to another target. In this case, therefore, the fixation point jumps from a visual target to another target. Consequently, the movement is rapid in healthy subjects, but in some patients the saccade may become very slow. By contrast, smooth pursuit is induced when the eyes maintain fixation to a slowly moving visual target, and its speed depends on the speed of the target movement. As a visual target is usually moved slowly for inducing the smooth pursuit, the induced eye movement is slow and smooth in healthy subjects. However, if a visual target is moved rapidly, the induced ocular movement can be as fast as the saccade.

through the cerebellar nuclei to the saccadic burst neurons in the midbrain and pons (Figure 9-6). The cerebellum acts to accurately control the amplitude of saccades, and its dysfunction causes instability of the saccadic amplitude and impairment of VGS. Within the cerebellum, among others, flocculus and paraflocculus play an important role in stabilizing the visual image on the fovea of retina.

Output from the basal ganglia is inhibitory and acts to select necessary movements by suppressing unnecessary movements (see Chapter 16-2B). In Parkinson disease, the reaction time with saccades is delayed and the speed of saccade becomes slow in proportion to the reaction time of the hand ipsilateral to the side of gaze (Shibasaki et al, 1979). As the striatum is functionally connected to the supplementary motor area, it is considered to be especially important for the control of MGS. In Parkinson disease, MGS is mainly impaired, but VGS was also shown to be impaired, though to a relatively mild degree, from the early clinical stage (Terao et al, 2011).

5. EXAMINATION OF EXTRAOCULAR MUSCLES, GAZE, AND EYE MOVEMENTS

As gaze and eye movements cannot be tested if the extraocular muscles are paralyzed, it is reasonable to test the extraocular muscles first before testing the gaze and eye movements.

A. PTOSIS

Although the levator muscle of the upper eyelid is not directly related to eye movement, it is useful to observe the presence or absence of **ptosis (blepharoptosis)** to start with. This can be done by comparing the palpebral fissure between the two eyes.

Bilateral Ptosis

Bilateral ptosis is seen in disorders of muscles or neuromuscular junctions. In particular, it is important to think about the possibility of **myasthenia gravis** (MG). The cardinal feature of this condition is **easy fatigability**, which is usually suggested by the history. When examining the patient, ptosis may be noticeable several seconds after the patient arises from the lying position and it may return to normal once the patient lies down again.

When there is a possibility of MG, the diagnosis can be confirmed according to the following tests. First, the effect of cholinesterase inhibitor should be tested (**Tensilon test**) (see Chapter 29-1). Then, the response of a skeletal muscle to 3 Hz repetitive electrical stimulation of the corresponding motor nerve should be examined. In case of ocular MG, either the orbicularis oculi or the oris muscle can be studied by stimulating the facial nerve. Decrement of the muscle evoked potentials by more than 10% is judged to be positive (**waning**). Single fiber EMG may be also applied. Then, the serum should be tested for the antibody against acetylcholine receptor. This test is positive in the majority of patients with MG, but in a small proportion of patients, antibodies against muscle specific kinase (MuSK) and low density receptor-related protein 4 (Lrp4) might be positive instead (Vincent, 2014, and Ha & Richman, 2015, for review). Furthermore, as thymoma is present in about 15% of MG patients, X-ray and CT of the chest should be obtained.

Bilateral lesion of the brainstem tegmentum may cause bilateral ptosis as a part of Horner syndrome. In this case, however, it is extremely rare to show ptosis to equal degree in both eyes. In bilateral Horner syndrome, the ptosis is more conspicuous on the side of the smaller pupil. By contrast, in case of bilateral oculomotor nerve palsy, the ptosis is more conspicuous on the side of the larger pupil. Bilateral lesion of the brainstem tegmentum can be judged from other accompanying signs.

In aged subjects, the tissue of the upper eyelids may become loose and result in apparent ptosis. In this case, lifting of the slackened upper eyelid may disclose its real position.

Unilateral Ptosis

Unilateral ptosis of marked degree is usually caused by a lesion of the ipsilateral oculomotor nerve, because ptosis in Horner syndrome is usually mild in its degree. In unilateral ptosis of mild degree, its cause could be either oculomotor nerve palsy or Horner syndrome. Observation of pupils is of utmost importance for distinction of the two conditions (see Chapter 8-2).

Blepharospasm

When a patient complains of difficulty in seeing because of the eyelid drop, it may be also due to blepharospasm instead of ptosis. Since blepharospasm is caused by excessive contraction of the orbicularis oculi muscle (see Chapter 11-1A), the position of the lower eyelid is elevated in blepharospasm, which is not the case in ptosis. Furthermore, in blepharospasm, contraction of the orbicularis oculi muscle is enhanced either continuously (tonic contraction) or repetitively (phasic contraction), and blinks might be increased in intensity and frequency.

In case intermittent eye closure is limited only to one eye, it could be a part of **hemifacial spasm**, which is due to hyperexcitation of the facial nerve. In this case, however, contraction may also be seen in the ipsilateral orbicularis oris muscle either continuously or repetitively in synchrony with the contraction of the orbicularis oculi muscle (Chapter 11-1A). On the other hand, blepharospasm may look asymmetric in some cases. In this case, again observation of the orbicularis oris muscle is important for the distinction.

Blepharospasm is considered to be a kind of focal dystonia (see Chapter 18-6). The condition in which blepharospasm is accompanied by dystonia of the jaw and pharynx used to be called Meige syndrome.

B. EXAMINATION OF EXTRAOCULAR MUSCLES

Examination of the extraocular muscles can be effectively started by observing the eyes in the primary position when the subject spontaneously looks straight ahead. If an eye is deviated either medially or laterally, it may not necessarily be paralysis of extraocular muscles but it may be congenital strabismus (squint) or due to other ophthalmological causes. In congenital strabismus, the patient rarely complains of double vision (diplopia), and paralysis of extraocular muscles can be excluded by the examination as described below.

In paralysis of an extraocular muscle, the involved eye is deviated to the side of the opposing muscle. For example, in paralysis of the medial rectus muscle, the affected eye is deviated laterally in the primary position, and in paralysis of the lateral rectus muscle, the eye is deviated medially. In case one eye is deviated upward or downward, a pair of muscles rotating the eye either downward or upward may be affected, or one muscle of each pair may be affected.

Vertical Paralysis of One Eye

If one eye is rotated upward in the primary position, it suggests paralysis of either the superior oblique muscle or the inferior rectus muscle, or both, of that eye. In **unilateral paralysis of the superior oblique muscle**, the patient complains of diplopia (double vision) when looking downward, and the degree of diplopia (distance between the real image from the intact eye and the false image from the paralyzed eye) is increased when the visual target placed downward is moved laterally away from the side of the affected eye. In unilateral paralysis of the inferior rectus muscle, by contrast, the diplopia is increased in its degree when the visual target is moved toward the side of the affected eye. Furthermore, the patient with unilateral superior oblique muscle palsy tends to tilt his/her head toward the side of the intact eye. This is because the patient is spontaneously (involuntarily) trying to compensate for the relative position of the affected eye, which is otherwise rotated upward due to the downward paralysis of that eye. This phenomenon can be tested by tilting the patient's head toward the side of the affected eye, which will elevate the relative position of the eye further, resulting in an increase in the degree of diplopia. This phenomenon is called the **Bielschowsky sign**.

If one eye is rotated downward in the primary eye position, it suggests paralysis of either the superior rectus muscle or the inferior oblique muscle, or both, of that eye. The patient complains of diplopia when looking at an object placed upward. If the diplopia is increased by shifting the visual target from there to the side of the affected eye, it suggests impairment of the superior rectus muscle. Likewise, if the diplopia is increased by shifting the target to the side away from the affected eye, it suggests impairment of the inferior oblique muscle. In fact, as these two muscles are innervated by the same (oculomotor) nerve, they are often paralyzed together.

In case one eye is rotated either upward or downward in the primary position, it is important to observe the position of the other eye, because it might be skew deviation and not extraocular muscle palsy. In **skew deviation**, one eye is rotated upward while the other eye is rotated downward, producing a diagonal position. This phenomenon is seen in some lesions of either cerebellum or brainstem.

Congenital Disorders of Extraocular Muscles

Congenital paralysis of bilateral abducens nerves and/or bilateral facial nerves is called **Möbius syndrome** (see Box 20). These conditions are due to hypoplasia or aplasia of neurons of the abducens nucleus or the facial nucleus. Therefore, the signs are present from birth and not progressive. Möbius syndrome may also present with lateral gaze palsy due to hypoplasia of neurons in the lateral gaze center.

In another congenital condition known as **Duane syndrome**, the affected eye is medially rotated because of disturbance of lateral rotation, and an attempt to medially rotate the eye produces retraction of the eyeball associated with narrowing of the palpebral fissure. This phenomenon can be seen bilaterally. By using MRI with high spatial resolution, marked hypoplasia of the extramedullary fibers of the abducens nerve was demonstrated in this condition (Denis et al, 2008). It was thought that this condition was due to the histological reorganization of the abducens muscle itself, but it is now believed to be secondary to abducens nerve palsy.

Causes of Diplopia or Extraocular Muscle Paralysis

Causes of diplopia or extraocular muscle paralysis can be grouped into four main conditions (Table 9-1). Namely, diplopia may be caused by a lesion involving any part of the final common pathway extending from the relevant brainstem motor nuclei to the extraocular muscles. For the patients complaining of diplopia, therefore, it is useful to consider each possibility systematically throughout the history taking and the physical examination. The tests for MG, one of the most common causes of diplopia, were previously explained. Diplopia can occur in a lesion involving one or more of the three cranial nerves (oculomotor, trochlear, abducens) or those nuclei or fiber pathways within the brainstem (Box 13).

In relation to the above, some patients with a lesion in the occipital lobe may complain that a single object looks like more than one to them. In this case, it is not just double

TABLE 9-1 CAUSES OF EXTRAOCULAR MUSCLE PARALYSIS

1. Muscle disease
Ocular myopathy
Mitochondrial encephalomyopathy (among others Kearns-Sayre syndrome)
Myopathy associated with thyroiditis (so-called thyrotoxic ophthalmoplegia)
2. Disorders of neuromuscular junction
Myasthenia gravis
3. Cranial nerve lesion (III, IV, VI)
Cranial neuritis
Miller Fisher syndrome (Box 13)
Painful ophthalmoplegia (Tolosa-Hunt syndrome)
Diabetic neuropathy
Sarcoidosis
Aneurysm (internal carotid artery, basilar artery)
Metastatic brain tumor
Sphenoidal ridge meningioma
Tumor of the paranasal sinus (especially mucocele)
Trauma
4. Brainstem lesion
Multiple sclerosis
Angioma
Infarction
Hemorrhage
Tumor
Wernicke encephalopathy
Brainstem encephalitis

> **BOX 13 MILLER FISHER SYNDROME**
>
> A combination of ophthalmoplegia, trunk ataxia, and loss of tendon reflexes of acute onset following the symptoms of upper respiratory or gastrointestinal infection is called Miller Fisher syndrome. In spite of severe involvement of the oculomotor nerve, trochlear nerve, and abducens nerve, consciousness is preserved and there is no evidence of long tract signs, which suggests the extramedullary, inflammatory involvement of those cranial nerves. In this condition, the antibody against GQ1b is often elevated in the serum (Kusunoki et al, 2008). Some patients may have a combination of clinical features of Guillain-Barré syndrome, brainstem encephalitis of Bickerstaff, and Miller Fisher syndrome. Those cases might be regarded as a syndrome of anti-GQ1b antibody.

vision but more often multiple vision (**polyopia**), and the degree of polyopia does not change by moving eyes or by changing the position of object. Furthermore, it is often associated with disturbance of other visual cognitive functions (see Chapter 23-2C). Therefore, this condition can be easily distinguished from diplopia caused by a lesion of the final common pathway.

Ocular Myopathy

Ocular myopathy associated with thyrotoxicosis used to be called **thyrotoxic myopathy**, but this condition may not be directly related to the thyroid hormone. It is most likely that the extraocular muscles and the thyroid gland happen to be affected independently by an autoimmune process. Temporally, therefore, these two conditions do not always change in parallel.

A group of conditions due to abnormality of mitochondria-related genes and manifesting progressive external ophthalmoplegia in young adults is called **ophthalmoplegia plus** or p**rogressive external ophthalmoplegia** (Copeland, 2014, for review) (see Box 57). The most representative form of this condition is **Kearns-Sayre syndrome**, which is characterized by age at onset before 20 years, progressive external ophthalmoplegia, retinal pigment degeneration, cardiac conduction block, cerebellar ataxia, and increased protein in the cerebrospinal fluid. It is usually sporadic in its occurrence and is due to deletion of the mitochondrial DNA (mtDNA). Another condition of this group is mitochondrial neurogastrointestinal encephalomyopathy, which is characterized by progressive external ophthalmoplegia, motor and sensory polyneuropathy, chronic diarrhea, recurrent intestinal obstruction, and malnutrition. This condition is inherited in an autosomal recessive trait and is due to multiple deletion of mtDNA.

C. EXAMINATION OF FIXATION, GAZE, AND EYE MOVEMENTS

After having confirmed that the extraocular muscles are intact, or at least not markedly paralyzed, it is possible to test the gaze and eye movements. First, the primary position of eyes is observed while the patient is looking straight ahead. In case the eyes are unstable, associated with small rapid horizontal movements, the electronystagmogram

(ENG) may show small square waves. This phenomenon is called **square-wave jerks** and is seen in patients with cerebellar lesions. Then, for testing fixation, the patient is asked to look at an object placed in the central visual field and saccade to small shifts of the target. If the eyes miss the target and show several small oscillations before fixating on the target, it is called **ocular dysmetria**. In this case, the ENG shows a short burst of several rapid decrescendo beats before catching the target. **Flutter-like oscillations** may look like ocular dysmetria, but in this condition there is no decline of the ENG amplitude in the burst.

Lateral Gaze Palsy and Conjugate Deviation of Eyes

Deviation of the two eyes to either left or right to equal angle is called **conjugate deviation of eyes**. This is caused by a lesion involving either the cerebral hemisphere, especially the frontal lobe, ipsilateral to the side of deviation or the pontine tegmentum contralateral to the side of deviation. In the former case, it is usually seen in association with disturbance of consciousness as in acute stroke. If the head is also rotated to the same direction as the eyes, it is usually due to a lesion of the parieto-occipital lobe ipsilateral to the side of deviation. This condition is associated with either homonymous hemianopsia or hemispatial neglect on the side contralateral to the lesion. As visual spatial attention is mainly controlled by the right cerebral hemisphere in right-handed subjects, the above-described conjugate deviation of eyes and head is commonly seen in patients with right hemispheric lesions. Upward or downward deviation of eyes suggests the presence of downward gaze palsy or upward gaze palsy, respectively.

When there is lateral or vertical gaze palsy, it is important to examine the presence or absence of **oculocephalic reflex**. For this purpose, the head is passively rotated, and if the eyes change their relative position toward the opposite side of passive rotation, then the oculocephalic reflex is judged to be present. The presence of the oculocephalic reflex when there is a gaze palsy suggests **supranuclear paralysis**, and its absence suggests nuclear or infranuclear paralysis. In the latter case, the lateral gaze center in the pons (PPRF) or the vertical gaze center in the midbrain is directly involved by a lesion, and in the former case, the lesion is present central to the gaze centers. Progressive supranuclear palsy (see Box 79) is a typical example of supranuclear gaze palsy. The oculocephalic reflex is also called **doll's eye sign**, and it is an important test for examining a patient with possible brain death (see Chapter 29-5C).

Oculogyric Crisis

Upward or oblique upward deviation of eyes may not be due to downward gaze palsy but could be due to an **oculogyric crisis**. Oculogyric crisis was first described in patients with postencephalitic parkinsonism. Nowadays this phenomenon can be seen in a residual state of acute encephalitis or in the chronic phase of anoxic encephalopathy. Similar phenomena might be encountered during epileptic attacks, but the diagnosis of epileptic attacks can be easily made by taking into account other manifestations associated with epilepsy (see Chapter 24-1).

In healthy subjects, closure of eyelids is accompanied by upward rotation (elevation) of eyes, which is called the **Bell phenomenon**. In patients with a unilateral cerebral hemispheric lesion, elevation of the eyes produced by strong eyelid closure is deviated to either left or right. In 70% of cases, the eyes are deviated away from the side of the hemispheric lesion (Cogan sign), and in 20% of cases, they are deviated toward the side of the lesion (Sullivan et al, 1991).

Gaze Paralysis and Ocular Motor Apraxia

Examination of gaze can be done while examining the extraocular muscles, but as the patients with intact extraocular muscles may still have gaze disturbance, it is better to pay attention to the extraocular muscles and gaze separately. Gaze can be tested, with the eyes placed in the primary position, by asking the patient to look at either side or up and down without showing any visual target. If a patient is unable to look at any direction, it may be due to either gaze palsy or disturbance of even higher cortical functions. For distinguishing these two conditions, it is useful to observe spontaneous eye movements while the patient is talking for example. In **ocular motor apraxia**, eye movements may occur randomly in all directions in the spontaneous condition, but once the patient is asked to fixate on an object placed in the lateral visual field, then he/she is unable or finds it difficult to move the eyes to that direction. In this case, the head first rotates promptly and overshoots the target, and then it returns so that both the head and eyes catch the object. This phenomenon is called **head thrust**.

In **gaze palsy**, in contrast to the ocular motor apraxia, eye movements to the paralyzed direction are absent even in the spontaneous condition. In fact, ocular motor apraxia is much less common than gaze palsy. Gaze palsy is divided into two types: supranuclear and infranuclear. Infranuclear gaze palsy is caused by a lesion involving the gaze center in the midbrain or the pons or its efferent nerve fibers innervating the extraocular muscles. In contrast to the other skeletal muscles, neither the muscle volume nor the tendon reflex can be examined in the gaze palsy. Therefore, the oculocephalic reflex (see Chapter 9-5C) and other accompanying signs provide important clues to distinction of the supranuclear and infranuclear ophthalmoplegia. The presence of the oculocephalic reflex (doll's eye sign) suggests supranuclear palsy. In incomplete gaze paresis or during the recovery phase from the acute stage, gaze may be no longer paralyzed, but it may manifest itself as a slow speed of saccades. When testing the gaze, involuntary movements of eyes (to be described in the next section) can be also observed, if any.

Eye-Tracking Test

It is important to test saccades and smooth pursuit separately for horizontal as well as vertical gaze. For testing horizontal saccades, the examiner sits about 50 cm in front of the patient and holds visual targets (usually the examiner's hands) horizontally with the visual angle of about 30 degrees while the patient is asked to fixate at each target alternately. By this maneuver, approximate information is obtained as to the speed of saccades and how accurately the eyes can fixate on the target. For obtaining more detailed information, the patient is asked to look at a target placed in the central visual field and to promptly look at another target placed in the lateral field. If the eyes cannot fixate their gaze to the target accurately, it is called **dysmetria**. There are two types of dysmetria. In **hypermetria** or **hypermetric saccades**, the eyes overshoot and then return to the target, which is considered to be characteristic of cerebellar lesion, especially a lesion involving the dorsal vermis and fastigial nucleus. In **hypometria** or **hypometric saccades**, the eyes stop before reaching the target and then proceed further to catch the target. This condition is less lesion-specific than hypermetria, and is seen in disorders of cerebellum or basal ganglia, or the supranuclear ocular motor system.

Smooth pursuit can be tested by moving a visual target smoothly over the visual angle of about 30 degrees and by asking the patient to follow the moving target. If small saccades are superimposed on the smooth movement, the phenomenon is called **saccadic pursuit** or **catch-up saccades**. This phenomenon is also seen in cerebellar lesions, but its specificity to any site or any nervous system is relatively low.

Optokinetic Nystagmus

Optokinetic nystagmus (OKN) is produced by asking patients to watch a tape with a series of alternating stripes (or other objects). The tape can be moved horizontally or vertically. The eyes should move at the speed of the tape in the direction of the tape and then have periodic saccades in the opposite direction. OKN is a nice way of assessing whether saccades are present and symmetrical.

D. INVOLUNTARY MOVEMENTS OF EYES

The most common involuntary movement of eyes is nystagmus. In most cases of nystagmus, both eyes move to the same direction to the same degree and with the same speed (**conjugate nystagmus**). Exception to this is dissociated nystagmus, seen in INO, and seesaw nystagmus. Nystagmus may be seen in the primary position of eyes (**spontaneous nystagmus**), but it is often induced or increased by gaze (**gaze nystagmus**). Depending on the direction of involuntary movements, it is classified into **horizontal nystagmus**, **vertical nystagmus**, and **rotatory nystagmus**. The patients having nystagmus often complain of **oscillopsia**, but they may not complain of any symptoms. In order to diagnose ocular oscillations accurately, it is important to take a careful history and to perform a systematic examination of vision and each functional class of eye movement (Thurtell & Leigh, 2011, for review).

Spontaneous Nystagmus

Nystagmus is commonly formed by quick phase and slow phase, but some nystagmus may move with the same speed to both directions. This is called **pendular nystagmus** and is commonly seen in patients with congenital nystagmus. **Congenital nystagmus** is characterized by horizontal pendular nystagmus of large amplitude, its suppression by eyelid closure, and a reversed direction of OKN. As noted above, in healthy subjects, the quick phase of OKN is induced in the direction away from the side of the target movement, but in congenital nystagmus, it is induced toward the side of target movement. Moreover, congenital nystagmus is often associated with amblyopia from childhood, and the patient may not be aware of any oscillopsia or unsteadiness in spite of the presence of conspicuous nystagmus. Suppression of congenital nystagmus by eyelid closure may not be caused by masking of visual stimulus but may be related to the voluntary attempt to close eyes (Shibasaki et al, 1978).

In some cases of spontaneous nystagmus, its quick phase might change its direction from one to the other periodically. This phenomenon is called **periodic alternating nystagmus** and is typically seen in a lesion of cerebellum, especially the nodulus.

Gaze Nystagmus

Horizontal nystagmus is commonly induced or enhanced by lateral gaze. The quick phase is induced toward the side of gaze in most cases, but in some cases it may be to the opposite direction. Lateral gaze may also induce vertical nystagmus or rotatory nystagmus. In patients with cerebellar lesions, the quick phase of nystagmus induced by lateral gaze may change its direction when the eyes return to the primary position. For example, the gaze nystagmus that is induced by lateral gaze to the right with its quick phase directed to the right changes its quick phase to the left as soon as the eyes are returned to the primary position. This phenomenon is called **rebound nystagmus**, and is seen in a lesion of the cerebellum, especially the flocculus and paraflocculus.

Vertical gaze nystagmus is commonly induced to the direction of vertical gaze, but it may be induced to the reverse direction. Namely, upward gaze commonly induces **up-beat nystagmus**, but it may induce **down-beat nystagmus** and vice versa. Down-beat nystagmus is seen in patients with Arnold-Chiari malformation, paraneoplastic syndrome, and intoxication with lithium, carbamazepine, or amiodarone. This is also believed to be caused by involvement of the flocculus and paraflocculus. **Arnold-Chiari malformation (Chiari malformation)** is a congenital condition in which the cerebellar tonsils, and in severe cases the inferior vermis and lower medulla as well, are displaced below the foramen magnum.

In patients with the **sylvian aqueduct syndrome, convergence-retraction nystagmus** may be induced by vertical gaze, especially by upward saccade provoked by downward movement of the OKN stimulus. In this condition, pupillary abnormality may be also seen.

Superior oblique myokymia is a burst of rotatory pendular rapid small movements seen in one eye. This condition can be only recognized with a slit lamp examination, because each movement is quite small. The patient with this condition may complain of rotatory oscillopsia when looking at an object monocularly.

Ocular Myoclonus

Rhythmic vertical oscillation of eyes at a frequency of about 3 Hz used to be called **ocular myoclonus**, but its mechanism seems to be similar to that of tremor. In most cases of this condition, the ocular movements are associated with synchronous vertical movements of the soft palate. The latter phenomenon also used to be called palatal myoclonus, but it is now more often called **palatal tremor. Symptomatic oculopalatal tremor** is caused by a lesion involving any part of the Guillain-Mollaret triangle, but most commonly by a lesion of the central tegmental tract in the pons, and then by a cerebellar lesion (see Box 60).

Opsoclonus

Opsoclonus is seen in the spontaneous eye position and is characterized by irregular gross quick conjugate movements of the eyes to various directions. Each movement is shock-like and resembles myoclonus of the extremities (Figure 9-8). In fact, opsoclonus is often associated with myoclonus in the trunk or extremities. However, unlike myoclonus of cortical origin, opsoclonus is not preceded by EEG spikes. It is postulated that the saccadic burst neurons in the brainstem gaze centers generate bursts of discharges as a result of a cerebellar lesion.

Opsoclonus-myoclonus syndrome is seen in children with cerebellar neuroblastoma and is also seen in adults with autoimmune or infectious cerebellitis. It is also known to occur as a paraneoplastic syndrome. Opsoclonus has also been reported in cases of neuroborreliosis due to infection with borrelia burgdorferi.

In some cases, opsoclonus may need distinction from ocular flutter. **Ocular flutter**, also called **flutter-like oscillation**, is a short burst of horizontal rhythmic quick movements and is enhanced by gaze. It is distinguished from opsoclonus in that flutter is a burst of rhythmic beats whereas opsoclonus is irregular, but the two conditions can be seen in the same patient at the same time or at different stages of the clinical course.

Ocular Bobbing and Ocular Dipping

Quick sinking of both eyes followed by slow return to the primary position is called **ocular bobbing**, and slow sinking

Saccadic lateral gaze to right by 20 degrees

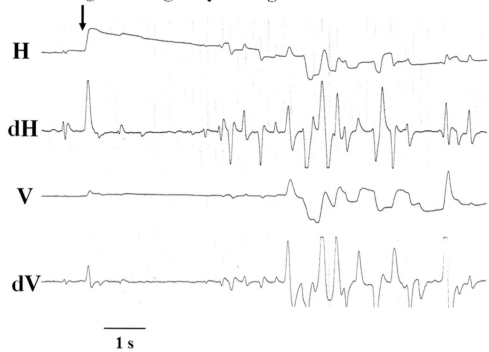

H

dH

V

dV

1 s

Figure 9-8 Electronystagmogram of opsoclonus. H: original waveform (horizontal), V: original waveform (vertical), dH: differential waveform (horizontal), dV: differential waveform (vertical).

of both eyes followed by quick return to the primary position is called **ocular dipping**. Both conditions are seen in bilateral massive lesion of the pontine tegmentum.

BIBLIOGRAPHY

Bienfang DC. Crossing axons in the third nerve nucleus. Invest Ophthalmol 14:927–931, 1975.

Chusid JG, McDonald JJ. Correlative Neuroanatomy and Functional Neurology. 12th ed. Lange, Maruzen Asian Edition, Tokyo, 1964.

Claude H. Syndrome pédonculaire de la région du noyau rouge. Rev Neurol (Paris) 23:311–313, 1912.

Claude H, Loyez M. Ramollissement du noyau rouge. Rev Neurol (Paris) 24: 49–51, 1912.

Copeland WC. Defects of mitochondrial DNA replication. J Child Neurol 29:1216–1224, 2014. (review)

Denis D, Dauletbekov D, Girard N. Duane retraction syndrome: Type II with severe abducens nerve hypoplasia on magnetic resonance imaging. J AAPOS 12:91–93, 2008.

Girard B, Berthoz A. From brainstem to cortex: computational models of saccade generation circuitry. Prog Neurobiol 77:215–251, 2005. (review)

Ha JC, Richman DP. Myasthenia gravis and related disorders: pathology and molecular pathogenesis. Biochim Biophys Acta 1852:651–657, 2015. (review)

Kusunoki S, Kaida K, Ueda M. Antibodies against gangliosides and ganglioside complexes in Guillain-Barre syndrome: new aspects of research. Biochim Biophys Acta 1780:441–444, 2008.

Kwon J-H, Kwon SU, Ahn H-S, Sung K-B, Kim JS. Isolated superior rectus palsy due to contralateral midbrain infarction. Arch Neurol 60:1633–1635, 2003.

Lencer R, Trillenberg P. Neurophysiology and neuroanatomy of smooth pursuit in humans. Brain Cogn 68:219–228, 2008. (review)

Liu GT, Crenner CW, Logigian EL, Charness ME, Samuels MA. Midbrain syndromes of Benedikt, Claude, and Nothnagel: setting the record straight. Neurology 42:1820–1822, 1992.

Matsumoto R, Ikeda A, Nagamine T, Matsuhashi M, Ohara S, Yamamoto J, et al. Subregions of human MT complex revealed by comparative MEG and direct electrocorticographic recordings. Clin Neurophysiol 115:2056–2065, 2004.

Mustari MJ, Ono S, Das VE. Signal processing and distribution in cortical-brainstem pathways for smooth pursuit eye movements. Ann NY Acad Sci 1164:147–154, 2009.

Parinaud H. Paralysis of the movement of convergence of the eyes. Brain 9:330–341, 1886.

Pierrot–Deseilligny CH, Chain F, Gray F, Serdaru M, Escourolle R, Lhermitte F. Parinaud's syndrome: electro-oculographic and anatomical analyses of six vascular cases with deductions about vertical gaze organization in the premotor structures. Brain 105:667–696, 1982.

Ramat S, Leigh RJ, Zee DS, Optican LM. What clinical disorders tell us about the neural control of saccadic eye movements. Brain 130:10–35, 2007.

Shibasaki H, Yamashita Y, Motomura S. Suppression of congenital nystagmus. J Neurol Neurosurg Psychiatry 12:1078–1083, 1978.

Shibasaki H, Tsuji S, Kuroiwa Y. Oculomotor abnormalities in Parkinson's disease. Arch Neurol 36:360–364, 1979.

Sullivan HC, Kaminski HJ, Maas EF, Weissman JD, Leigh RJ. Lateral deviation of the eyes on forced lid closure in patients with cerebral lesions. Arch Neurol 48:310–311, 1991.

Terao Y, Fukuda H, Yugeta A, Hikosaka O, Nomura Y, Segawa M, et al. Initiation and inhibitory control of saccades with the progression of Parkinson's disease—changes in three major drives converging on the superior colliculus. Neuropsychologia 49:1794–1806, 2011.

Thurtell MJ, Leigh RJ. Nystagmus and saccadic intrusions. In Kennard C, Leigh RJ (eds.). Handbook of Clinical Neurology, Vol 102 (3rd series), Neuro-ophthalmology, Elsevier, Amsterdam, 2011, pp.333–378.

Tsukamoto T, Yamamoto M, Fuse T, Kimura M. A case of isolated crossed paralysis of the superior rectus muscle. Clin Neurol 45:445–448, 2005 (abstract in English).

Vincent A. Autoantibodies at the neuromuscular junction—link to the central nervous system. Rev Neurol 170:584–586, 2014. (review)

Weber H. A contribution to the pathology of the crura cerebri. Medico Chirurg Trans 46:121–139, 1863.

10.

TRIGEMINAL NERVE

1. STRUCTURES AND FUNCTIONS

The fifth cranial nerve (trigeminal nerve) innervates facial sensation and jaw movement. Anatomically the nerve consists of three branches: the first branch (ophthalmic nerve), the second branch (maxillary nerve), and the third branch (mandibular nerve).

A. SOMATOSENSORY PATHWAY

Sensory nerves of the trigeminal nerve innervate skin of the face and forehead, a part of the oral mucosa, and a large part of the meninges. The primary neurons are in the **semilunar ganglion (gasserian ganglion)**, which is located in the middle cranial fossa (Figure 10-1, see also Figure 8-2a).

The **ophthalmic nerve** transmits sensory impulses from the skin of the frontal scalp (supraorbital nerve) and the nasal ala. The nerve fibers arising from the sensory receptors of those areas pass posteriorly below the superior wall of the orbit, and together with the fibers coming from the orbital mucosa, exit from the orbit through the superior orbital fissure (see Figure 8-2a) to enter the anterior cranial fossa. Then they pass further posteriorly through the cavernous sinus (see Figure 8-1) to enter the middle cranial fossa, where they project to the semilunar ganglion. Intracranially, the ophthalmic nerve transmits nociceptive impulse from the meninges of the anterior cranial fossa and the cerebellar tent. In relation to this tentorial branch, the frontal headache occasionally complained of by a patient with posterior fossa lesion is explained as a referred pain. The patient feels as if the pain is coming from the frontal region because the tentorial branch enters the ophthalmic nerve.

The **maxillary nerve** transmits sensory impulses from the skin of the upper lip and cheek and from the mucosa of the nose and the upper oral cavity. It enters the middle cranial fossa through the foramen rotundum (see Figure 8-2a), and after being joined by the nociceptive input from the middle cranial fossa, it projects to the semilunar ganglion. The **mandibular nerve** transmits sensory impulses from the skin of the jaw and temple and the mucosa of the lower oral cavity. It enters the middle cranial fossa through the foramen ovale (see Figure 8-2a) and projects to the semilunar ganglion.

The primary sensory neuron of the trigeminal nerve, like other primary somatosensory neurons, is a bipolar cell (see Figure 19-1). The impulse generated at the peripheral receptors is conducted through the peripheral axon to the semilunar ganglion and enters the lateral pons through its central axon. Soon after entering the pontine tegmentum, the fibers separate into two groups as follows.

Small nociceptive fibers form the **spinal tract of the trigeminal nerve** and descend through the lateral tegmentum of pons and medulla oblongata to reach the upper cervical segments (see Figures 5-2, 5-3 and 5-5). As the impulses descend through the spinal tract, they are transmitted to the secondary neurons at each level in the **spinal nucleus of the trigeminal nerve**, which is located just medial to the spinal tract (Figure 10-1). The secondary sensory fibers cross to the other side at each level and join the medial part of the contralateral spinothalamic tract to form the **trigeminothalamic tract**. This tract ascends to reach the **ventral posteromedial nucleus (VPM) of the thalamus**, where the third sensory neurons originate. As described in Chapter 5-5, the spinal nucleus of the trigeminal nerve extends from the middle pons to the upper cervical segments, and thus is the longest nucleus among the cranial nerve nuclei.

Large sensory fibers related to tactile sensation enter the **main sensory nucleus of the trigeminal nerve**, which is located in the middle part of the pontine tegmentum (Figure 10-1). The secondary fibers originating from the main sensory nucleus cross to the other side to join the medial lemniscus, and project to the VPM of the thalamus.

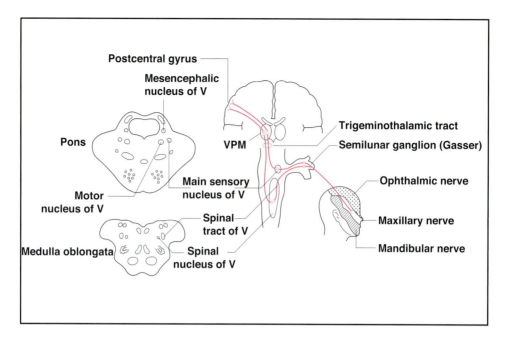

Figure 10-1 Schematic illustration of composition of the trigeminal nerve (V) and its branches.

As expected from the above, if one of the three branches is affected, the patient suffers from superficial sensory loss and/or complains of pain or numbness localized to the area of the skin and mucosa innervated by that branch. If a lesion involves the main trunk of the trigeminal nerve (central to the semilunar ganglion), then the sensory impairment occurs in the whole area innervated by the whole nerve.

An extramedullary lesion of the trigeminal nerve usually affects both nociceptive and tactile sensation. As for intramedullary lesions, a lesion located at the entrance area is expected to disturb all kinds of sensation, but after the fibers are separated into the nociceptive group and the tactile group, either of the two senses might be selectively affected (**dissociated sensory loss**). Furthermore, as the spinal nucleus of the trigeminal tract extends for a long distance, the sensory impairment caused by the lesion may not involve the whole face. However, correlation between the site of the lesion and the distribution of sensory impairment has not been clearly established.

In lateral medullary syndrome (Wallenberg syndrome) (see Box 21), the spinal tract is damaged at the upper medullary level, but the pain and temperature senses are usually lost over the whole area of the ipsilateral face. On the other hand, it is expected theoretically that a lesion of the upper cervical cord might cause sensory symptoms on the face, but this phenomenon is extremely rare.

B. CORTICAL RECEPTION OF SOMATOSENSORY INPUT FROM FACE

The third sensory fibers originating from the VPM of the thalamus ascend through the internal capsule and the corona radiata, and project to the face area of the **primary somatosensory cortex** (SI) in the postcentral gyrus. In the postcentral gyrus, the receptive area of impulses arising from the face is located over the lateral convexity, whereas that from the foot is located over the mesial area, forming an upside down homunculus (Figure 10-2). Regarding specific parts of the face, however, there is no upside down somatotopy, and the area for the eyes is located dorsal to that for the jaw. Functional localization in the SI is described in the chapter on the somatosensory system (Chapter 19-1) (see Figure 19-3).

Nerve fibers originating from the SI project bilaterally to the **secondary somatosensory cortex** (SII), located in the superior bank of the sylvian fissure, and also to the ipsilateral areas 5 and 7 located posterior to the SI. There is some somatotopic organization also in the SII, with the face area being located more anteriorly and the foot area more posteriorly.

C. NERVE INNERVATION OF MASTICATORY MUSCLES

The **motor nucleus of the trigeminal nerve** is located in the middle of the pontine tegmentum just medial to the

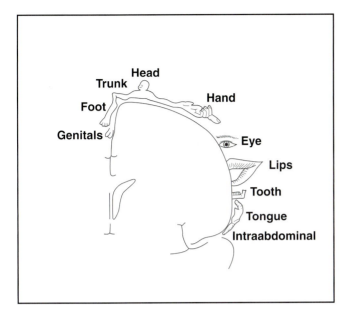

Figure 10-2 Schematic illustration of somatotopic organization of the primary somatosensory cortex. Frontal view of the left hemisphere.

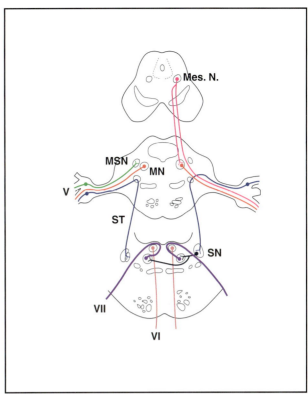

Figure 10-3 Schematic diagram showing nuclei of the trigeminal nerve (V) and neuronal circuits of the corneal reflex and the masseter reflex (jaw jerk). The polysynaptic reflex arc of the corneal reflex is shown in purple with the spinal tract (ST) projecting to the motor nucleus of the facial nerve (VII) via the spinal nucleus (SN). The monosynaptic reflex arc of the masseter reflex is shown in pink with the mesencephalic nucleus (Mes.N.) sending its efferent nerve to the ipsilateral motor nucleus of the trigeminal nerve (MN). MSN: main sensory nucleus, VI: abducens nerve.

main sensory nucleus (Figures 10-1 and 10-3). Its efferent fibers exit the pons from its lateral rim and pass through the semilunar ganglion to form the mandibular nerve. After exiting from the middle cranial fossa through the foramen ovale, the motor fibers separate into three branches to innervate the temporal muscle, masseter, and pterygoid muscles. In a lesion of the mandibular nerve, atrophy and weakness can be seen or palpated in the temporal muscle and masseter. As the lateral pterygoid muscle acts to open the mouth by protruding the mandible forward and downward, its unilateral paralysis pushes the jaw to the paralyzed side when opening the mouth, causing deviation of the jaw to the affected side. As the lateral pterygoid muscle also acts to push the jaw to the other side, its weakness can be felt by palpation by asking the patient to push the jaw to the side contralateral to the weakened muscle. As the motor nucleus of the trigeminal nerve is bilaterally innervated by the corticobulbar tract, a unilateral lesion of the corticobulbar tract does not cause paralysis of the masticatory muscles.

Motor fibers of the mandibular nerve also innervate the tensor tympani muscle. As this muscle acts to control the tonus of the tympanic membrane, its paralysis is theoretically considered to decrease the tonus of the tympanic membrane. However, hearing deficit due to trigeminal nerve lesion is not encountered in the clinical setting.

D. REFLEX PATHWAY OF JAW JERK

As the masseter is bilaterally innervated by the corticobulbar tracts, its tendon reflex is not enhanced with a unilateral lesion. The **masseter reflex (jaw jerk)** is elicited by tapping the jaw downward with the mouth gently opened. Its afferent neuron is in the **mesencephalic nucleus of the trigeminal nerve,** which is located in the midbrain (Figures 10-1 and 10-3). Unlike other tendon reflexes, which are monosynaptic with the afferent neuron situated in the sensory ganglion, the afferent neuron of this particular monosynaptic reflex is situated in the brainstem. An afferent impulse generated by stretch of the masseter muscle spindle is conducted through the afferent axon of the mandibular nerve and is projected to the bipolar neuron in the mesencephalic nucleus, where the impulse is reflected through its efferent axon and monosynaptically transmitted to the ipsilateral motor nucleus of the trigeminal nerve, which then causes contraction of the masseter.

In patients with dysphagia and dysphonia or dysarthria, the jaw jerk is used to distinguish between bulbar palsy and pseudobulbar palsy (see Chapter 14-7 for definition), because it is impossible to test the tendon reflex in the bulbar muscles such as soft palate and tongue (see Chapter 14-1). Although the reflex center is located in the pons, enhancement of jaw jerk in those patients suggests pseudobulbar palsy due to bilateral lesions of the corticobulbar tracts. However, in a condition in which the upper and lower motor neurons are both affected, as in amyotrophic lateral sclerosis, the jaw jerk might be enhanced with the presence of muscle atrophy of the tongue.

E. NEURAL PATHWAY OF CORNEAL REFLEX

The **corneal reflex** is a polysynaptic reflex with the trigeminal nerve forming its afferent arc and the facial nerve forming its efferent arc (see Chapter 11-1A). An impulse generated in the nociceptive receptors of the cornea is conducted through the ophthalmic nerve to the spinal tract of the trigeminal nerve. Then an impulse arising from the spinal nucleus of the trigeminal nerve is conducted to the ipsilateral as well as the contralateral facial nucleus (Figure 10-3). Thus, a nociceptive stimulus given to the cornea of one eye causes the eyelid closure bilaterally.

The blink reflex, a reflex closely associated with the corneal reflex, can be tested electrophysiologically by presenting an electric shock to the ophthalmic nerve (usually the supraorbital branch) and by recording the surface electromyogram (EMG) from the orbicularis oculi muscles (**blink reflex**). The initial response (R1) is recorded from the muscle ipsilateral to the stimulus at a latency of about 10 ms, and the second response (R2) is recorded bilaterally at a latency of about 30 ms (see Kimura, 2013). As only R2 can be recognized on clinical observation, the corneal reflex is seen bilaterally in healthy subjects.

2. EXAMINATION OF FUNCTIONS RELATED TO THE TRIGEMINAL NERVE

A. MOTOR NERVE

First, volume of the masticatory muscles (masseter and temporal) should be observed by visual inspection and palpation. In case of atrophy of these muscles, the zygomatic bone of the affected side appears protruded. Even when the muscle atrophy is not visible, palpation of those muscles while clenching the teeth might disclose the atrophy on the affected side.

Next, the position of the jaw can be observed while the patient opens the mouth. In unilateral paralysis of the lateral pterygoid muscle, jaw is deviated to the affected side upon the mouth opening because the muscle of the intact side pushes the jaw forward and downward. Furthermore, palpation of the jaw on both sides while the patient tries to shift the jaw laterally might disclose weakness of the lateral pterygoid muscle contralateral to the direction of shifting.

The temporal muscle and masseter are commonly affected in **myotonic dystrophy**. Because these muscles are bilaterally affected in this condition, the zygomatic bones appear bilaterally protruded (**hatchet face**). Early frontal baldness is also commonly seen in this condition (see Chapter 16-3F).

Trismus (Lockjaw)

When a patient complains of difficulty in opening the mouth, it could be the initial symptoms of **tetanus**. Therefore, **trismus (lockjaw)** of acute onset should be considered with caution. Tetanus is caused by a toxin produced by anaerobic bacteria *Clostridium tetani*. Infection occurs from an injury wound, and the toxin produced at the injury site is transported through the motor nerve axon to the spinal cord and brainstem, where inhibition is blocked by the toxin, leading to excessive activity of the motor neuron and severe spasm of the corresponding muscles. The motor nucleus of the trigeminal nerve is commonly affected in this condition, resulting in trismus. The trismus may continue and look like a smiling face (**risus sardonicus**). In the patient with tetanus, any external stimulus causes generalized muscle spasm and **opisthotonus**, an abnormal posture in which the trunk is markedly bent backward due to excessive spasm of the spinal muscles. It could be fatal and requires intensive treatment (see Chapter 29-3).

Difficulty in jaw opening can be caused by local inflammatory as well as noninflammatory diseases of the temporomandibular joints and peritonsillar or retropharyngeal abscess, but tetanus is the most important differential diagnosis from a neurological point of view.

Jaw-Winking Phenomenon

In this condition, chewing movements are associated with opening and closure of one eye (**Marcus Gunn phenomenon**) (Box 14). Marcus Gunn in 1883 reported a 15-year-old girl who had drop of the left upper eyelid, which quickly elevated when she opened the mouth or moved the jaw to the right (Marcus Gunn, 1883). The left upper eyelid

Regarding the hypothesis of possible misconnection between the motor fibers of the mandibular nerve targeting at the lateral pterygoid muscle and those of the oculomotor nerve targeting at the levator muscle of the upper eyelid, these two nerves or their nuclei are never located in any proximity. Moreover, if the above theory is correct, voluntary elevation of the upper eyelid is also expected to open the mouth, which is not the case.

In view of the fact that the mesencephalic nucleus is the only component of the trigeminal nerve located in the midbrain, Shimono et al. (1975) studied possible participation of the proprioceptive afferents from either the masseter or the lateral pterygoid muscle. Namely, the isometric contraction of the lateral pterygoid muscle induced by asking the patient to open the mouth while the jaw was fixed from below also elevated the upper eyelid. This finding was interpreted to exclude participation of the stretch afferent from the masseter, but to suggest a proprioceptive afferent from the lateral pterygoid muscle through the group Ib fibers. It was thus postulated that fibers of the mesencephalic tract of the trigeminal nerve and fibers of the oculomotor nerve targeting at the levator muscle of the upper eyelid might be misconnected. However, a question as to why, among other fibers of the oculomotor nerve, only the nerve fibers targeting the levator muscle of the upper eyelid are affected remains to be solved.

remained elevated as long as the patient kept the new position of the jaw. However, voluntary opening of the left eye did not cause either opening of the mouth or deviation of the jaw. This phenomenon was noted about 5 weeks after birth and slightly improved at age 12 years. Regarding the mechanism underlying this phenomenon, Marcus Gunn postulated the presence of hypoplasia in the motor fibers of the left oculomotor nerve targeting at the levator muscle of the upper eyelid and its compensatory innervation by fibers of the left trigeminal nerve targeting the lateral pterygoid muscle, thus causing elevation of the upper eyelid upon voluntary contraction of the lateral pterygoid muscle (Box 14 for discussion).

The Marcus Gunn phenomenon can be either congenital or acquired, and its familial occurrence has also been reported. Marin Amat, a Spanish ophthalmologist, reported in 1919, in addition to a typical case of Marcus Gunn phenomenon, a 56-year-old man with inverse Marcus Gunn phenomenon (**Marin Amat syndrome**) (Marin Amat, 1919). That patient suffered from severe trauma on the left face resulting in atrophy of the left optic disc and right facial palsy and deafness, and 45 days later he was treated with palpebral suture for right lagophthalmos (failure to close eyelids) (see Chapter 11-2A). About a year and a half later, it was noted that opening the mouth or shifting the jaw to the left closed the right eye. The right eye remained closed as long as the right lateral pterygoid muscle was kept contracted, and it was also accompanied by lacrimation and nasal discharge on the right. It was postulated that the motor fibers of the mandibular nerve and those of the facial nerve might have been misconnected.

B. SENSORY NERVE

Impairment of the sensory fibers of the trigeminal nerve causes numbness of the face and the anterior half of the scalp on the affected side. Pain, temperature, and tactile senses can be tested by using sterile pins, flasks filled with hot or cold water, and tissue paper, respectively. It is important to compare the two sides for each test. If any sensory abnormality is found, it is important to know the affected area of the skin precisely, so as to determine whether the abnormality is restricted to a region corresponding to any of the three branches or involves the whole unilateral face. It is useful to note that the ophthalmic nerve shares a border with the greater occipital nerve of cervical origin at the vertex of the head and that the mandibular nerve shares a border with the third cervical nerve at the chin. As the trigeminal nerve also innervates the mucosa of the oral cavity including the tongue, namely the maxillary nerve for the upper oral mucosa and the mandibular nerve for the lower oral mucosa, it is important to pay attention to the oral mucosa as well, including the teeth. Numbness of either half of the tongue suggests the impairment of the corresponding branch of the trigeminal nerve. Toothache is felt through either the maxillary nerve or the mandibular nerve.

Trigeminal Neuralgia

Shock-like shooting pain in the face is known as **trigeminal neuralgia** (**tic douloureux**). A territory of the maxillary nerve is most commonly involved, but **postherpetic neuralgia** is more common in the territory of the ophthalmic nerve. In neuralgia of the maxillary nerve, pain shoots up laterally from the maxilla toward the temple, and several beats of radiating pain tend to occur as a cluster. It is often triggered by stimulating the skin or mucosa (**trigger zone**). Trigeminal neuralgia is mostly considered to result from compression of the trigeminal nerve by tortuous branches of the vertebrobasilar artery. Thus this type of neuralgia is common in the aged population. It is postulated that the pain is not directly caused by mechanical compression but is due to secondary demyelination of the nerve trunk. However, in view of the fact that surgical decompression of the nerve can remove the pain immediately, demyelination may not be the sole mechanism.

Trigeminal neuralgia may also occur in an intramedullary brainstem lesion. In fact, multiple sclerosis is one of the common causes of trigeminal neuralgia in young subjects. It has been reported based on an MRI study that, among patients with trigeminal neuralgia, an organic lesion is found in about 15% (Gronseth et al, 2008). Association of trigeminal neuralgia with Horner syndrome is known as **paratrigeminal syndrome (Raeder syndrome)** (Box 15).

C. JAW JERK (MASSETER REFLEX)

The jaw jerk is the only tendon reflex that can be tested for the muscles innervated by cranial nerves. To elicit this reflex, the jaw is tapped downward while the mouth is kept gently open (see Figure 17-2a). The response can be seen as jaw elevation or masseter contraction. This reflex may not be very conspicuous even in healthy subjects, and therefore loss of this reflex cannot be confirmed clinically.

BOX 15 RAEDER (PARATRIGEMINAL) SYNDROME

Raeder in 1924 reported five cases of neuralgia or sensory disturbance in a territory of the trigeminal nerve associated with ipsilateral Horner syndrome (Raeder, 1924). The etiology was trauma in two cases, tumor of the middle cranial fossa in one, and undetermined in two. Motor fibers of the trigeminal nerve were also affected in one case, and optic neuropathy and external ophthalmoplegia were also seen each in two cases. The neuralgia most commonly affected the ophthalmic nerve. In all cases, responsible lesions were localized at or around the semilunar ganglion in the middle cranial fossa, and extended to the internal carotid artery to involve the sympathetic nerve fibers (see Chapter 8-1). Regarding Horner syndrome in those cases, only ptosis and miosis were seen, but enophthalmos, conjunctival hyperemia, hypohidrosis (decreased sweating), and increased temperature of the facial skin were not present. This is considered to be due to the fact that the sympathetic fibers innervating those functions other than the eyelid elevation and pupillary dilation bifurcate before the internal carotid artery enters the cranial fossa.

Enhancement of this reflex suggests hyperexcitability of motor neurons in the motor nucleus of the trigeminal nerve in the pons as a result of bilateral lesion of the corticobulbar tracts or of impairment of the upper motor neurons innervating those motor nuclei. In patients with bulbar symptoms such as dysphagia and dysphonia/dysarthria, enhancement of jaw jerk serves as a supplementary evidence for **pseudobulbar palsy** (see Chapter 14-7).

D. CORNEAL REFLEX

This reflex is generally tested only when it is judged necessary from the history and other neurological findings. In order to elicit this reflex, a twisted string of tissue paper can be used to gently touch the cornea from the lateral visual field, and the response can be judged by observing closure of eyelids. Coming in from the lateral side, rather than from directly in front, reduces the chances of a visual response to the stimulus. Touching the sclera is not effective because there are no nociceptive receptors in the sclera. In patients who have too frequent blinks or who are unable to keep the eyes open, the eye to be stimulated is held open by the examiner and the response of the stimulus eye can be judged by observing contraction of the orbicularis oculi muscle in the other eye. The same technique can be used to examine comatose patients.

A similar reflex can be elicited by touching the cilia (eyelash) and may be called the "ciliary reflex," but this terminology is more properly used for the accommodation reflex of the ciliary muscle (see Chapter 8-1). As the corneal reflex is more sensitive than the ciliary reflex, it should be tested even when the ciliary reflex is absent.

Loss of the corneal reflex suggests either impairment of the ophthalmic nerve of the stimulated side or bilateral paralysis of the orbicularis oculi muscles. When the corneal reflex is lost in one eye regardless of the side of stimulation, it suggests paralysis of the facial nerve on that side. In this case, spontaneous blinking is either incomplete or lost in the affected eye. Likewise, the blink reflex elicited by tapping the glabella is either lost or slower on the side of the affected facial nerve.

As the trigeminothalamic tract ascends through the pontine tegmentum along the lateral edge, it can be affected by extramedullary compression (see Figure 5-5). For example, in a large cerebellopontine angle tumor like acoustic neurinoma compressing the pons, loss of the corneal reflex is an important sign in addition to sensorineural deafness and cerebellar ataxia.

Enhancement of Blink Reflex

In some cases of degenerative diseases involving basal ganglia, blink reflex (glabellar tap reflex) may be exaggerated or may respond to repetitive stimuli continuously. This phenomenon is called **Myerson sign**.

E. PRIMITIVE REFLEXES

In patients with cerebral hemispheric lesions, especially with bilateral frontal lobe lesions, stimuli given to the skin or mucosa innervated by the trigeminal nerve may elicit reflexes that are seen only in infants (primitive reflex) (Schott & Rossor, 2003, for review). Gentle stroking of the upper lip will elicit a sucking movement in the lips (**sucking reflexes**), and gentle tapping of the upper lip will elicit pouting of lips (**snout reflex**). Stimuli presented to the cornea might elicit contraction in the mental muscles or even might move the jaw (**corneomandibular reflex**).

Other primitive reflexes may be elicited by stimulating the skin of the upper extremity. Stroking the thenar aspect of the palm might cause contraction in the mental muscles (**palmomental reflex**). In extreme cases, this reflex might be induced by stroking the forearm. Furthermore, **forced grasping** (Boxes 16 and 17)

BOX 16 FORCED GRASPING

In infants, stroking the palm or sole toward the tips causes flexion of the fingers or toes, which is called **palmar grasp** and **plantar grasp**, respectively. The grasp reflex disappears in adults, but may reappear in special pathological conditions. **Forced grasping** is considered to be an exaggerated state of this grasp reflex, but it might be overlooked unless specifically examined. In forced grasping of severe degree, the patient might forcefully grasp the caregiver's hand or object and be unable to let it go, which will cause significant disability of daily living (Schott & Rossor, 2003, and Mestre & Lang, 2010, for review). This phenomenon is especially common in neurodegenerative diseases presenting with parkinsonism and dementia, such as corticobasal degeneration and progressive supranuclear palsy (Mestre & Lang, 2010, for review). Forced grasping might also be seen in vascular lesions of the frontal lobe, in the hand contralateral to the lesion. Which structures of the frontal lobe are important for this phenomenon has not been precisely elucidated, but the supplementary motor area and the cingulate gyrus contralateral to the grasp have been incriminated. Forced grasping might be also seen in response to visual stimulus (**forced groping**).

BOX 17 HEAD RETRACTION REFLEX AND OPISTHOTONUS

Touching the upper lip might cause retraction of the head. The **head retraction reflex** might be seen in neurodegenerative diseases presenting with parkinsonism. Among others, this sign is especially common in progressive supranuclear palsy and corticobasal degeneration, but it has been reported also in patients with stiff-person syndrome and other related conditions (Berger & Meinck, 2003). Head retraction after tapping the nose is a feature of hereditary startle syndrome (hyperekplexia). **Opisthotonus** seen in patients with stiff-person syndrome and tetanus may appear similar to the head retraction reflex, but in opisthotonus, not only the head but also the trunk is retracted. In opisthotonus, therefore, the lower motor neurons of the whole body are considered to be hyperexcitable (see Chapter 29-3), while the neck extensors are selectively involved in the head retraction reflex.

---

and **utilization behavior** (see Chapter 23-1B) are also regarded as primitive reflexes. Primitive reflexes may be also induced by visual stimulus. For example, reaching out the examiner's hand toward the patient's face might make the patient open the mouth, or touching the cheek or just showing an object visually might make the patient reach out his/her face and mouth toward the object (**rooting reflex**).

BIBLIOGRAPHY

Berger C, Meinck H-M. Head retraction reflex in stiff-man syndrome and related disorders. Mov Disord 18:906–911, 2003.

Gronseth G, Cruccu G, Alksne J, Argoff C, Brainin M, Burchiel K, et al. Practice parameter: the diagnostic evaluation and treatment of trigeminal neuralgia (an evidence-based review): report of the Quality Standards Subcommittee of the American Academy of Neurology and the European Federation of Neurological Societies. Neurology 71:1183–1190, 2008. (review)

Kimura J. Electrodiagnosis in Diseases of Nerve and Muscle: Principles and Practice. 4th ed. Oxford University Press, New York, 2013.

Marcus Gunn R. Congenital ptosis with peculiar associated movements of the affected lid. Trans Ophthalmol Soc UK 3:283–287, 1883.

Marin Amat M. Sur le syndrome ou phénomène de Marcus Gunn. Ann Oculist 156:513–528, 1919.

Mestre T, Lang AE. The grasp reflex: a symptom in need of treatment. Mov Disord 25:2479–2485, 2010. (review)

Raeder JG. "Paratrigeminal" paralysis of oculo-pupillary sympathetic. Brain 47:149–158, 1924.

Schott JM, Rossor MN. The grasp and other primitive reflexes. J Neurol Neurosurg Psychiatry 74:558–560, 2003. (review)

Shimono M, Soezima N, Shibasaki H, Shida K, Kuroiwa Y. The pathogenesis of Marcus Gunn phenomena. Clin Neurol 15:347–354, 1975. (abstract in English)

11.

FACIAL NERVE

The seventh cranial nerve (facial nerve) contains four different groups of nerve fibers: motor, somatosensory, gustatory, and autonomic (parasympathetic).

1. STRUCTURES AND FUNCTIONS

A. MOTOR NERVE

The facial motor nucleus is located in the pontine tegmentum, anterior and lateral to the abducens nucleus on each side. Its nerve fibers first run posteromedially toward the fourth ventricle and, after having encircled the abducens nucleus, they run anterolaterally and exit the pons through its lateral edge (see Figure 5-2). In the cerebellopontine angle of the posterior cranial fossa, they enter the internal auditory meatus of the temporal bone, pass through the **geniculate ganglion** in the facial canal, and exit from the stylomastoid foramen (Figure 11-1). After passing through the parotid gland, they separate to project to the frontal, orbicularis oculi, and orbicularis oris muscles and platysma. If the facial nerve is affected by infectious or autoimmune inflammation, these muscles are paralyzed to various degrees (**Bell palsy**) (Box 18).

When the facial nerve is in a hyperexcitable state, the orbicularis oculi muscle and/or the orbicularis oris muscle twitches repetitively or continuously, resulting in the eyelids closure or lateral upward pulling of the oral angle. This condition is called **hemifacial spasm**, which is, like trigeminal neuralgia (see Chapter 10-2B), considered to be due to demyelination of the nerve fibers secondary to its compression by tortuous branches of the vertebrobasilar artery. However, as this phenomenon is not due to direct compression by the arteries, the twitches seen in those muscles are not synchronous with cardiac pulsation. As the result of electrophysiological studies by stimulating the facial nerve and by recording the evoked EMG from the corresponding muscle (F-wave), motor neurons of the facial nucleus were shown to be hyperexcitable (Ishikawa et al, 2010). The spasms, however, may arise from ectopic activity in the demyelinated segment of the nerve.

In the facial canal, the facial nerve sends a branch also to the stapedius muscle, which acts to relieve tension of the tympanic membrane. In Bell palsy, therefore, the tympanic membrane becomes hypertensive, causing **hyperacusis**.

Somatotopic Organization of Motor Cortex and Its Face Area

The face area of the primary motor cortex (MI) is located at the lateral convexity of the precentral gyrus and, like the primary somatosensory cortex (SI), there is somatotopic organization in MI showing the upside down homunculus (Figure 11-2). However, just like SI, the organization within the face area is not upside down, and the eye area is located dorsal to the mouth area. The MI is mostly located in the anterior wall (area 4) of the central sulcus, and at least for the face and hand areas, the crown of the precentral gyrus is occupied by the premotor area (area 6) (Figure 11-3). For the upper part of the face, in addition to MI, the cingulate area sends a strong projection to the facial nucleus (Hanakawa et al, 2008).

Corticospinal tracts and corticobulbar tracts are made of nerve fibers directly projecting from the pyramidal tract cells of the MI and the premotor area. As for the nerve fibers originating from the supplementary motor area (SMA), at least as far as those projecting to the anterior horn cells related to the distal extremity muscles are concerned, they join the corticospinal tract via MI or the premotor area. Electrophysiologically, an electrical shock presented to the hand area of the MI or the premotor area evokes a phasic contraction in the contralateral hand muscle at a latency of 20 ms, while an electric shock given to SMA evokes slow muscle contraction bilaterally. Thus, for the extremity muscles, the MI and the premotor area innervate contralaterally and the SMA innervates bilaterally.

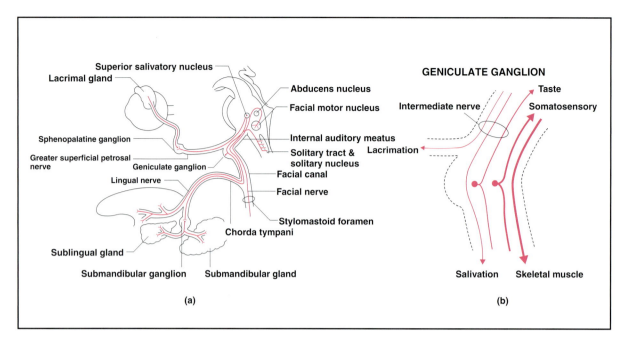

Figure 11-1 Structures of the facial nerve (a) and magnified view of the geniculate ganglion to show fiber compositions in it (b).

B. SOMATOSENSORY NERVE

Somatosensory fibers of the facial nerve transmit impulses arising from the skin of the inner aspect of the earlobe and the external auditory meatus. The primary sensory neuron is a bipolar cell of the geniculate ganglion (Figure 11-1b). Its peripheral axon conducts impulses from the above skin area, and through the central axon, the nociceptive input is conducted through the spinal tract of the trigeminal nerve to its nucleus, while the tactile input projects to the main sensory nucleus of the trigeminal nerve. Nerve fibers originating from the secondary neuron cross and ascend through the trigeminothalamic tract to reach the VPM of the contralateral thalamus (see Chapter 10-1).

When the geniculate ganglion is infected with **varicella zoster virus**, the somatosensory fibers are primarily affected because varicella zoster virus has a strong affinity to the sensory ganglion. In this condition, a vesicular skin rash is observed in the inner earlobe and the external auditory

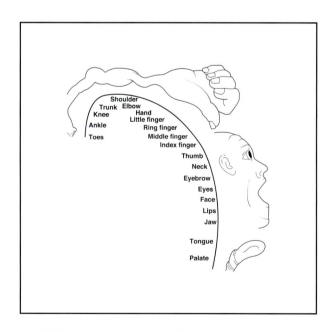

Figure 11-2 Somatotopic organization of the primary motor cortex.

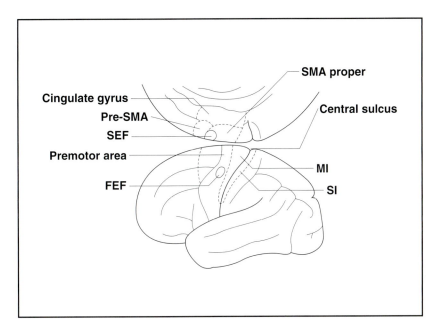

meatus associated with neuralgia, numbness, and sensory loss in that region (see Figure 3-7). Motor fibers are also affected by inflammation in the geniculate ganglion, causing motor paralysis (**Ramsay Hunt syndrome, Hunt syndrome**). Although other conditions including deep palmar branch ulnar neuropathy, dyssynergia cerebellaris myoclonica, juvenile Parkinson disease, and dentato-rubro-pallido-luysian atrophy might also be referred to as Ramsay Hunt syndrome, only the geniculate zoster is called Ramsay Hunt syndrome in this book to avoid confusion.

C. TASTE SENSE

Special nerve fibers for taste sense conduct impulses from the anterior two-thirds of the tongue. The primary neuron is a bipolar cell in the geniculate ganglion. Impulses arising from the taste buds are conducted through the peripheral axon as the lingual nerve and chorda tympani into the geniculate ganglion. The central axon conducts impulses to the **solitary nucleus** in the pontine tegmentum (Figure 11-1, see also Figures 5-3 and 5-5). In Bell palsy, the facial nerve is usually affected central to the bifurcation of chorda tympani from the facial nerve, thus involving the gustatory fibers, and therefore taste sense is lost in the anterior two-thirds of the tongue unilaterally.

The secondary gustatory fibers originating from the solitary nucleus project to the VPM of the thalamus, and the third fibers project to the tongue area of the SI and the anterior insula. In relation to this, some patients with mesial temporal lobe epilepsy complain of unusual taste as an aura. In addition, some fibers originating from the solitary nucleus project to the salivatory nucleus, the dorsal motor nucleus of the vagus nerve and hypothalamus, and they control digestion in a reflexive way. Taste sense of the posterior third of tongue is innervated by the glossopharyngeal nerve (see Chapter 14-3).

D. LACRIMATION AND SALIVATION

Parasympathetic efferent fibers of the facial nerve control secretion of the lacrimal gland and salivary gland. The nucleus innervating salivation is the **superior salivatory nucleus** situated in the pontine tegmentum, and that for lacrimation is the **lacrimal nucleus**. These two nuclei are attached together and may be considered as a single nuclear group (see Figure 5-2). The preganglionic fibers emerging from the nucleus form the **intermediate nerve** and enter the facial canal as a part of the facial nerve (Figure 11-1b).

The preganglionic fibers from the lacrimal nucleus bifurcate from the facial nerve just before they reach the geniculate ganglion and form the greater superficial petrosal nerve to project to the sphenopalatine ganglion. The postganglionic fibers emerging from the ganglion innervate the lacrimal gland (Figure 11-1a). The neurotransmitter of the preganglionic fibers is acetylcholine for nicotinic receptors and that of the postganglionic fibers is acetylcholine for muscarinic receptors. This system acts to facilitate lacrimation (Box 19).

The preganglionic fibers from the salivatory nucleus bifurcate from the facial nerve after it emerges from the geniculate ganglion and form the chorda tympani to project to the submandibular ganglion (Figure 11-1a). The postganglionic fibers emerging from the ganglion project to the sublingual gland and submandibular gland to facilitate salivation. The synaptic transmitters for this system are the same as for lacrimation.

In Bell palsy, if the inflammation involves the facial nerve before (proximal to) the bifurcation of the greater superficial petrosal nerve, the preganglionic fibers related to lacrimation are involved, which will cause loss of lacrimation. Furthermore, as the orbicularis oculi muscle is paralyzed to various degrees, it worsens the dryness of eyes and necessitates protection of the cornea and conjunctivae from excessive dryness. Theoretically, unilateral involvement of the facial nerve before the bifurcation of the chorda tympani will cause loss of salivation on the affected side, but this is compensated for by the intact salivation of the opposite salivary glands.

E. PARASYMPATHETIC INNERVATION OF FACIAL SKIN AND MUCOSA

In contrast with the sympathetic nervous system, the parasympathetic innervation of the facial skin and mucosa is not precisely known. However, it is most likely that the parasympathetic pathway goes through the facial nerve. If that is the case, lesion of the facial nerve is expected to show, contrary to Horner syndrome (see Chapter 8-1), anemic palpebral conjunctiva, decreased skin temperature, and decreased nasal discharge; however, these findings are not detected on routine clinical examination.

2. EXAMINATION OF FUNCTIONS RELATED TO THE FACIAL NERVE

Functions of the facial nerve can be examined by paying attention to the following five aspects.

A. MOTOR FUNCTION

First, it is important to observe the face closely, paying special attention to possible asymmetry in the forehead furrows, palpebral fissure, nasolabial folds, and level of oral angles. In peripheral facial paralysis, the furrows in the forehead look shallower on the affected side, and weakness of the frontal muscle can be confirmed by asking the patient to raise the eyebrows. The palpebral fissure on the affected side may be larger due to paralysis of the orbicularis oculi muscle. Complete failure to close the eyelids is called **lagophthalmos**. It should be kept in mind, however, that, in the chronic stage of Bell palsy, the palpebral fissure may be even smaller on the affected side due to abnormal electric discharge of the facial nerve causing repetitive or continuous contraction of the orbicularis oculi muscle. Furthermore, attempt to contract the orbicularis oris muscle may narrow the palpebral fissure of the affected side due to synkinesis of the orbicularis oculi muscle (Box 18).

It is also important to pay attention to blinks. In unilateral facial nerve palsy, blinks might decrease in amplitude and speed, and may even be completely absent on the affected side. When the patient is asked to close the eyes tight, cilia on the affected side might protrude forward (**ciliary sign**). Furthermore, the blink reflex elicited by tapping the glabella may be incomplete, slower or even absent on the affected side.

When the orbicularis oris muscle is paralyzed, the nasolabial fold is shallower and the oral angle might be lower on the affected side compared with the intact side. However, since even healthy subjects might show some asymmetry in the nasolabial folds and oral angles, their asymmetry has to be confirmed by muscle testing and other accompanying signs. Strength of the orbicularis oris muscle can be tested by asking the patient to move the mouth to various directions, whistle, and blow. If the patient is asked to pronounce a long 'i' sound, contraction of the platysma can be observed in the neck.

Paralysis of the stapedius muscle can be tested by checking hearing with a tuning fork. The hearing threshold is decreased because the paralyzed stapedius muscle cannot relieve the tension of the tympanic membrane (**hyperacusis**).

Central Facial Paralysis and Peripheral Facial Paralysis

In most cases, distinction of the central versus peripheral facial paralysis is not difficult from the history and the accompanying symptoms and signs. In case the motor paralysis is restricted to unilateral face without involving extremities, relative impairment of the orbicularis oris and oculi muscles provides a clue for the distinction. Paralysis of the orbicularis oris muscle with no associated paralysis, or only mild if any, of the orbicularis oculi muscle usually suggests **central facial paralysis**, because the upper facial muscles

are bilaterally innervated from the motor cortex and probably also because the facial subnucleus corresponding to the upper part of face receives projection from the cingulate motor area (Hanakawa et al, 2008) (Box 18).

Unilateral involvement of all facial muscles suggests a **peripheral facial paralysis**. Theoretically, there is no stretch reflex in the orbicularis oris muscle, because muscle spindles are not known to exist in this muscle. However, tapping the lips occasionally cause a twitch in the muscle. Like the blink reflex (see Chapter 10-1), this reflex is considered to be a polysynaptic reflex in response to activation of the skin receptors. On some occasions, it is also difficult to distinguish it from the snout reflex. In peripheral facial paralysis, all these reflexes are expected to be lost.

In central facial paralysis, it is often associated with deviation of the tongue to the side of facial paralysis when voluntarily protruded, because the mouth and the tongue areas are represented close to each other both in the motor cortex and the corticobulbar tracts (Box 20, see Box 22).

Crossed Hemiplegia of Facial Muscle

A combination of unilateral peripheral facial paralysis with contralateral hemiplegia is called **Millard-Gubler syndrome**, and further addition of lateral gaze palsy to the side of facial palsy is called **Foville syndrome** (see Table 8-1). Both conditions are crossed syndromes due to an intramedullary lesion in the pons (Silverman et al, 1995, for review). Millard in 1856 reported autopsy findings of one of two cases reported by Senac and a case reported by Poisson in

---

BOX 20 BILATERAL FACIAL PARALYSIS

Bilateral peripheral facial paralysis is not very common, but if it is seen, the following causes are considered. Bilateral peripheral facial paralysis of acute or subacute onset suggests systemic conditions including sarcoidosis, Lyme disease, and leprosy. In **sarcoidosis**, the facial nerves are involved by granulomatous inflammation. Both facial nerves may be affected simultaneously or independently, one after the other. Association of facial nerve palsy with uveitis and parotid swelling is known as **Heerfordt disease**. **Lyme disease** is caused by infection with a spirochete *Borrelia burgdorferi*, which is mediated by tics. In facial palsy due to tuberculoid leprosy, the frontal and orbicularis oculi muscles are commonly involved. As described in Chapter 9-5B, congenital bilateral facial nerve paralysis (Möbius syndrome) is due to hypoplasia of the corresponding neurons in the facial motor nucleus.

the *Bulletin of the Anatomical Society of Paris*, and ascribed the former combination to a pontine hemorrhage (Millard, 1856). Foville in 1858 reported a 43-year-old man with possible pontine hemorrhage manifesting the latter combination (Foville, 1858). He postulated the presence of some mechanism in the pons that controls abduction of one eye and adduction of the other eye. There was no concept of lateral gaze center at that time.

Mimetic Muscles

Mimetic muscles employed for laughing and crying are also involved in peripheral facial paralysis, but are not much impaired in central facial paralysis. Facial muscles related to emotional expression might be also controlled by the basal ganglia, hypothalamus, and cingulate gyrus, either directly or indirectly. In fact, those muscles are affected in basal ganglia disorders, and the facial expression is lost contralateral to the lesion. A **mask-like face** is often seen in patients with Parkinson disease.

B. SOMATOSENSORY FUNCTION

If there is any possibility of herpes zoster infection as a cause of peripheral facial paralysis, it is important to look for vesicular rash on the skin of the inner earlobe and the external auditory meatus (**Ramsay Hunt syndrome**). It is usually associated with sensory impairment in that region.

C. TASTE SENSE

Loss of taste sense (**ageusia**) is noticed by the patient only when the taste buds are totally damaged as in the case of side effects of drugs and zinc deficiency. Unilateral loss of taste sense due to a facial nerve lesion can be detected by comparing the taste sense between two sides of the anterior two-thirds of the tongue. Taste sense can be tested by touching each side of the tongue with a wet swab soaked in salt or sugar, while the tongue is gently protruded. The patient is asked to show by hand if the taste is felt and to tell later what kind of taste it was. Then the other half of the tongue is tested after washing out the mouth.

D. LACRIMATION AND SALIVATION

In unilateral peripheral facial paralysis the patient often complains of dryness in the affected eye. This is tested by measuring the volume of tears with a piece of filter paper placed on the lower eyelid (**Schirmer test**). In Bell palsy, as described above, dryness of the affected eye becomes even worse due to paralysis of the orbicularis oculi muscle. In the recovery phase from Bell palsy, the crocodile tears syndrome (Box 19) may be confirmed by the history taking or by actual observation while the patient is eating.

Dryness in the mouth is a complaint of a patient with a **sicca syndrome** like Sjögren syndrome and Mikulicz syndrome. In this case, eyes are also found to be dry. In unilateral lesion of the facial nerve, unilateral loss of salivation is never noticed by the patient because of normal salivation from the intact side and also because of the intact glossopharyngeal nerve, which innervates salivation of the parotid gland (see Chapter 14-4).

E. FACIAL SKIN AND MUCOSA

In relation to the autonomic nervous functions, attention might be paid to the color of the facial skin, palpebral conjunctiva, and oral mucosa, and temperature and moisture of the facial skin. In Horner syndrome, conjunctival hyperemia, decreased sweating, and elevated temperature might be observed on the affected side (see Chapter 8-1). In peripheral facial paralysis, although the parasympathetic fibers are considered to be contained in the facial nerve, abnormalities of the skin and mucosa are not usually observed. Occasionally, peripheral facial paralysis might be accompanied by edema of the ipsilateral tongue and face (**Melkersson-Rosenthal syndrome**) (Hallett & Mitchell, 1968).

BIBLIOGRAPHY

Foville A. Note sur une paralysie peu connue de certains muscles de l'oeil, et sa liaison avec quelques points de l'anatomie et la physiologie de la protubérance annulaire. Bull Soc Anat Paris 33:393–414, 1858.

Hallett JW, Mitchell B. Melkersson-Rosenthal syndrome. Am J Ophthalmol 65:542–544, 1968.

Hanakawa T, Dimyan MA, Hallett M. The representation of blinking movement in cingulate motor areas: a functional magnetic resonance imaging study. Cereb Cortex 18:930–937, 2008.

Ishikawa M, Takashima K, Kamochi H, Kusaka G, Shinoda S, Watanabe E. Treatment with botulinum toxin improves the hyperexcitability of the facial motoneuron in patients with hemifacial spasm. Neurol Res 32:656–660, 2010.

Millard M. Extrait du rapport de M. Millard sur les observations précédentes. Bull Soc Anat Paris 31:217–221, 1856.

Silverman IE, Liu GT, Volpe NJ, Galetta SL. The crossed paralyses. The original brain-stem syndromes of Millard-Gubler, Foville, Weber, and Raymond-Cestan. Arch Neurol 52:635–638, 1995. (review)

12.

AUDITORY FUNCTION

1. STRUCTURES OF THE AUDITORY PATHWAY

Receptors of auditory sense are hair cells in the organ of Corti of the cochlea. The primary neuron is a bipolar cell in the **spiral ganglion**, and its peripheral axon is very short. Its central axon (**cochlear nerve** or **acoustic nerve**) forms, together with the vestibular nerve, the eighth cranial nerve (**vestibulocochlear nerve**), which passes medially through the internal auditory meatus to enter the cerebellopontine angle in the posterior cranial fossa and enters the lateral posterior part of the medulla oblongata (Figure 12-1). The secondary neuron is in the **dorsal and ventral cochlear nucleus**, located in the upper lateral part of the medullary tegmentum.

Most of the secondary nerve fibers originating from the ventral cochlear nucleus run ventrally, and after crossing in the trapezoid body, they go through the contralateral **superior olive** to form the **lateral lemniscus** (Figure 12-2). Some fibers form synaptic connections to the tertiary neurons in the superior olive and ascend through the lateral lemniscus. Some fibers from the ventral cochlear nucleus also project to the ipsilateral superior olive, and the tertiary fibers from there join the ipsilateral lateral lemniscus. The **lateral lemniscus** projects to the **inferior colliculus** in the midbrain. The secondary fibers originating from the dorsal cochlear nucleus cross in the tegmentum and join the contralateral lateral lemniscus. Some of the third or fourth order neurons originating from the inferior colliculus send their axons to the ipsilateral **medial geniculate body**, and the fibers of the other group cross and project to the contralateral medial geniculate body. The fibers originating from the medial geniculate body project through the acoustic radiation of the cerebral white matter to the ipsilateral **auditory cortex (Heschl gyrus)** located in the inferior bank of the sylvian fissure (Figure 12-2).

As the auditory pathways cross partially at the upper part of the medulla oblongata, and again partially after the inferior colliculus, each auditory cortex receives the input from both ears. However, based on studies using magnetoencephalography and neuroimaging techniques, it is known that the input to the auditory cortex from the contralateral ear is greater compared to the ipsilateral ear. In sensory systems in general, it is the tertiary neurons that project to the cortical receptive areas, but in the auditory system, it is mediated by more than three steps.

Brainstem Auditory Evoked Potentials

Based on the concept of far-field potentials, which can be recorded from the electrodes placed on the head surface, it is possible to follow the conduction of auditory impulses through the brainstem pathways noninvasively. In brainstem auditory evoked potentials (BAEPs), seven small surface-positive peaks can be identified within 10 ms after presentation of a click stimulus (Figure 12-3). The generator sources of those peaks are postulated to be the acoustic nerve for peak I, acoustic nerve or cochlear nucleus for II, superior olive for III, lateral lemniscus for IV, inferior colliculus for V, medial geniculate body for VI, and auditory radiation for VII. The BAEPs are used as a method to assess the integrity of parts of the brainstem, including confirmation of loss of brainstem functions in possible cases of brain death (see Chapter 29-6).

Cognitive Functions Related to the Auditory Sense

By magnetoencephalographic studies, **tonotopic organization** was demonstrated in the primary auditory cortex. Namely, the auditory input is received in sequentially different areas of the cortex depending on its frequency. **Spatial perception of auditory input** or the information as to where a sound has come from is achieved based on a subtle difference in the arrival time of the sound to both ears and consequently on a subtle difference in the arrival time of impulses to the cortices on both sides. Regarding **selective attention**, if special attention is paid to a particular

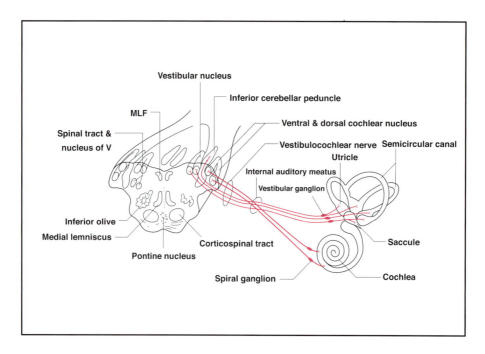

Figure 12-1 Schematic diagram to show the neural pathways of auditory and vestibular senses. MLF: medial longitudinal fasciculus, V: trigeminal nerve.

voice among others at a party, that voice can be heard even in noisy circumstances. This so-called cocktail party effect has been shown to occur also in the primary auditory cortex (see Box 87). Thus, the primary auditory cortex plays an important role in the cognitive auditory functions.

2. EXAMINATION OF AUDITORY FUNCTION

Hearing of each ear is tested by using, for example, a vibrating tuning fork. If hearing is decreased in one ear, the **Weber test** can be done by placing a vibrating tuning fork on the

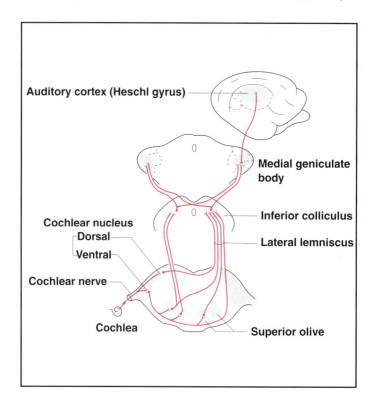

Figure 12-2 Central pathway of the auditory sense. (Modified from Brodal, 2010, with permission)

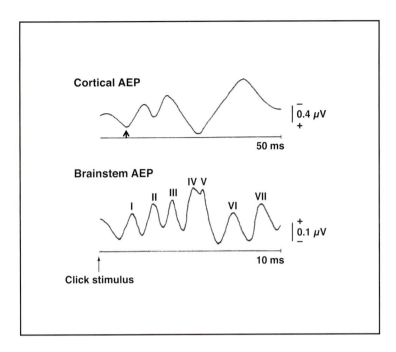

Figure 12-3 Auditory evoked potentials (AEP) in response to click stimulus (arrow). In the cortical AEP shown on the top, the initial impulse arrives at the cortex at latency of about 17 ms (arrowhead). The brainstem AEP shown on the bottom is generated in deep structures but can be recorded from the electrodes placed on the scalp as far-field potentials due to volume conduction. See text for the generator source of each peak.

midline forehead and by asking the patient to judge on which side he/she hears the sound of the tuning fork. For this test, it is important to specify in which ear the patient hears, but not on which side he/she feels the vibration of the tuning fork. If the patient hears on the side of hearing loss, it suggests **conductive deafness**. In that case, the tympanic membrane should be checked. If the patient hears on the intact side, it suggests **sensorineural deafness**. As some patients might predict that they should be able to hear on the intact side, if there is any question as to the results of Weber test, they should be well informed that they might hear more on the affected side. If some question still remains in the interpretation of the results, it is useful to mask one ear and confirm that it is heard on the masked side. Sometimes, this maneuver might help obtain some clue to possible diagnosis of psychogenic disorders. In case of bilateral hearing loss, the Weber test can be still applied. If the patient hears the tuning fork better on the more severely affected side, it suggests conductive deafness, and vice versa.

Alternatively, a vibrating tuning fork can be placed on the retroauricular part of the temporal bone to compare bone conduction to air conduction (**Rinne test**). The bone conduction is preserved in conductive deafness whereas, in sensorineural deafness, both air conduction and bone conduction are lost.

As described in Chapter 10-2D, if unilateral sensorineural deafness is associated with cerebellar ataxia and loss of the ipsilateral corneal reflex, it suggests acoustic neurinoma occupying the cerebellopontine angle, compressing the pons.

Tinnitus

Tinnitus is a common complaint related to hearing disturbance. Sound produced intracranially can be heard continuously or intermittently in one ear or in both ears. Usually it is heard only in the patient's own ears, but occasionally it can be heard by other nearby people. Causes of the latter condition include disturbance of intracranial blood circulation, some types of palatal tremor, or abnormalities of temporomandibular joints. Subjective tinnitus occurs in organic disorders of any of the outer, middle, and inner ears, and any part of the auditory pathway, but it is particularly common in association with sensorineural deafness. However, tinnitus is extremely rare in disorders of the central nervous system even if the auditory pathway is involved. Unilateral tinnitus might be an initial symptom of acoustic neurinoma.

Sensorineural Deafness

Sensorineural deafness is caused by a number of conditions. It may be seen as a sequel of inflammatory diseases such as meningitis, mumps, and syphilis. It may be also seen in drug intoxication, organic mercury poisoning (Minamata disease), and Ménière disease. A typical case of progressive unilateral sensorineural deafness is acoustic neurinoma.

In some neurodegenerative diseases, sensorineural deafness may be seen as one of its cardinal symptoms. Among others, **Refsum disease** (heredopathia atactica polyneuritiformis due to phytanic acid oxidase deficiency) and **Kearns-Sayre syndrome** (see Box 57) are well known. **Susac syndrome** occurs in women of age 20–40 years, and is characterized by acute encephalopathy with headache and psychiatric symptoms, occlusion of retinal arteries, and sensorineural deafness. In some cases of Susac syndrome, cranial MRI shows a white matter change like acute disseminated encephalitis, probably suggesting an autoimmune disorder (Rennebohm et al, 2008, for review). In Susac syndrome, retinal pathology can be detected by spectral-domain optical coherence tomography (Ringelstein et al, 2015). **Superficial siderosis** occurs in the aged population and is characterized by progressive bilateral sensorineural deafness, cerebellar ataxia, and pyramidal signs (Kumar et al, 2009; Vernooij et al, 2009). This condition is thought to be due to repetitive subarachnoid hemorrhage of mild degree or amyloid angiopathy.

Auditory pathways may be involved by intramedullary lesions of the brainstem, but as the input arising from each ear ascends bilaterally in the brainstem, this does not manifest hearing deficit in the clinical setting. As the lateral lemniscus ascends through the lateral part of the pons, its bilateral involvement is rarely encountered. Bilateral involvement of the lateral lemniscus may occur in a massive pontine lesion, but in that case the patient may not be in a sufficiently alert condition for the hearing test.

BIBLIOGRAPHY

Brodal P. The Central Nervous System: Structure and Function. 4th ed. Oxford University Press, New York, 2010.

Kumar N, Lane JI, Piepgras DG. Superficial siderosis: sealing the defect. Neurology 72: 671–673, 2009.

Rennebohm RM, Egan RA, Susac JO. Treatment of Susac's syndrome. Curr Treat Options Neurol 10:67–74, 2008. (review)

Ringelstein M, Albrecht P, Kleffner I, Bühn B, Harmel J, Müller A-K, et al. Retinal pathology in Susac syndrome detected by spectral-domain optical coherence tomography. Neurology 85:610–618, 2015.

Vernooij MW, Ikram MA, Hofman A, Kreslin GP, Breteler MM, van der Lugt A. Superficial siderosis in the general population. Neurology 73:202–205, 2009.

13.

SENSE OF EQUILIBRIUM

1. STRUCTURES AND FUNCTIONS OF THE PATHWAYS RELATED TO EQUILIBRIUM

Receptors of the sense of equilibrium are hair cells located in the semicircular canals, saccule, and utricle of the labyrinth. The **semicircular canals** receive input related to rotatory acceleration of head, and the saccule and utricle receive input related to the position and rectilinear acceleration of head. Among the latter two receptors, the **saccule** is sensitive to the acceleration of gravity while the **utricle** is sensitive to horizontal acceleration. For example, when riding a roller coaster, sudden acceleration forward is received by the utricle, and when taking an elevator, sudden vertical acceleration is received by the saccule.

The primary neuron of the vestibular system is a bipolar cell located in the **vestibular ganglion (Scarpa's ganglion)**. Its peripheral axon conducts impulses from the receptors to the central axon (**vestibular nerve**), which, along with the cochlear nerve, passes through the internal auditory meatus. In the posterior cranial fossa, they enter the dorsolateral tegmentum of the medulla oblongata and project to the vestibular nuclei (vestibular complex) (see Figure 12-1).

The **vestibular complex** is made of four nuclei: medial, lateral, upper, and inferior. Most nerve fibers originating in the semicircular canals project to the superior vestibular nucleus and the rostral part of the medial vestibular nucleus. Nerve fibers originating in the saccule and utricle mainly project to the lateral vestibular nucleus (Deiters nucleus). In addition, the vestibular complex receives input from the spinal cord, brainstem reticular formation, superior colliculus, and flocculus, nodulus, and anterior lobe of the cerebellum.

The secondary nerves originating in the vestibular complex ascend through the ipsilateral vestibulothalamic tract in the medial brainstem (Yang et al, 2014) and they project to the ventral posterolateral nucleus of thalamus (VPL), from which the tertiary nerves project to the cortex. Based on the results of evoked potential recording and direct stimulation study, the cortical receptive areas of the vestibular input are postulated to be a region posterior to the face area of the postcentral gyrus and the parietal insular vestibular cortex located in the junction between the parietal lobe and insula (Mazzola et al, 2014). In relation to this, some patients with temporal lobe epilepsy complain of vertigo as an aura (**vertiginous seizure, epileptic vertigo**) (Tarnutzer et al, 2015, for review).

In addition to the above pathways directly related to the sense of equilibrium, nerve fibers originating in the vestibular complex also project to motor nuclei targeting the extraocular muscles, cerebellum, and anterior horn of the spinal cord. Those fibers targeting at the spinal cord originate mainly in the lateral nucleus and form the **lateral vestibulospinal tract**, which projects to the α and γ motor neurons at the anterior horn. The vestibulospinal tract is considered to give a facilitatory effect on the muscle tone of extensors. This pathway is considered to be significant in the pathophysiology of **decerebrate posture** and **decerebrate rigidity** seen in tentorial herniation. Namely, as the inhibitory pathway projecting to the vestibular complex is impaired due to midbrain compression, it disinhibits the facilitatory vestibulospinal input to the extensor muscles, causing the extensor posture in all extremities (see Chapter 29-5C). If the herniation progresses to compress the lower brainstem, the vestibular complex itself is also damaged, resulting in total loss of muscle tone.

Nerve fibers related to eye movements originate mainly in the superior and medial vestibular nuclei. Most of them ascend through the ipsilateral medial longitudinal fasciculus (MLF), but some fibers cross and ascend through the contralateral MLF (see Chapter 9-2). In addition, some other fibers form synaptic connection to the tertiary neurons in the ipsilateral as well as contralateral paramedian pontine reticular formation (PPRF) and then join the MLF. The latter pathway controls conjugate lateral gaze.

The vestibulocerebellar tract originates from the medial and inferior (descending) vestibular nuclei and projects via the inferior cerebellar peduncle to the vestibulocerebellum (see Figure 16-18). This pathway plays an important role in the control of equilibrium. Some patients with localized cerebellar lesion may complain of vertigo, most likely due to involvement of the vestibulocerebellum.

2. EXAMINATION OF THE SENSE OF EQUILIBRIUM

Whenever a patient complains of "dizziness," it is important to judge whether it is vertigo in the narrow sense or dizziness in general (Figure 13-1). Dizziness is a common symptom in patients having syncope. It is usually described as a feeling of fainting or even blackout in a severe case. A variety of systemic conditions can cause dizziness, including cardiovascular insufficiency, postural hypotension, pulmonary diseases, and severe anemia (see Table 4-1).

By contrast, vertigo is commonly associated with oscillopsia because of the presence of nystagmus. **Oscillopsia** is a phenomenon in which the patient sees the visual scene moving, and with vertigo, it might be rotating. If it is accompanied by tinnitus or hearing disturbance, it suggests vertigo rather than pre-syncope. This is because the vestibular pathway and the cochlear pathway are anatomically close to each other all the way from the inner ear to the brainstem nuclei. A typical example is **Ménière disease**, which presents with attacks of vertigo and slowly progressive sensorineural hearing disturbance due to dysfunction of the labyrinth.

Benign paroxysmal positional vertigo is a common disease that is characterized by vertigo of sudden onset triggered by changing the head position, especially upon awakening in the morning. Vertigo in this condition lasts for several hours to several days and tends to relapse frequently. Its commonest cause is considered to be a fall of an otolith (small stone) from the utricular macula into the space of posterior semicircular canal, which produces the flow of endolymph and pathologically excites the cupula ampularis. As it often resists drug treatment, various maneuvers have been applied to restore the otolith position (Epley maneuver) (Fife et al, 2008; Kerber et al, 2012; Kim et al, 2012).

Vertigo is a common symptom encountered in an ischemic condition of **vertebrobasilar artery territory**, especially in the **lateral medullary syndrome (Wallenberg syndrome)** (see Box 21). Wallenberg syndrome is commonly caused by infarction in the territory of the posterior inferior cerebellar artery, but vertigo is also seen in infarction of the territory of the anterior inferior cerebellar artery. By contrast with Wallenberg syndrome, the latter infarction is characterized by peripheral facial paralysis and hearing deficit of the affected side in addition to vertigo. As the fibers targeting at the solitary nucleus are not affected in this case, the peripheral facial paralysis is not associated with loss of taste.

Examination of vestibular functions depends on the history and other accompanying signs. If the vestibular system is expected to be impaired, detail examination is needed. The most essential test of vestibular functions is observation of the standing posture and gait, which may be done after other neurologic examinations are completed (see Chapter 21).

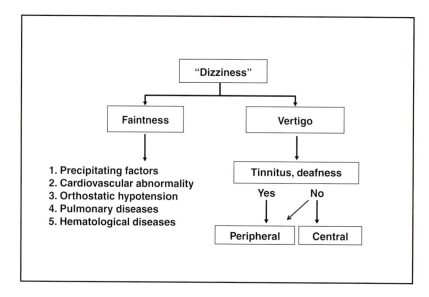

Figure 13-1 Flow chart used for the diagnosis of "dizziness." It is practical to distinguish faintness and vertigo.

In the standing position, the trunk may be tilted, usually toward the side of the affected vestibular system. Upon walking or on tandem gait, the body tends to fall to the affected side (**body lateropulsion**, **axial lateropulsion**). In a medullary lesion like Wallenberg syndrome, the lateropulsion occurs on the affected side, but in a lesion of the paramedian region of the rostral midbrain, it occurs on the side contralateral to the lesion. In Wallenberg syndrome, lateropulsion may be also observed in the eye movement (**saccadic lateropulsion**). Namely, lateral saccadic movement of the eyes to the affected side causes their overshoot, and upon the vertical saccadic movement, the eyes may be pulled toward the affected side during the saccade.

If stability of the trunk position could be confirmed even with the eyes closed, then the past pointing test may be done. With the eyes closed in the standing position, the patient is asked to hold his/her arms straight ahead so that each hand can touch the examiner's opposing hand, and after raising both arms above, to return them to touch the examiner's hands again. Deviation of the patient's arms to either side is called **past pointing**, and usually it deviates to the side of the affected vestibular system. If a Bàràny chair (a chair used for turning the patient for testing vestibular function) is available, it might be used to induce vertigo and nystagmus. If a Bàràny chair is not available, it may be possible to ask the patient to turn around in the standing position, but this maneuver should be avoided in order to prevent falling.

Vestibular Nystagmus

Close observation of nystagmus is very important for testing vestibular functions. **Rotatory nystagmus** and **positional nystagmus** are suggestive of vestibular dysfunction.

During bedside testing of vestibular functions, the first thing to do is to see whether there is any involuntary movement in the eyes in the primary spontaneous position. Then in the supine position, with the head tilted either up by 30 degrees or down by 60 degrees, the presence or absence of nystagmus is checked. If there is no nystagmus induced in the above positions, then the patient is requested to do lateral gaze to either side in each of the head positions. Then with the head returned to the original flat position, the patient is asked to take the recumbent position on each side, to see whether any vertigo or nystagmus is induced or not.

Some patients with cervical spondylosis may complain of vertigo when rotating the head on either side. In this case, the vertebral artery might be compressed during its passage through the transverse foramen at the upper cervical level, and this may cause vertigo as a result of ischemia. Vertigo and/or consciousness disturbance induced by the head rotation is known by the name of **bow hunter's stroke**. Vestibular nystagmus is usually enhanced by blocking fixation, such as closing the eyes or applying Frenzel glasses (lenses for inhibiting fixation), which is contrary to congenital nystagmus (see Chapter 9-5D).

Caloric Test

The most objective test of vestibular function available at the bedside is the caloric test, although its execution requires some expertise. With the patient placed in a supine position with the head extended by 60 degrees, 100 to 200 mL of cold water (or 5–10 mL of ice water) is injected into the external auditory meatus while the patient is asked to indicate as soon as vertigo or nausea is felt, and the induced nystagmus is observed. In healthy subjects, this procedure induces nausea and horizontal nystagmus with the quick phase directed toward the side contralateral to the injection. If the vestibular system is totally damaged, neither nausea nor nystagmus is induced. In case of mild impairment, the response to stimulation of the affected side is weaker compared with the intact side. If only nausea is induced while no nystagmus is induced, it might be due to external ophthalmoplegia or lateral gaze palsy.

In case of abnormally enhanced excitability of the vestibular system, the response to the water injection might occur earlier and stronger as compared with the intact side. The caloric test is one of the most valuable tests in the diagnosis of brain death as it is a very good probe for brainstem function (see Chapter 29-5C).

BIBLIOGRAPHY

Fife TD, Iverson DJ, Lempert T, Furman JM, Baloh RW, Tusa RJ, et al. Practice parameter: therapies for benign paroxysmal positional vertigo (an evidence-based review): report of the Quality Standards Subcommittee of the American Academy of Neurology. Neurology 70:2067–2074, 2008. (review)

Kerber KA, Burke JF, Skolarus LE, Callaghan BC, Fife TD, Baloh RW, et al. A prescription for the Epley maneuver. Neurology 79:376–380, 2012.

Kim JS, Oh SY, Lee SH, Kang JH, Kim DU, Jeong SH, et al. Randomized clinical trial for geotropic horizontal canal benign paroxysmal positional vertigo. Neurology 79:700–707, 2012.

Mazzola L, Lopez C, Faillenot I, Chouchou F, Mauguière F, Isnard J. Vestibular responses to direct stimulation of the human insular cortex. Ann Neurol 76:609–619, 2014.

Tarnutzer AA, Lee S-H, Robinson KA, Kaplan PW, Newman-Toker DE. Clinical and electrographic findings in epileptic vertigo and dizziness: a systematic review. Neurology 84:1595–1604, 2015. (review)

Yang T-H, Oh S-Y, Kwak K, Lee J-M, Shin B-S, Jeong S-K. Topology of brainstem lesions associated with subjective visual vertical tilt. Neurology 82:1968–1975, 2014.

14.

SWALLOWING, PHONATION, AND ARTICULATION

1. INNERVATION OF SWALLOWING, PHONATION, AND ARTICULATION

The final common pathway related to swallowing (deglutition), phonation (vocalization), and articulation are the ninth cranial nerve (glossopharyngeal nerve), the tenth cranial nerve (vagus nerve), and the twelfth cranial nerve (hypoglossal nerve).

A. GLOSSOPHARYNGEAL NERVE AND VAGUS NERVE

The motor nucleus of the glossopharyngeal and vagus nerves is the **nucleus ambiguus**, located in the center of the tegmentum of the medulla oblongata on each side (see Figure 5-3). These two nerves pass behind the spinal tract of the trigeminal nerve and exit the medulla oblongata from its lateral edge. Then they exit the posterior cranial fossa through the **jugular foramen** just lateral to the foramen magnum (see Figure 8-2).

As motor fibers of the glossopharyngeal nerve control swallowing and phonation by innervating the soft palate and pharyngeal muscles, their bilateral lesion causes marked **nasal voice (rhinolalia)** and **dysphagia**. In a unilateral lesion of the glossopharyngeal nerve, the soft palate of the affected side appears as a curtain because of its paralysis (**curtain sign**), and the uvula is pulled toward the intact side. Nasal voice and dysphagia can be quite severe even in unilateral bulbar palsy, as in **Wallenberg syndrome** (Box 21, Figures 14-1, 14-2 and 14-3).

Motor fibers of the vagus nerve innervate not only pharyngeal muscles but also laryngeal muscles, including the vocal cord. In a severe unilateral lesion of the vagus nerve, both abductor and adductor muscles of the vocal cord are paralyzed so that the affected vocal cord becomes immobile and fixed in the intermediate position, causing **hoarseness** or **aphonia**, and even difficulty in breathing. As the **recurrent laryngeal nerve** innervates all laryngeal muscles other than the cricothyroid muscle, its unilateral lesion causes hoarseness, but it could well be asymptomatic as movement of the unaffected contralateral laryngeal muscles could be adequate. Bilateral lesions of the recurrent laryngeal nerve are seen in lead poisoning and may cause stridor and dyspnea. Bilateral complete lesions of the vagus nerve impair all the parasympathetic nerve supply to the visceral organ in addition to dyspnea.

As the glossopharyngeal nerve and the vagus nerve take the same course within and outside of the brainstem, they are often impaired together. When hoarseness and dyspnea are seen in addition to nasal voice and dysphagia, it suggests an impairment of not only the glossopharyngeal nerve but also the vagus nerve.

B. HYPOGLOSSAL NERVE

All the tongue muscles are innervated by the hypoglossal nerve, which is purely made of motor fibers. The **hypoglossal nucleus** is located in the medial part of the medullary tegmentum just anterior to the fourth ventricle (see Figure 5-3). Fibers emerging from the nucleus pass anteriorly all the way through the medial part of the medulla and exit the medulla just lateral to the pyramid. Then they turn laterally and exit the posterior cranial fossa through the **hypoglossal canal** just lateral to the foramen magnum (see Figure 8-2a).

In a unilateral lesion of the hypoglossal nerve, muscle atrophy is seen in the affected half of the tongue. In its acute lesion like hypoglossal neuritis, however, muscle atrophy may not be recognized until about a week after the clinical onset. Unilateral weakness of the tongue muscle can be detected by asking the patient to push the tongue against the cheek and by palpating its force from the cheek skin, but it can be confirmed more efficiently by demonstrating deviation of the protruded tongue to the affected side. This is due to the fact that the genioglossus muscle acts to protrude the tongue forward and thus the muscle on the intact side overcomes that on the affected side, causing the tongue to deviate to the affected side on protrusion.

WALLENBERG SYNDROME AND RELATED CONDITIONS

This is a good example to demonstrate how many symptoms/signs may be produced even by a small lesion depending on its anatomical compactness.

The symptomatology of the **lateral medullary syndrome** (Wallenberg syndrome) is systematically composed of **bulbar palsy** due to a lesion of the nucleus ambiguus, **crossed analgesia** on the ipsilateral face due to a lesion of the spinal tract and nucleus of the trigeminal nerve and on the contralateral limbs and trunk due to a lesion of the spinothalamic tract, **vertigo and loss of equilibrium** due to a lesion of the vestibular nucleus, **cerebellar ataxia** of the ipsilateral limbs due to a lesion of the cerebellar hemisphere, and ipsilateral **Horner syndrome** due to a lesion of the descending sympathetic tract (Figures 14-1 and 14-2, see Table 8-1). This syndrome is caused by an infarction of the lateral part of the medullary tegmentum due to thrombosis of the posterior inferior cerebellar artery. Regarding the above, if a lesion also involves the trigeminothalamic tract, which crosses from the contralateral spinal nucleus of the trigeminal nerve, the hemianalgesia contralateral to the lesion involves the face as well.

Babinski and Nageotti in 1902 reported a 50-year-old man who suddenly presented with vertigo, ataxic gait, dysphagia, and dysphonia and showed soft palate paralysis and loss of gag reflex, Horner syndrome and cerebellar ataxia on the left, hemiparesis and decreased tactile and pain sense on the right, and sensory loss on bilateral face. At autopsy, four lesions were found in the left medulla oblongata, the largest occupying nearly the whole area of the left rostral medulla (Babinski & Nageotti, 1902). In the same paper, they also reported two other clinical cases in which the crossed sensory disturbance was seen only for pain but sparing touch and proprioception. Thus, Babinski-Nageotti syndrome consists of symptoms/signs seen in Wallenberg syndrome plus hemiplegia (Figure 14-3). A condition similar to Babinski-Nageotti syndrome but without vertigo and cerebellar ataxia is called Cestan-Chenais syndrome (Figure 14-3) (Krasnianski et al, 2006).

If the hypoglossal nerve is affected at the pyramid together with the corticospinal tract, hypoglossal nerve palsy might be associated with contralateral spastic hemiplegia (**hypoglossal crossed hemiplegia**).

C. CORTICAL INNERVATION OF BULBAR MUSCLES

The cortical area related to movements of the pharynx, larynx, and tongue is located in the ventral part of the face

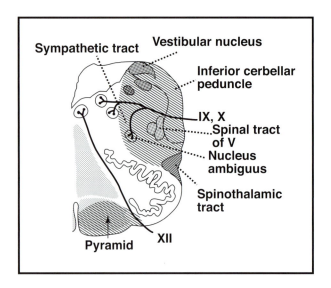

Figure 14-1 Schematic diagram of medulla oblongata indicating a lesion of the lateral medullary syndrome (Wallenberg syndrome). The lesion is indicated by striped lines on the lateral medulla. V: trigeminal nerve, IX: glossopharyngeal nerve, X: vagus nerve, XII: hypoglossal nerve. (Modified from Chusid & McDonald, 1964)

area of the primary motor cortex (see Figure 11-2). The nucleus ambiguus and the hypoglossal nucleus are bilaterally innervated by motor cortices with one exception (Box 22 for the exception). Therefore, only bilateral lesions of the corticobulbar tracts cause functional disturbance

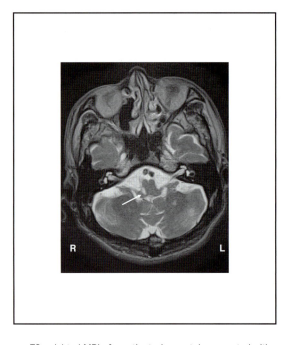

Figure 14-2 T2-weighted MRI of a patient who acutely presented with dysphagia, vertigo, nystagmus, left hemianalgesia including the left face, and Horner syndrome and cerebellar ataxia on the right (Wallenberg syndrome). A localized area of increased signal intensity is seen in the lateral part of the right medullary tegmentum (arrow). (Courtesy of Dr. Masutaro Kanda, Ijinkai Takeda General Hospital, Kyoto)

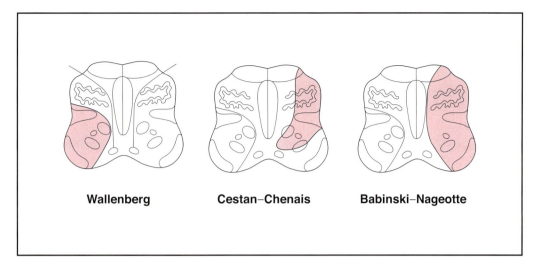

such as dysphagia and dysarthria. This condition is called **pseudobulbar palsy**.

Even in a unilateral vascular lesion of the frontal lobe, mild dysphagia might be occasionally seen. This is explained by the hypothesis that there is some hemispheric dominance in terms of swallowing, although the dominant side seems to differ among subjects. Furthermore, if there was a latent ischemic lesion in one cerebral hemisphere in the past, the new vascular lesion in the other hemisphere might cause pseudobulbar palsy.

BOX 22 WHY THE TONGUE DEVIATES ON PROTRUSION EVEN IN A UNILATERAL HEMISPHERIC LESION

In patients with hemiplegia due to a unilateral vascular lesion of the cerebral hemisphere, the tongue often deviates to the hemiplegic side on protrusion in spite of bilateral cortical innervation of the bulbar muscles. This is due to the fact that, unlike other bulbar muscles, the genioglossus muscle is unilaterally innervated by the contralateral motor cortex. As the genioglossus muscle acts to protrude the tongue forward, a lesion of the left cerebral hemisphere, for example, causes paralysis of the right genioglossus muscle so that the left genioglossus muscle overcomes the right to push the tongue toward the right. Thus, this phenomenon is similar to the peripheral hypoglossal paralysis, but muscle atrophy does not appear in the supranuclear lesion. Moreover, central hypoglossal palsy is commonly associated with central paralysis of the orbicularis oris muscle, because of the anatomical proximity of the central pathways related to the two muscles.

D. INVOLVEMENT OF THE CRANIAL NERVES INNERVATING BULBAR MUSCLES

As the jugular foramen and the hypoglossal canal are closely located at the exit from the posterior cranial fossa, the last four cranial nerves (IX to XII) tend to be affected together, the condition called **Collet-Sicard syndrome** (Table 14-1). Furthermore, the IXth and Xth cranial nerves may be affected together with the XIth cranial nerve (accessory nerve) at the exit from the jugular foramen (**jugular foramen syndrome**, **Vernet syndrome**) (see Chapter 15-1 for the accessory nerve). These syndromes can be caused by a mechanical injury or tumor, but can be also due to inflammation (**multiple cranial neuritis**). Jackson in 1886 reported a patient with syphilis who presented with tongue muscle atrophy and paralysis of the soft palate and vocal cord on the right and a left brachial plexus lesion (Jackson, 1886). Consequently,

TABLE 14-1 SYNDROME DUE TO LESIONS OF MULTIPLE CRANIAL NERVES

Syndrome	Affected Nerves	Sites of Lesion
Gradenigo	V, VI	Tip of petrous pyramid
Vernet	IX, X, XI	Jugular foramen
Collet-Sicard	IX, X, XI, XII	Jugular foramen, hypoglossal canal
Raeder*	V, sympathetic nerve	Semilunar ganglion
Villaret	IX, X, XII, sympathetic trunk	Retroparotid skull basis

(Roman letters indicate the number of cranial nerves.)

* See Box 15.

similar conditions have been reported with various names such as Schmidt syndrome, resulting in some confusion.

Villaret in 1916 reported two cases of trauma in the mastoid process, manifesting ipsilateral tongue atrophy, Horner syndrome, and paralysis of vocal cord and soft palate, and additional facial palsy in one of the cases. Villaret postulated an extracranial involvement of the ninth, tenth, and twelfth cranial nerves and the sympathetic trunk, and named this condition "le syndrome nerveux de l'espace rétro-parotidien postérieur" (Villaret, 1916) (Box 23).

2. SOMATOSENSORY INNERVATION OF PHARYNX AND LARYNX

As described in relation to the trigeminal nerve (Chapter 10-2B), the somatic sense of the oral cavity and tongue is mostly innervated by the trigeminal nerve, but the pharynx, uvula, tonsils, posterior two-thirds of the tongue, eustachian tube, and mucosa of the epiglottis are innervated by the sensory fibers of the glossopharyngeal nerve. Somatosensory impulses arising from the larynx are conveyed through the vagus nerve, and those from the inner aspect of the tympanic membrane and the tympanic cavity are conveyed through the tympanic nerve (Jacobson's nerve), which joins the vagus nerve.

The primary sensory neurons are in the two small ganglia located just outside of the jugular foramen: the superior ganglion and the petrous (petrosal) ganglion (Figure 14-4). Their central axons enter the spinal nucleus and the main sensory nucleus of the trigeminal nerve in the medulla oblongata. Neuralgia of these sensory nerves is called **glossopharyngeal neuralgia**. In an attack of this neuralgia, lightning pain starts from the root of tongue or the lateral wall of the pharynx and radiates toward the inner ear.

This sensory pathway also acts as an afferent arc of the **pharyngeal reflex (gag reflex)** with the reflex center being in the solitary nucleus and with its efferent arc formed by motor fibers of the glossopharyngeal and vagus nerves. A typical example of this reflex is a vomiting reflex elicited when a toothbrush happens to touch the pharynx. The presence or absence of this reflex is also important for testing the integrity of the medullary function in the examination of comatose patients (see Chapter 29-5C).

3. TASTE SENSE

Gustatory impulses from the posterior third of the tongue are conducted through the glossopharyngeal nerve (Figure 14-4), while those from the anterior two-thirds are conveyed through the facial nerve (see Chapter 11-1C). The primary neurons are in the superior or petrous ganglion, and their central axons enter the solitary tract and solitary nucleus in the medulla oblongata along with the gustatory fibers of the facial nerve. The central pathway from the solitary nucleus is the same as that originating from the facial nerve.

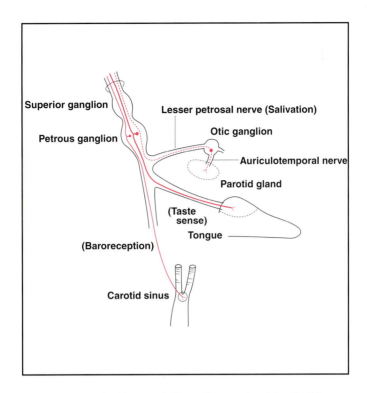

Figure 14-4 Autonomic efferent and afferent fibers, and gustatory (taste) fibers of the glossopharyngeal nerve.

4. SALIVATION

Parasympathetic efferent fibers of the glossopharyngeal nerve act to facilitate salivation of the parotid gland. Its nucleus is the inferior salivatory nucleus located in the medullary tegmentum, and the preganglionic fibers bifurcate from the glossopharyngeal nerve as the lesser petrosal nerve to project to the otic ganglion (Figure 14-4). The postganglionic fibers arising from the otic ganglion pass through the auriculotemporal nerve, which is a branch of the trigeminal nerve, and innervate the parotid gland (Box 24). The synaptic transmitter for the preganglionic fibers is acetylcholine (nicotinic) and that for the postganglionic fibers is acetylcholine (muscarinic).

5. AUTONOMIC INNERVATION OF VISCERAL ORGANS

Parasympathetic efferent fibers of the vagus nerve innervate the visceral organs such as cardiovascular system, bronchus and lung, esophagus, small intestine, large intestine proximal to the middle of the transverse colon, liver, gallbladder, pancreas, and others (Figure 14-5). The preganglionic fibers arise from the **dorsal motor nucleus of the vagus**, which is located in the medullary tegmentum anterior to the fourth ventricle and just lateral to the hypoglossal nucleus

(see Figure 5-3). Recently, this particular nucleus has drawn an increasing attention as one of the earliest nervous systems to be affected by Lewy bodies in Parkinson disease (see Box 26). This autonomic pathway is also called the **visceral efferent** or **visceromotor nerve**. Postganglionic neurons are located in close proximity to their target organs,

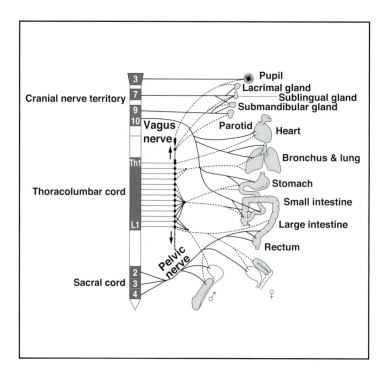

Figure 14-5 Parasympathetic efferent innervation of visceral organs. (Reproduced from Haymaker, 1969, with permission)

and their fibers innervate each target organ by acetylcholine (muscarinic) as the neurotransmitter (see Figure 20-2). Their action for the cardiovascular system is to slow down the pulse rate, to dilate the vessels, and to lower the blood pressure, but for the gastrointestinal system they act to facilitate intestinal peristalsis.

6. AFFERENT PATHWAY FROM THE VISCERAL ORGANS

The glossopharyngeal and vagus nerves play an important role in conveying the afferent input from visceral organs. Visceral afferents from the **baroreceptor of the carotid sinus (carotid body),** which is situated in the wall of the internal carotid artery, pass through the glossopharyngeal nerve and convey impulses to the visceral afferent bipolar neurons in the superior and petrous ganglia (Figures 14-4 and 14-6). The central axons of those neurons enter the solitary nucleus in the medulla oblongata and form a reflex arc with the dorsal motor nucleus of the vagus. On the other hand, the afferents from the **aortic receptors (aortic body)** in the aortic arch pass through the vagus nerve and project to the visceral afferent bipolar neurons in the nodose ganglion, and the central axons also project to the solitary nucleus to form a reflex arc like the baroreceptors from the carotid sinus (Figure 14-6).

The above two pathways play an important role in the regulation of blood pressure. For example, if blood pressure changes rapidly, the baroreceptors sense the change and, via the medullary reflex arc, regulate the blood pressure automatically. If this reflex pathway is impaired, it becomes difficult to control the blood pressure upon sudden arising **(orthostatic hypotension).**

Visceral sensation from the pharynx, larynx, bronchus, esophagus, and abdominal visceral organs is conveyed to the central nervous system through the vagus nerve. Typical examples of visceral sensation are a feeling of satiety and a feeling of hunger. These visceral afferent neurons are also in the nodose ganglion, and the central axons convey impulses to the solitary nucleus. The efferents from the solitary nucleus are conducted to the cerebral cortex via the thalamus on one hand and form a reflex arc with the autonomic efferent pathway in the brainstem on the other hand (see "Autonomic Nervous System," Chapter 20-2). As visceral pain is conveyed through the sympathetic fibers, it is discussed in Chapter 20-2.

7. EXAMINATION OF SWALLOWING, PHONATION, AND ARTICULATION

Swallowing, phonation and articulation can be examined in the following order.

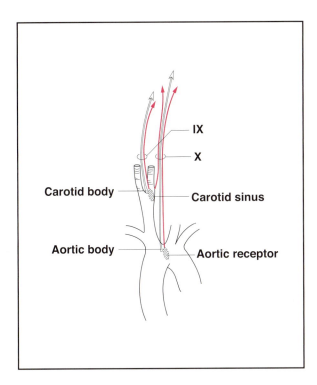

Figure 14-6 Afferent fibers related to baroreception. IX: glossopharyngeal nerve, X: vagus nerve.

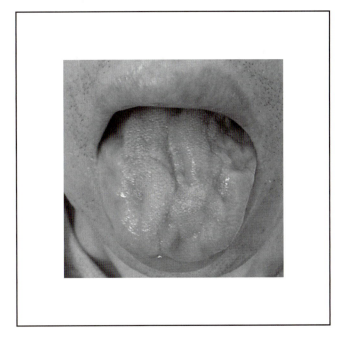

Figure 14-7 Muscle atrophy of the tongue in a patient with bulbospinal muscular atrophy (Kennedy disease). (Courtesy of Dr. Masutaro Kanda, Ijinkai Takeda General Hospital, Kyoto)

A. EXAMINATION OF THE TONGUE

If there is muscle atrophy and/or fasciculation (see Chapter 16-3B for fasciculation) on one side of the tongue, it suggests involvement of either the ipsilateral medulla oblongata or the hypoglossal nerve. As the genioglossus muscle acts to protrude the tongue forward, the tongue will deviate to the affected side upon protrusion. By contrast, bilateral involvement of the tongue with muscle atrophy or fasciculation suggests degenerative diseases of the motor neurons (Figure 14-7). As described in Box 22, among other tongue muscles, only the genioglossus muscle receives unilateral innervation from the contralateral motor cortex. Therefore, even in a unilateral hemispheric lesion, the tongue deviates to the side contralateral to the lesion upon protrusion.

B. EXAMINATION OF THE SOFT PALATE AND SWALLOWING

In a unilateral lesion of the medullary tegmentum or the ninth/tenth cranial nerves, the affected soft palate drops and moves incompletely (**curtain sign**). If the patient is asked to pronounce an "Ah" sound loudly with the mouth kept open, the intact soft palate is seen to rise, whereas the affected side only incompletely, if any. The **gag reflex** elicited by touching the lateral pharyngeal mucosa with

a swab may be lost on the affected side. As the gag reflex causes bilateral contraction of the relevant muscles, loss of gag reflex only on one side suggests impairment of the afferent reflex arc on the affected side. Bilateral loss of gag reflex suggests bilateral impairment of the ninth/tenth cranial nerves, but it should be kept in mind that this reflex may not be clearly observable in normal aged subjects and even in some young subjects.

Spasm of the Deglutition Muscles

Dysphagia in some patients might be due to excessive contraction or spasm of the deglutition muscles instead of their paralysis. This condition is called **spasmodic dysphagia**. In patients with dysphagia, therefore, it is useful to observe how they actually swallow a cup of water during the physical examination, and it is especially so for a possible case of spasmodic dysphagia.

Dysphonia

For testing phonation, it is useful to ask the patient to pronounce the same sound repeatedly including a labial sound (mi-mi-mi), palatal sound (ga-ga-ga), and lingual sound (la-la-la). Paralysis of the soft palate is manifested as **nasal voice (rhinolalia)**, that of the vocal cord as **hoarseness** and, when sound is lost completely, **aphonia**. Although nasal voice and hoarseness are commonly seen in common cold, the distinction is not difficult from the history and other accompanying symptoms. Furthermore, like dysphagia, spasm of the articulatory muscles may cause dysphonia (**spasmodic dysphonia**). Spasmodic dysphonia is most commonly an adult onset focal dystonia, but may be seen as a manifestation of autosomal dominant hereditary dystonia ("whispering dysphonia," DYT4 dystonia) (Lohmann et al, 2013). Spasmodic dysphonia may be due to spasm, not just of the vocal cord but of the respiratory muscles as a whole (**laryngeal dystonia**) (Payne et al, 2014).

Dysarthria

A condition in which a patient cannot speak properly or fluently is called **dysarthria**. Dysarthria characterized by prolonged and irregular intervals and variable loudness among syllables is called **scanning speech** or **slurred speech**. This kind of speech is also characterized by an abrupt increase in loudness (**explosive speech**). Dysarthria with these characteristics is commonly seen in patients with cerebellar ataxia. In disorders of the basal ganglia like Parkinson disease, speech is characterized by low-pitched and monotonous voice, and intervals between syllables become increasingly shorter while speaking. This speech is compared to propulsion or festination seen in parkinsonian gait (see Chapter 21-2), and may be called **oral festination** (Moreau et al, 2007). It is important to know that dysarthria due to pseudobulbar palsy is usually accompanied by severe dysphagia.

C. BULBAR PALSY AND PSEUDOBULBAR PALSY

When muscle atrophy and/or fasciculation are seen in the tongue in patients with dysphagia, dysphonia, and/or dysarthria, it suggests **bulbar palsy**, and if the jaw jerk is clearly enhanced, it suggests **pseudobulbar palsy**. The term "pseudobulbar palsy" comes about because it looks like a lesion of the medulla, but it is not. However, bulbar palsy may not necessarily be accompanied by tongue atrophy, and the jaw jerk may not necessarily be enhanced even in pseudobulbar palsy. If there is a clear asymmetry in paralysis of the soft palate or if there are nasal voice and/or hoarseness of marked degree, then it more likely suggests the presence of bulbar palsy. **Amyotrophic lateral sclerosis** is characterized by a coexistence of bulbar palsy and pseudobulbar palsy. In this condition, therefore, there is muscle atrophy in the tongue and yet the jaw jerk is hyperactive.

Patients with pseudobulbar palsy occasionally tend to cry or laugh for no reasonable cause. These are called **forced crying** and **forced laughing (forced laughter)**, respectively. The pseudobulbar affect is commonly seen in motor neuron diseases (Floeter et al, 2014). In most cases, the facial expressions are not accompanied by emotional changes (mirthless crying, mirthless laughter), and they are considered to be due to paroxysmal involuntary contractions of emotional muscles.

Somatic sense of the soft palate and pharynx can be tested by using swabs only when judged necessary based on the history and other physical signs. The gag reflex can also be tested by the same maneuver. Taste sense of the posterior third of the tongue may also be tested, but this is more difficult to test than the anterior two-thirds of the tongue. As was described in relation to the facial nerve, salivation of the parotid gland is not tested in the ordinary clinical setting (see Chapter 11-2D). Autonomic reflexes of the cardiovascular system will be explained in the chapter on the autonomic nervous system (Chapter 20-3). During the bedside examination, we can test whether the pulse rate changes with deep breathing or not, whether the blood pressure drops by standing up from the supine position, and whether the bowel sounds are hyperactive or hypoactive.

BIBLIOGRAPHY

Babinski J, Nageotte J. Hémiasynergie, latéropulsion et myosis bulbaires avec hémianesthésie et hémiplegie croisées. Rev Neurol (Paris) 10: 358–365, 1902.

Chusid JG, McDonald JJ. Correlative Neuroanatomy and Functional Neurology. 12th ed. Lange, Maruzen Asian Edition, Tokyo, 1964.

de Bree R, van der Waal I, Leemans CR. Management of Frey syndrome. Head Neck 29:773–778, 2007. (review)

Floeter MK, Katipally R, Kim MP, Schanz O, Stephen M, Danielian L, et al. Impaired corticopontocerebellar tracts underlie pseudobulbar affect in motor neuron disorders. Neurology 83:620–627, 2014.

Haymaker W. Bing's Local diagnosis in neurological diseases. 5th ed. Mosby, St Louis, 1969.

Jackson JH. Paralysis of tongue, palate, and vocal cord: treatment of obscure forms of metrorrhagia. Lancet 130:689–690, 1886.

Krasnianski M, Müller T, Stock K, Zierz S. Between Wallenberg syndrome and hemimedullary lesion: Cestan-Chenais and Babinski-Nageotte syndromes in medullary infarctions. J Neurol 253:1442–1446, 2006.

Lohmann K, Wilcox RA, Winkler S, Ramirez A, Rakovic A, Park J-S, et al. Whispering dysphonia (DYT4 dystonia) is caused by a mutation in the TUBB4 gene. Ann Neurol 73:537–545, 2013.

Moreau C, Ozsancak C, Blatt JL, Derambure P, Destee A, Defebvre L. Oral festination in Parkinson's disease: biomechanical analysis and correlation with festination and freezing of gait. Mov Disord 22:1503–1506, 2007.

Payne S, Tisch S, Cole I, Brake H, Rough J, Darveniza P. The clinical spectrum of laryngeal dystonia includes dystonic cough: observations of a large series. Mov Disord 29:729–735, 2014.

Pearce JMS. Vagal-accessory-hypoglossal syndrome: Schmidt's or Jackson's? Eur Neurol 55:118–119, 2006. (review)

Schoenberg BS, Massey EW. Tapia's syndrome: the erratic evolution of an eponym. Arch Neurol 36:257–260, 1979. (review)

Villaret M. Le syndrome nerveux de l'espace rétro-parotidien postérieur. Rev Neurol (Paris) 29:188–190, 1916.

15.

NECK AND TRUNK

1. EXAMINATION OF THE NECK

The following points should be checked during the examination of the neck.

A. POSTURAL ABNORMALITY OF THE NECK

Posture of the neck can be observed in the sitting or standing position. Stooped posture of the neck may be physiologically seen in the aged population. Two abnormal postures of the neck are **flexed posture**, seen in patients with Parkinson disease or parkinsonism, and dropped head syndrome. In Parkinson disease and parkinsonism, not only the neck but also the whole upper trunk is commonly flexed. Moreover, tone of the neck muscle is often increased and there is resistance against passive lateral flexion and rotation. Occasionally, cogwheel rigidity might also be found in the neck muscles (see Chapter 16-2B).

In the **dropped head syndrome**, flexed posture is almost restricted to the neck muscles. Two conditions are conceivable for this syndrome: weakness of the neck extensors and excessive contraction (dystonia) of the neck flexors. In order to distinguish between these two conditions, it is useful to test the strength of the neck extensor muscles by asking the patient to lift up the head in a prone position. Weakness of the neck extensors in this condition is thought to be myogenic rather than neurogenic, and is seen in parkinsonism, especially multiple system atrophy (see Box 69).

Extended posture of the neck (**retrocollis**) is commonly seen in patients with progressive supranuclear palsy. However, absence of retrocollis does not completely exclude a possibility of this disease.

Rotated posture of the neck to either side is called **torticollis**. As this condition is considered to be caused by a mechanism of focal dystonia, it is also called **cervical dystonia**. It is often a partial manifestation of generalized dystonia, and it could be its initial manifestation, although generalized dystonia more commonly begins in the leg. As the postural abnormality of neck may almost disappear in the supine position, it is important to observe the neck in the upright position. In the early stage of torticollis, it may not stay with the rotated posture, but it may present with repetitive rotatory phasic movements of the neck to one side, resembling tremor. In the continuously rotated state of the neck, examination of the neck tone might show increased resistance to passive rotation to the normal position. This is in contrast with the neck tone in generalized dystonia, because muscle tone is not increased in most cases of generalized dystonia. In torticollis of long duration, the sternocleidomastoid muscle contralateral to the side of neck rotation is often hypertrophic. Usually the patient cannot return the neck to the normal position, and even if it is possible to do so to some degree, it tends to return to the rotated posture soon.

Sensory trick is a characteristic sign of focal dystonia, especially torticollis (see Chapter 18-6). Typically, the neck returns to the normal position as soon as the cheek or other part of the head is touched by the patient's own hand or by another person's hand. In standing posture against a wall, the neck may return to the normal position as soon as the posterior head touches the wall, but it rotates back again as soon as the patient steps away from the wall. In this case, the sensory trick seems to occur even before the posterior head is actually touched if the patient could anticipate the touch in advance. A mechanism underlying the sensory trick has not been fully elucidated, but this is an example of sensorimotor integration that serves favorably for the patient.

B. EXAMINATION OF MUSCLES INNERVATED BY THE ACCESSORY NERVE

The muscles innervated by the eleventh cranial nerve (accessory nerve), namely the **sternocleidomastoid** muscle (SCM) and the **trapezius muscle**, can be tested when examining the neck. The SCM acts to rotate the neck to the opposite side. Therefore, when testing the left SCM, for example, that muscle should be observed as well as palpated by asking the patient to turn the neck to the right. The two SCM muscles activate together to flex the neck. The SCM is considered to be innervated by the ipsilateral motor cortex, because, in a focal motor seizure, the neck rotates to the side contralateral to the epileptogenic focus. The trapezius muscle can be observed and palpated while the patient is asked to raise the shoulders. In unilateral trapezius palsy, the shoulder of the affected side is lower compared with the intact side when the patient in a standing position is observed from behind.

C. CERVICAL SPONDYLOSIS

In radiculopathy (disorders of nerve roots) due to cervical spondylosis, radiating pain might be induced in the arm by tilting the neck posteriorly and laterally to the affected side (**Spurling sign**). This maneuver makes the intervertebral foramen even narrower so that the nerve root is compressed to produce "root pain."

Other causes of **neck pain** include whiplash injury, intervertebral disc protrusion, ossification of the posterior longitudinal ligament, atlantoaxial dislocation, and Klippel-Feil syndrome. Severe neck pain of acute onset associated with limited range of motion in aged subjects is seen in the **crowned dens syndrome**. In this case, computed tomography (CT) of the neck shows calcification around the odontoid process (dens), and C-reactive protein (CRP) is elevated in the serum. It is important to consider this condition because it sometimes resembles meningitis and also because it responds well to nonsteroidal anti-inflammatory agents (Taniguchi et al, 2010).

In addition to radiculopathies due to abnormalities of the cervical spine as listed above, it should be kept in mind that systemic diseases such as thyroiditis, lymphadenitis and vascular diseases may also cause neck pain.

Lhermitte Sign

Lhermitte sign is a radiating pain starting from the upper back down to the dorsal aspects of lower limbs upon neck flexion. This phenomenon is commonly encountered in an intramedullary lesion of the cervical cord, especially in multiple sclerosis or neuromyelitis optica. The underlying mechanism is thought to be due to abnormal impulse transmission within the posterior column.

D. MENINGEAL IRRITATION

When the history suggests a possibility of meningitis or subarachnoid hemorrhage with severe headache and nausea, the presence or absence of **nuchal stiffness** is important. This is tested by observing the range of neck flexion by raising the head passively in the supine position. If one of the examiner's hands is placed behind the neck during this maneuver, it may be able to feel a reflex contraction of the nuchal muscle. This reflex spasm is considered to be due to inflammatory involvement of the posterior cervical roots as they pass through the meninges. It is important to keep in mind that, in subarachnoid hemorrhage, nuchal stiffness is not detectable until about 24 hours after the onset.

The **Kernig sign** is also well known as a sign of meningeal irritation. This is tested by passively raising a lower limb with the knee flexed in the supine position and then by extending the knee joint. If the angle of knee extension is limited or if the patient complains of pain on the posterior aspect of the thigh, the Kernig sign is judged positive. Sometimes, this test might be confused with the **Lasègue sign**, seen in patients with lumbar radiculopathy upon the straight leg raising test (see below). Moreover, the Kernig sign may be negative while nuchal stiffness is present, and thus nuchal stiffness is more sensitive to the state of meningeal irritation.

For the **straight leg raising test**, the relaxed and extended lower extremity is slowly lifted passively in a supine position, and the patient is instructed to report whether pain occurs or not. If this maneuver causes radiating pain downward along the back of the leg (Lasègue sign), it suggests the presence of lumbar radiculopathy.

2. EXAMINATION OF THE TRUNK

Observation of posture in the standing position provides important information. Flexed posture of the neck and upper trunk is commonly seen in patients with Parkinson disease or parkinsonism. Marked flexion of the trunk to 45 degrees or even more in the standing position is called **camptocormia (bent spine syndrome)**. This postural abnormality becomes less pronounced in the recumbent position. There are a variety of etiologies, both peripheral and central, for this condition (Srivanitchapoom & Hallett, 2015, for review), but there are two main hypotheses: dystonia or rigidity of the truncal muscles on one hand and myopathy of the paraspinal muscles on the other (von Coelln et al, 2008; Jankovic, 2010, for review). In addition, scoliosis is also common in Parkinson disease.

In patients with Parkinson disease or parkinsonism, movement in general is slower than normal, especially in turning around or sitting up on bed, and standing on the floor (**bradykinesia**).

Muscle tone of the truncal muscles is difficult to test, but tone of the paraspinal muscles can be estimated by the following maneuver. With a patient placed in the supine position with the knees flexed and with the examiner's hands holding the lateral aspect of the knees, the examiner rotates the patient's trunk to each side and feels the resistance. In healthy subjects, there is little, if any, resistance against this maneuver, but in patients with Parkinson disease, resistance can be felt, often with significant asymmetry. In patients with rigidity of limbs more on one side than on the other, the resistance against the trunk rotation away from the more rigid side is greater than that toward the more rigid side. In this case, the trunk often shows scoliosis concave to the more rigid side.

The above postural abnormality of the cervical or thoracic spine is seen in disorders of the spine itself, such as kyphosis, lordosis, and scoliosis of the spine. Usually, differentiation of neurological disorders from these spine disorders is not difficult from the history and other accompanying signs, but it is helpful to compare the postural abnormality during wakefulness and sleep. Abnormalities of the spine are persistent during sleep while abnormality of muscle tone tends to diminish during sleep. Furthermore, abnormality of muscle tone may change depending on posture of the patient.

BIBLIOGRAPHY

Jankovic J. Camptocormia, head drop and other bent spine syndromes: heterogeneous etiology and pathogenesis of parkinsonian deformities. Mov Disord 25:527–528, 2010. (review)

Srivanitchapoom P, Hallett M. Camptocormia in Parkinson's disease: definition, epidemiology, pathogenesis and treatment modalities. J Neurol Neurosurg Psychiatry 87:75–85, 2016. (review)

Taniguchi A, Ogita K, Murata T, Kuzuhara S, Tomimoto H. Painful neck on rotation: diagnostic significance for crowned dens syndrome. J Neurol 257:132–135, 2010.

Von Coelln R, Raible A, Gasser T, Asmus F. Ultrasound-guided injection of the iliopsoas muscle with botulinum toxin in camptocormia. Mov Disord 23:889–892, 2008.

16.

MOTOR FUNCTIONS

1. FINAL COMMON PATHWAY OF THE MOTOR SYSTEM

The final common pathway for movement consists of the central motor pathway, which projects from the motor cortex through the corticobulbar tract to the brainstem motor nuclei or through the corticospinal tract to the anterior horn of the spinal cord and the peripheral motor pathway, which projects from the brainstem motor nuclei or the anterior horn cells by means of the α motor fibers to the skeletal muscles. Neurons of the cerebral cortex forming the corticobulbar and corticospinal tracts are called **upper motor neurons**, and neurons of the brainstem motor nuclei and the spinal anterior horn forming the α motor fibers are called **lower motor neurons**. A representative degenerative disease characterized by systematic involvement of the upper and lower, or either, motor neurons is **motor neuron disease**.

A. MOTOR CORTEX AND CORTICOSPINAL TRACTS

The motor cortex is formed of the **primary motor area (Brodmann area 4; MI)**, **supplementary motor area (SMA)**, **lateral premotor area**, and **cingulate gyrus**. The SMA is further divided into the **SMA proper** and the **pre-SMA** (see Figure 11-3). Electrophysiological and neuroimaging studies of cortical activities in humans suggest that voluntary unilateral simple movement of the hand is preceded by increasing activity first in the pre-SMA and SMA proper bilaterally, then in the lateral premotor area and the MI bilaterally but with contralateral predominance, and finally neurons primarily of the MI are activated so that their impulses descend through the fast-conducting corticospinal tract to activate the corresponding anterior horn cells (Shibasaki, 2012, for review). For the corticospinal tracts, all fibers originating

from the MI and most fibers from the lateral premotor area form the **direct corticospinal tract**, while the fibers originating from the SMA proper and some fibers from the lateral premotor area project to the spinal cord via the MI. In addition, some fibers from the SMA proper and the lateral premotor area descend to the spinal cord indirectly via brainstem nuclei such as the reticular formation and the vestibular nuclei (**indirect corticospinal tract**).

Pyramidal Tract and Upper Motor Neuron

The corticospinal tract in the narrow sense indicates a pathway directly projecting to the spinal cord, but in the wider sense it also includes fibers that do not arise in the cortex. The **pyramidal tract** was originally named to indicate fiber tracts passing through the medullary pyramid, and the term is used to mean the direct corticospinal tract. Fibers of the pyramidal tract originate not only from large neurons in the MI (pyramidal tract cell, Betz cell) but also from a much larger number of other neurons in the MI, neurons in the SMA proper, some neurons in the lateral premotor area, and in the postcentral gyrus. Clinically, signs due to involvement of the pyramidal tract are called **upper motor neuron signs** or **pyramidal tract signs (pyramidal signs)**.

Corticospinal Tract

Impulses conducted through the direct corticospinal tract are transmitted to the anterior horn cells either directly (monosynaptically) or via spinal interneurons. Neurotransmission at the nerve terminal is mostly glutamatergic. Especially, most impulses targeting intrinsic hand muscles are transmitted monosynaptically, which is thought to be effective for quick and precise movement of the fingers. In fact, in a relatively mild or

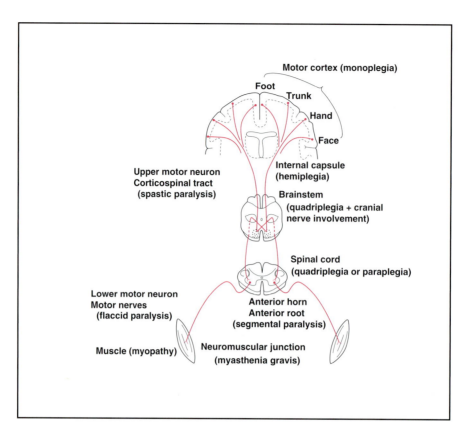

Figure 16-1 Schematic illustration of motor pathways from the motor cortex to the muscles. Distribution of motor paralysis is shown in the parenthesis for each site of lesion.

early lesion of the motor cortex or corticospinal tract, the initial sign is disturbance of fine finger movement rather than weakness.

About 85% of fibers constituting the pyramidal tract cross at the **pyramidal decussation** of the medulla, and descend through the contralateral **lateral corticospinal tract**. The remaining 15% of fibers descend through the ipsilateral **anterior corticospinal tract** (Figures 16-1, 16-2 and 16-3). However, the ratio of the crossing fibers is known to vary considerably among subjects, and it is known that in some exceptional cases all fibers cross. The anterior corticospinal tract terminates at the lower cervical level.

In unilateral infarction of the medulla, ipsilateral hemiplegia may be seen occasionally (Opalski syndrome). This is explained by an involvement of the corticospinal tract after crossing (distal to the pyramidal decussation) in the medulla (Nakamura et al, 2010). Furthermore, in mechanical compression of the craniocervical junction, spastic paralysis of unusual distribution may be seen (Yayama et al, 2006). For example, bilateral weakness of upper limbs is called cruciate paralysis, and a combination of spastic paralysis of the ipsilateral upper limb and

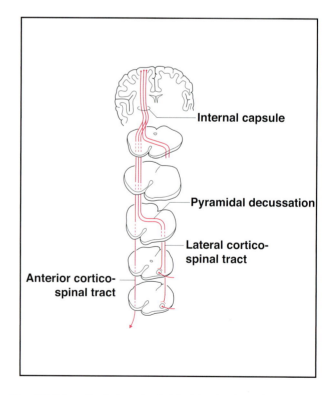

Figure 16-2 Schematic diagram showing the lateral and anterior corticospinal tracts.

THE NEUROLOGIC EXAMINATION

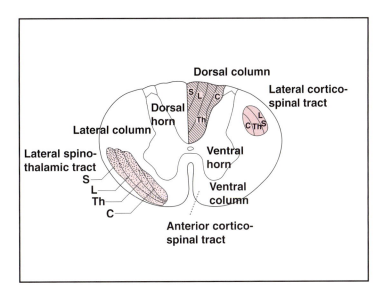

Figure 16-3 Laminar structures of the lateral corticospinal tract and somatosensory pathway in the cervical cord. C (cervical), Th (thoracic), L (lumbar), and S (sacral) in the descending lateral corticospinal tract indicate the target segments and those in the ascending lateral spinothalamic tract and dorsal column indicate the segments of origin. (Modified from Haymaker, 1969, with permission)

pyramidal signs of the contralateral lower limb may be called hemiplegia cruciata. Structural or functional misinnervation of the corticospinal tracts may present itself as mirror movements (Box 25).

Lesion of the Corticospinal Tract and Distribution of Motor Paralysis

As described in Chapter 11 (see Figure 11-2), there is somatotopic organization in MI. Different body parts are quite

---

BOX 25 MIRROR MOVEMENT

In this condition, intended movement of one hand is accompanied by the same movement in the opposite hand. This phenomenon causes significant difficulty in daily life, especially in actions requiring movement of bilateral fingers like piano playing. Mechanisms underlying **congenital mirror movement** seem to differ among patients. In some cases, the uncrossed corticospinal tract is excessively developed, and activation of unilateral motor cortex may cause simultaneous activation of both the crossed and uncrossed corticospinal tracts. In other cases, the motor cortex ipsilateral to the intended movement might be coactivated with the contralateral motor cortex. By using the triple stimulation technique of transcranial magnetic stimulation (TMS) in a case of congenital mirror movement, Ueki et al. (2005) reported evidence for predominant ipsilateral innervation. In a patient with **Kallmann syndrome**, which is an X-linked hereditary disease characterized by anosmia, hypogonadotropic hypogonadism and mirror movement (see Chapter 6-2), the late phase of Bereitschaftspotential was distributed over the motor area not only contralateral but also ipsilateral to the intended unilateral hand movement, suggesting activation of bilateral motor cortices (Shibasaki & Nagae, 1984).

Mirror movement can be also seen in acquired conditions (**acquired mirror movement**). When a patient during the recovery phase from stroke moves the intact hand, similar movement may be seen in the paretic hand (Etoh et al, 2010). Additionally, an attempt to move the paretic hand may be associated with similar movement in the intact hand. The latter phenomenon might be related to the fact that, even in healthy subjects, an attempt to make a complex movement by one hand is associated with bilateral activation of motor cortices (Kitamura et al, 1993b; Shibasaki et al, 1993). Therefore, it is postulated that, in patients with severe motor disability irrespective of its etiology, even a simple movement of one hand might cause bilateral activation of motor cortices, thus resulting in mirror movement.

In relation to the above, when interpreting data of Bereitschaftspotential and neuroimaging studies for investigating a mechanism of motor recovery from stroke, increased activation of the motor cortex ipsilateral to the paretic limb might be due to subjective complexity of the motor task and it may have little to do with compensatory activation of the nonaffected cerebral hemisphere.

separate, but within a body part the muscle representations are intermixed. The corticospinal tract descends medially through the cerebral white matter and converges at the posterior limb of the internal capsule like the pivot of a fan (Figure 16-1). Thus, if the MI is affected focally, or if the corresponding group of the corticospinal fibers is subcortically affected, the resulting paralysis is limited to a part of the contralateral extremity or face innervated by the damaged area (**monoplegia**). For example, if the hand area of the left precentral gyrus is focally affected, motor paralysis or disturbance of fine finger movement may appear only in the right hand.

When the posterior limb of the internal capsule is affected, all fibers of the corticospinal tract are involved, causing weakness of all contralateral skeletal muscles including the lower face (**hemiplegia**). A typical example is lacunar infarction in the internal capsule. In this case, even a small lesion localized to the posterior limb of the internal capsule can cause complete hemiplegia involving the lower face and upper as well as lower extremities. As the somatosensory system is not involved in this case, it causes **pure motor hemiplegia** (see Box 3). Clinically, pure motor hemiplegia most likely suggests the presence of a small lesion in the posterior limb of the internal capsule.

By contrast with the above two examples, if the corticospinal tract is involved between the motor cortex and the internal capsule in the cerebral white matter, the resulting hemiplegia is incomplete in its distribution. Namely, if an infarction occurs in the deep cerebral white matter, weakness is often seen in the contralateral upper and lower limbs, sparing the face. In this case, the somatosensory impairment of various degrees may be also present.

In the brainstem, the corticospinal tract is located most anteriorly from the midbrain to the medulla. In the cerebral peduncle, fibers projecting to the brainstem motor nuclei are located medially, those projecting to the caudal spinal cord laterally, and those projecting to the rostral spinal cord in between. This arrangement is reasonable because the fibers targeting the more rostral motor nuclei can easily cross from the medial part of the tract. Most of the fibers project to the brainstem motor nuclei bilaterally, but those fibers innervating the lower facial muscles and the genioglossus muscle of the tongue project only to the contralateral facial motor nucleus and hypoglossal nucleus, respectively (see Boxes 18 and 22).

B. STRUCTURE AND FUNCTION OF SPINAL CORD

The spinal cord is formed of 30 segments: 8 cervical, 12 thoracic, 5 lumbar, and 5 sacral. There is no structural boundary dividing the segments, which are numbered according to the nerve root emerging from each segment. By contrast, there are 29 vertebrae: 7 cervical, 12 thoracic, 5 lumbar, and 5 sacral. In the cervical cord, therefore, the number of spinal segments is not the same as that of vertebrae. The first cervical nerve exits the spinal canal rostral to the first cervical vertebra, and the eighth cervical nerve exits the canal between the seventh cervical vertebra and the first thoracic vertebra. Thus, the cervical nerves emerge from the spinal canal rostral to each corresponding vertebra with the exception of the eighth cervical nerve. All other spinal nerves from the first thoracic nerve down emerge from the spinal canal caudal to each respective vertebra (Figure 16-4).

The caudal end of the spinal cord (**conus medullaris**) is located between the first and second lumbar vertebrae, and thus the spinal cord is shorter than the spinal canal. The lumbar cord is actually located at the level of the caudal end of the thoracic vertebrae, and the nerve roots originating in the lumbar cord (**cauda equina**) descend through the spinal canal for some distance and then emerge from each respective intervertebral foramen (Figure 16-4).

Laminar Structure of the Lateral Corticospinal Tract

Fibers of the lateral corticospinal tract and those of the anterior corticospinal tract targeting each segment of the spinal cord leave the tracts and turn anteromedially and posteriorly, respectively, so that they project to the anterior horn at each level. As seen in the transverse section of the lateral corticospinal tract (Figure 16-3), fibers projecting to the cervical segments are located medially and those projecting to the sacral segments are located laterally, so that the fibers targeting the more rostral segments can leave the tract easily. For the same anatomical reason, when the cervical cord is compressed from the lateral side, the pyramidal signs first appear in the ipsilateral lower extremity. When the lateral compression is strong, pyramidal signs also appear in the contralateral lower extremity because of a contrecoup effect against the opposite wall of the spinal canal and partly because the spinal cord is fixed to the lateral wall of the spinal canal by the denticulate ligament, which causes mechanical distortion of the cord. For the same reason, if the pyramidal signs are clearly limited to the ipsilateral extremities, it more likely suggests the presence of an intramedullary lesion.

Blood Perfusion of the Spinal Cord

The cervical cord receives blood perfusion mostly from the **anterior spinal artery**, which is formed by branches of

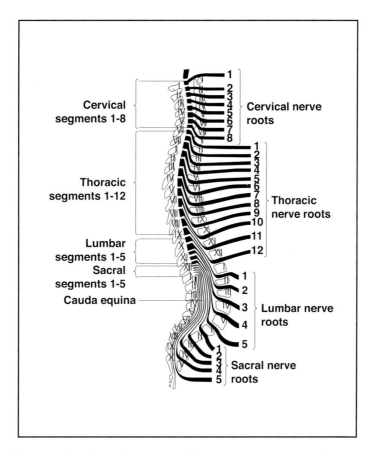

Figure 16-4 Anatomical interrelationship among the spinal cord segments, spinal nerve roots, and vertebrae. (Reproduced from Haymaker, 1969, with permission)

Cervical segments 1-8 — **Cervical nerve roots** (1–8)

Thoracic segments 1-12 — **Thoracic nerve roots** (1–12)

Lumbar segments 1-5
Sacral segments 1-5
Cauda equina — **Lumbar nerve roots** (1–5)

Sacral nerve roots (1–5)

vertebral arteries (see Figure 9-3). The thoracic cord is supplied by **radicular arteries**, which bifurcate from the aorta. Therefore, narrowing of the intervertebral foramen may compress not only the nerve roots but also the radicular arteries, causing ischemic damage to the cord. In relation to this, as surgical treatment of aortic diseases may cause ischemic lesion in the cord, intraoperative electrophysiological monitoring of spinal functions can be applied to detect any functional abnormality that otherwise may not be detected until the effect of anesthesia wears off. Caudal segments of the thoracic cord and the lumbar cord are supplied by the **Adamkiewicz artery**, which bifurcates from the aorta and enters the upper lumbar cord from the left.

The anterior spinal artery descends along the anterior aspect of the spinal cord at the midline, and its branches perfuse the anterior two-thirds of the cord (Figure 16-5). If the anterior spinal artery is occluded, the corticospinal tracts, spinothalamic tracts, and sympathetic nervous pathways are bilaterally affected, causing paralysis and loss of pain/temperature sense below the affected segment and sphincter disturbance, but sparing proprioceptive sensation because of intact posterior columns (see Chapter 19-1).

This condition is called **anterior spinal artery syndrome**. Posterior spinal arteries are located at the lateral posterior aspect of the spinal cord, and send their branches to the posterior column on each side. However, some patients who presented with bilateral impairment of proprioceptive sensation, pyramidal signs, and sphincter disturbance due to unilateral occlusion of the posterior spinal artery have been reported (Moriya et al, 2011).

Veins from the spinal cord exit the spinal canal along with the nerve roots and enter the corresponding venous plexus. Therefore, the radicular veins might be also compressed by the narrowed intervertebral foramen, thus causing a congestive lesion in the corresponding segments of spinal cord.

C. ANTERIOR HORN CELLS AND PERIPHERAL MOTOR NERVES

For voluntary movements of the extremities, the anterior horn cells receive excitatory impulses from the motor cortex through the corticospinal tract, and through their axons (**α motor fibers**) activate their innervated muscles.

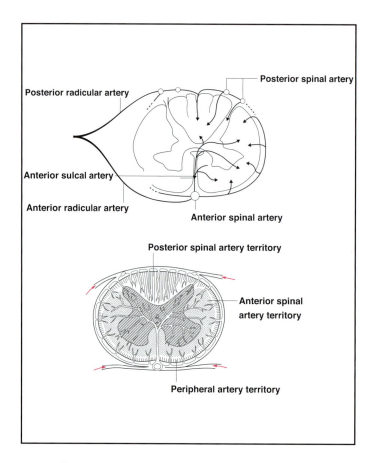

Figure 16-5 Transverse section of spinal cord showing its arterial supply.

α *Motor Fibers*

The intramedullary part of the α motor fibers histologically belongs to the central nervous system because the myelin sheath is derived from the cell membrane of oligodendroglia. The extramedullary axons are covered by myelin sheath that is derived from the cell membrane of Schwann cells, and thus they histologically belong to the peripheral nervous system (Figure 16-6). The α motor fiber is a large myelinated fiber with diameter of 12 ~ 21 μm, and its conduction velocity is about 50 m/s (see Table 19-2). These fibers exit the spinal cord at each segment as the **anterior root**, and along with the posterior root, they exit the spinal canal through the **intervertebral foramen** and innervate the corresponding muscle via the neuromuscular junction. The α motor fibers of cranial nerves exit the cranium through the foramen corresponding to each nerve (see Chapter 5-2).

In the α motor fibers, an electric impulse is conducted in the same direction as the axonal flow. Therefore, if its axon is damaged, the innervated muscle not only becomes paralyzed but also rapidly falls into atrophy due to deprivation of neurotrophic factors. As the α motor fibers innervating the distal extremities are as long as 1 meter, they are vulnerable to axonal damage.

Motor Unit and Reinnervation

The combination of a single anterior horn cell and all the skeletal muscle fibers innervated by that cell is called a **motor unit**, and its size is expressed by the number of muscle fibers innervated by that single anterior horn cell. The size ranges from less than 10 to more than 1,000, with the mean being about 150. Motor units of a muscle engaged in fine finger movement are small. In chronic neurogenic muscle atrophy, when a single anterior horn cell is degenerated and lost, the surviving anterior horn cells reinnervate those muscle fibers deprived of innervation, and this process is repeated so that the motor unit of the reinnervating cell keeps increasing. If this condition is recorded by needle electromyography (EMG), it shows **giant motor unit potentials**.

γ *Motor Fibers*

There is another kind of motor neuron in the anterior horn. That is a small neuron called the γ motor neuron, and its fiber runs along with the α motor fiber. While the α motor fiber innervates the main muscle fibers of a muscle, the extrafusal fibers, the γ motor fiber innervates the intrafusal fibers of the muscle spindle. The γ motor

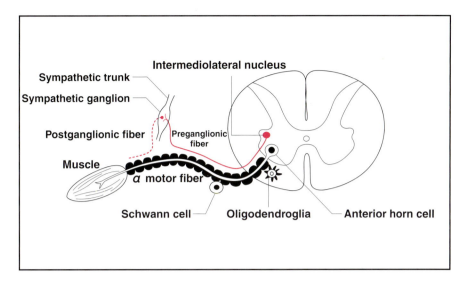

Figure 16-6 Schematic diagram of a transverse section of the thoracic cord to illustrate the anterior horn cell and anterior spinal root. Sympathetic preganglionic fiber (shown in red) exits the cord through the anterior spinal root. The γ motor fiber is not shown in this figure.

system plays an important role in the spinal reflexes (see Chapter 17-1).

D. NEUROMUSCULAR JUNCTION AND MUSCLE

An electric impulse of an α motor fiber is transmitted to a muscle fiber via the neuromuscular junction. Each muscle fiber has a single neuromuscular junction regardless of its length, and the junction is located in the middle of the fiber. Extraocular muscle fibers are an exception in this regard, because each fiber is known to have multiple junctions. The synaptic terminal of the α motor fiber is called the **motor end-plate**, from which synaptic vesicles release acetylcholine into the synaptic cleft. Then acetylcholine activates the acetylcholine receptor located in the junctional fold of the muscle fiber and opens sodium channels. Electrophysiologically, a **miniature end-plate potential** is recorded corresponding to each synaptic vesicle, but such events are generally due to spontaneous release when the nerve is not active. An action potential in the nerve will lead to the simultaneous release of many vesicles and is called the **end-plate potential**. Typically, end-plate potentials are large enough to trigger an action potential in the muscle cell membrane, which causes contraction of the muscle fiber (**excitation-contraction coupling**; **EC coupling**).

2. CENTRAL CONTROL OF VOLUNTARY MOVEMENT

The final common pathway for voluntary movement of extremities is formed of the motor cortices, corticospinal tract, anterior horn cells, α motor fibers, and muscles.

However, simple excitation of the upper motor neuron in the MI will produce just a simple twitch of the corresponding muscles, but no purposeful movement. In order to produce purposeful movement, the secondary motor cortices such as the SMA and lateral premotor area, the basal ganglia, and the cerebellum participate in controlling the excitability of the motor cortex neurons (Figure 16-7), and these structures are known to start functioning before the beginning of the movement and keep working throughout the motor execution. Control of the motor cortex neurons in advance of the actual movement is known as **feedforward control** as opposed to feedback control.

A. HIGHER FUNCTIONS OF MOTOR CORTICES

Voluntary unilateral simple movement of the hand is preceded by increasing activities first in the pre-SMA and the SMA proper bilaterally, then in the lateral premotor area and the MI bilaterally but with contralateral predominance, and finally in the contralateral MI (Shibasaki, 2012, for review). There is somatotopic organization in the SMA proper to some extent and in the lateral premotor area and the MI more precisely. In unilateral complex movement of the hand, the SMA is more activated than in simple movement, and the MI tends to be activated bilaterally just before movement onset (Kitamura et al, 1993b; Shibasaki et al, 1993). The SMA is also known to be activated when the subject just imagines movement without actual motor execution. Furthermore, an isolated discrete finger movement is preceded by larger activity of the contralateral MI compared with the simultaneous movement of more than one fingers (Kitamura et al, 1993a). This is in conformity

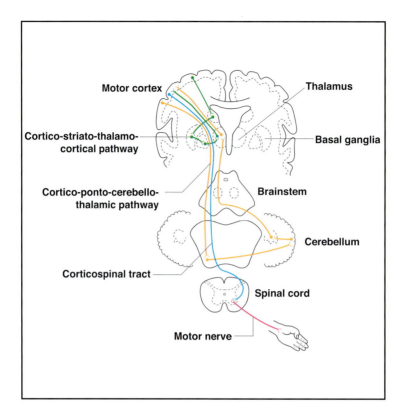

Figure 16-7 Schematic illustration of neural circuits involved in the central control of voluntary movement. The circuits involving the basal ganglia and cerebellum are shown in green and orange, respectively, and the corticospinal tract is shown in light blue.

with the clinical notion that the essential motor deficit of the MI lesion is a disturbance of fine finger movement.

In those movements employed for daily activities such as tool use and gesture, the parietal cortex of the dominant hemisphere is activated first, and then the frontal motor cortices are activated (Wheaton et al, 2005). In this case, the functional connectivity from the left inferior parietal cortex to the left premotor area plays an important role (Hattori et al, 2009). This is related to the clinical concept of ideational and ideomotor apraxia (see Chapter 23-1B).

B. BASAL GANGLIA

Basal ganglia are situated in the deep cerebral hemisphere and are formed of multiple nuclei (Figure 16-8). The main input from the cerebral cortex to the basal ganglia enters the **putamen** and **caudate nucleus**, and its synaptic transmitter is glutamate. The putamen and caudate nucleus together are called **corpus striatum** or **striatum**.

Cytoarchitecture of Striatum and Neural Circuits of Basal Ganglia

In the striatum, more than 90% of neurons are **medium spiny neurons** whose neurotransmitter is gamma-aminobutyric

acid (GABA). There are two classes of medium spiny neurons with two output; the **direct pathway** with GABA and substance P (SP) as the transmitter and the **indirect pathway** with GABA and enkephalin as the transmitter (Figures 16-9 and 16-10). The direct pathway projects directly to the internal segment of the globus pallidus (GPi), while the indirect pathway first projects to the external segment of the globus pallidus (GPe) and from there sends GABAergic fibers to the **subthalamic nucleus** (STN, also called the Luys body). The STN sends its glutamatergic output to the GPi. In effect, the direct pathway inhibits the GPi while the indirect pathway excites the GPi so that they maintain balance. This concept is known as the parallel pathway hypothesis. In fact, however, this neural circuit does not seem that straightforward. There are multiple other connections and pathways. One critical additional pathway is the excitatory hyperdirect pathway from the cortex to the STN; its action supplements that of the indirect pathway. It is noteworthy that GABA is produced from glutamate by glutamic acid decarboxylase (GAD), but the action of the glutamate pathway is excitatory whereas that of GABA is inhibitory to the target receptors.

Cholinergic interneurons represent a small percentage of all striatal neurons, but acetylcholine is believed to

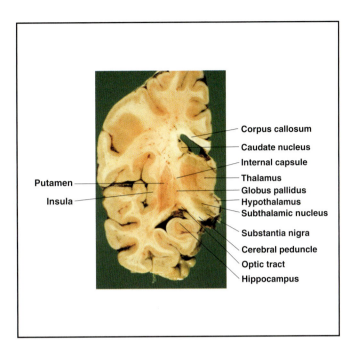

Putamen
Insula

Corpus callosum
Caudate nucleus
Internal capsule
Thalamus
Globus pallidus
Hypothalamus
Subthalamic nucleus
Substantia nigra
Cerebral peduncle
Optic tract
Hippocampus

Figure 16-8 Frontal section of the right cerebral hemisphere showing deep structures. (Courtesy of Dr. Jun Tateishi, Emeritus Professor of Kyushu University)

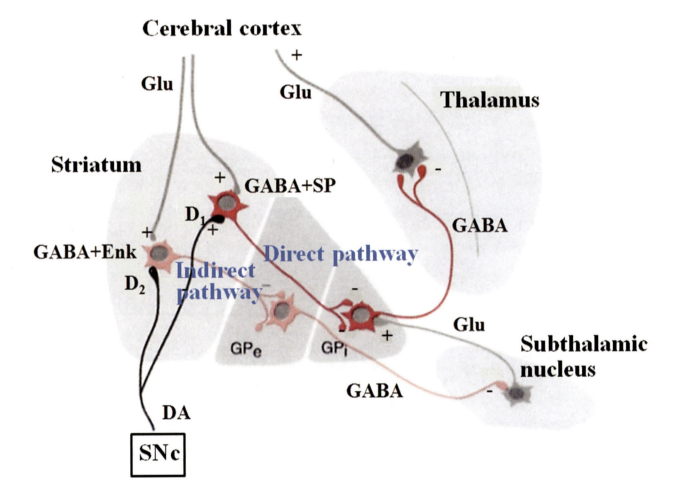

Figure 16-9 Cytoarchitecture of the striatum and neural circuits of basal ganglia with neurotransmitters. D1: D1 receptor, D2: D2 receptor, DA: dopamine, Enk: enkephalin, GABA: gamma-aminobutyric acid, Glu: glutamate, GPe: external segment of globus pallidus, GPi: internal segment of globus pallidus, SNc: substantia nigra pars compacta, SP: substance P. (Modified from Brodal, 2004, with permission)

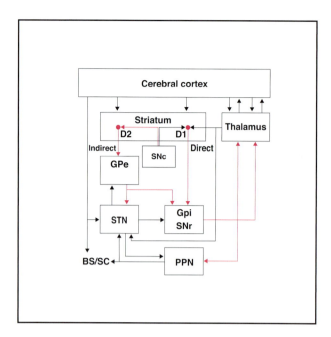

Figure 16-10 Neural circuit of basal ganglia and cerebral cortex. Excitatory pathways are shown in black arrows and inhibitory pathways are shown in red arrows. BS: brainstem, PPN: pedunculopontine nucleus, SC: spinal cord, SNc: substantia nigra pars compacta, SNr: substantia nigra pars reticulata, STN: subthalamic nucleus. Otherwise the same abbreviations as in Figure 16-9.

regulate the function of the striatal microcircuit and striatal output (Girasole and Nelson, 2015, for review).

Output from the basal ganglia is mostly through the GPi and projects the GABAergic pathway mainly to the **ventral anterior nucleus (VA)** and **ventral lateral nucleus (ventrolateral nucleus, VL)** of thalamus (see Figure 27-1). The receiving areas of the VL are considered to correspond to the **anterior oral ventral nucleus (Voa)** and **posterior oral ventral nucleus (Vop)** by Hassler's terminology (Krack et al, 2002, for review; Molnar et al, 2005).

In Figure 16-11 is introduced the center surround hypothesis, which takes into account the striatal function of motor selection (Mink, 2007, for review). According to this theory, there is some somatotopic organization in the striatum and GPi, and the GABAergic fibers from the striatum give rise to focal inhibition of the GPi. As a result, the GABAergic output from the GPi to the thalamic relay nuclei is focally disinhibited, and consequently the glutamatergic pathway from the thalamus to the cortex is focally facilitated. By contrast, as the glutamatergic excitatory projection from the STN to the GPi has no somatotopic organization, it excites the GPi rather diffusely. As a result, the thalamic relay nuclei are diffusely inhibited and serve to suppress unintended movement. The balance between these two systems is postulated to play a role in selecting the intended movement and suppressing other movements (**motor selection**). In this hypothesis, the direct glutamatergic projection from the frontal cortex to STN (**hyperdirect pathway**) also plays a significant role (Mink, 2007, for review).

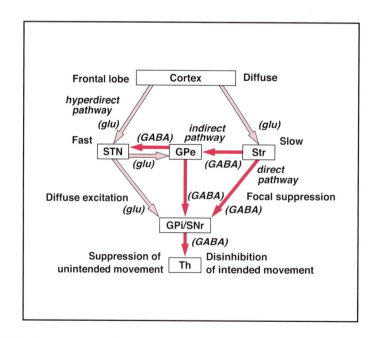

Figure 16-11 Schematic diagram to show the center surround hypothesis of basal ganglia. Excitatory pathways are shown in pink arrows, and inhibitory pathways are shown in red arrows. Str: striatum, SNr: substantia nigra pars reticulata, Th: Thalamus. Otherwise the same abbreviations as in Figure 16-9 and Figure 16-10. (Reproduced from Mink, 2007, with permission)

Nigrostriatal System

The dopaminergic pathway from the substantia nigra pars compacta (SNc) to the striatum is crucial in modulating the basal ganglia. Its degeneration is clinically important in Parkinson disease. Metabolism of dopamine is shown in Figure 16-12a. It excites the D1 receptors of the GABA/SPergic neurons in the striatum (direct pathway) and inhibits the D2 receptors of the GABA/enkephalinergic neurons (indirect pathway) (Figures 16-9 and 16-10). However, the distribution of these two receptors is not completely distinct, and many striatal neurons may have both types of receptors though with predominance of one of them.

In Parkinson disease, the dopaminergic neurons in SNc selectively degenerate resulting in dopaminergic deficiency (Figures 16-13, 16-14 and 16-15). The GABA/enkephalinergic medium spiny neurons are disinhibited, and through the indirect pathway they increase activities of the STN and GPi, which then inhibits activities of the thalamic relay nuclei. This results in a decrease in the glutamatergic thalamocortical projection, thus lowering the excitability of motor cortices (Figures 16-9 and 16-10). The direct pathway neurons are disfacilitated also leading to increased activity of the GPi. In confirmation, if electrical activities are recorded at the time of deep brain stimulation (DBS) in patients with Parkinson disease, neuronal discharge is abnormally increased in the STN and GPi. The projection from the basal ganglia to the motor cortex via the thalamus is believed to affect primarily the SMA.

Deep Brain Stimulation in Parkinson Disease

Recently DBS is commonly used for the symptomatic treatment of Parkinson disease (Katz et al, 2015). For DBS, microelectrodes are placed in the GPi or STN and are continuously stimulated at a frequency of about 130 Hz. In view of the fact that the neuronal discharge is increased in the two nuclei, it used to be believed that DBS has favorable effect by inhibiting the discharges, but its physiological mechanism has not been clearly elucidated. In a PET study using glucose metabolism, it has been reported that the metabolism is even increased in the STN and GPi by the stimulation of the STN (Hilker et al, 2008). In fact, it has been shown that the neural network in the basal ganglia is not a simple circuit of excitatory and inhibitory pathways, either in series or in parallel (Figure 16-10). Moreover, flow of impulses among different nuclei of basal ganglia is mostly bidirectional. Therefore, it may not be reasonable to ascribe the effect of DBS simply to excitation or inhibition.

Recently Brown and his colleagues, based on field potential recordings from deep structures in patients with Parkinson disease, have reported that oscillation in the β band at around 20 Hz shows high correlation among different basal ganglia nuclei as well as between the basal ganglia and the motor cortex. Clinically, it has been reported that the higher the interregional correlation, the more severe the bradykinesia, and that the correlation is suppressed when the patient improves by L-dopa medication or DBS (Hammond et al, 2007, for review). This theory that attaches importance to **synchronization** or **resonance** among neuronal activities is called the **temporal information processing hypothesis**. For this functional interrelationship between the basal ganglia and the motor cortex, the direct pathway from the frontal cortex to the STN (hyperdirect pathway) seems to play an important role in addition to the corticostriatal input and the striato-thalamo-cortical output (Figure 16-11).

Significance of Raphe Nucleus and Locus Coeruleus

The serotonergic raphe nucleus and the noradrenergic locus coeruleus are known to project to the SNc and striatum, and Lewy bodies have been shown to appear in both nuclei at an early stage of Parkinson disease (Box 26). Impairment of the raphe nucleus might be related to non-REM sleep disorder and depression, which are commonly encountered in patients with Parkinson disease, and that of the locus coeruleus might be related to sleepiness, REM sleep behavior disorder, and dysfunction of the autonomic nervous system, which are also common in this disease.

Parkinsonism

Clinical manifestations of basal ganglia disorders are diverse, but they can be largely divided into two groups. One group is characterized by an increase in muscle tone and a decrease in speed, size, and frequency of movement, and the other group is characterized by a decrease in muscle tone and frequent involuntary movements. A typical example of the former group is Parkinson disease or parkinsonism, in which movements are generally slow, small, and scanty. In particular, it takes time to initiate the intended movement, and the movement is slow throughout its execution (**bradykinesia**). In movements requiring repetition, like walking and speaking, each movement becomes increasingly small (sequence effect) and the repetition rate increases until it finally stops. This phenomenon is called **festination**; **festinating gait** for small and quick steps and **oral festination** for quick speech

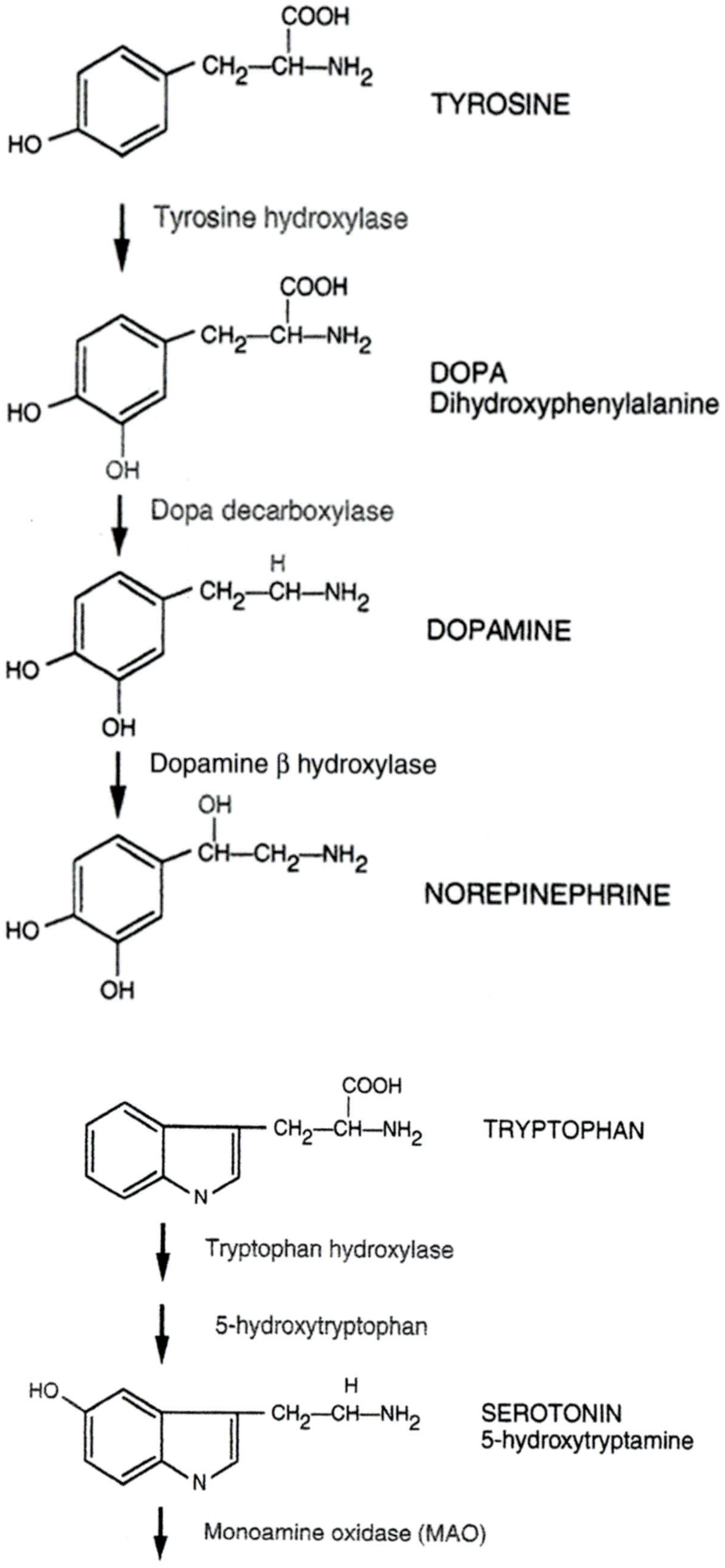

Figure 16-12 Synthesis of dopamine (top) and serotonin (bottom). (Reproduced from Brodal, 2010, with permission)

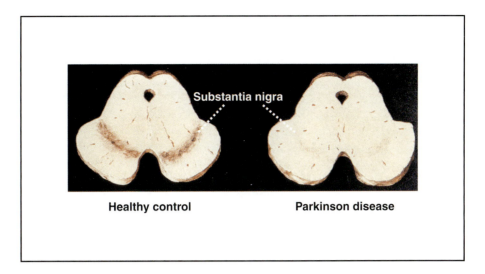

Substantia nigra

Healthy control   Parkinson disease

Figure 16-13 Transverse sections of midbrain from a patient with Parkinson disease and a healthy control. In Parkinson disease, melanin pigment is lost in the substantia nigra pars compacta. (Courtesy of Dr. Jun Tateishi, Emeritus Professor of Kyushu University)

resembling stuttering (Moreau et al, 2007). Once the patient stops walking, it is extremely difficult to start walking again (**freezing phenomenon, freezing of gait, start hesitation**). Likewise, hand-written letters become smaller toward the end of line (**micrographia**) (Figure 16-16), and the voice becomes softer while speaking (**hypophonia**).

Muscle tone is increased in Parkinson disease and parkinsonism. When a skeletal muscle is passively stretched by the examiner in a relaxed condition, resistance of various degrees is felt by the examiner's hand regardless of the speed of stretch (**rigidity**). Typically,

this resistance is felt as trembling and is called the **cog-wheel phenomenon**.

Considering the above symptomatology, it is postulated that the basal ganglia keep controlling the state of muscles so that a voluntary movement can be executed smoothly and quickly. As the basal ganglia are closely connected to the ipsilateral motor cortices, the clinical manifestations due to a basal ganglia lesion appear in the contralateral extremities (Figure 16-7). Furthermore, as the basal ganglia send their descending projections to the brainstem and spinal cord through the **pedunculopontine**

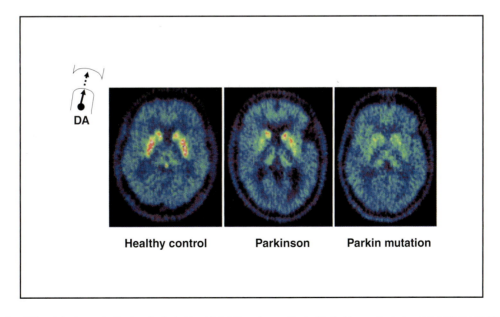

DA

Healthy control   Parkinson   Parkin mutation

Figure 16-14 Dopamine (DA) uptake image in the terminal of nigrostriatal fibers in a patient with Parkinson disease and a patient with Parkin gene mutation in comparison with a healthy control. Positron emission tomographic (PET) study with 18F-labeled DOPA. DA uptake is decreased in Parkinson disease and Parkin gene mutation. (Courtesy of Dr. David Brooks of Hammersmith Hospital, London, UK)

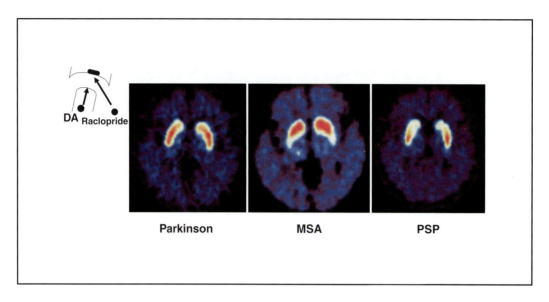

Figure 16-15 PET image of receptor binding with D2-selective ligand raclopride in a patient each with Parkinson disease, multiple system atrophy (MSA), and progressive supranuclear palsy (PSP). Binding of raclopride is partially decreased in the putamen of MSA and in the caudate of PSP, but preserved in the striatum of Parkinson disease. (Courtesy of Dr. Hidenao Fukuyama of Kyoto University)

nucleus (**PPN**) (Figure 16-17), a unilateral lesion of the basal ganglia is expected to cause motor disturbances bilaterally as seen in postural abnormality and gait disturbance (Box 27).

Causes of Parkinsonism

Parkinsonism is characterized by bradykinesia, rigidity, resting tremor, and disturbance of postural control. The most common cause of parkinsonism is idiopathic **Parkinson disease**, but many of these cases are now recognized to be caused by genetic mutations even without an obvious family history. A number of important dominant and recessive mutations have been identified. Parkinsonism can also be caused by a variety of conditions including vascular disease, side effects of drugs such as phenothiazine and sulpiride, intoxication with manganese and carbon monoxide, and sequel of acute encephalitis. Parkinsonism due to ischemic vascular disease (**vascular parkinsonism**) is commonly encountered, but its diagnostic criteria have not been fully established. By contrast with Parkinson disease, vascular parkinsonism commonly shows stepwise exacerbation of symptoms and poorly responds to L-dopa treatment. In addition, the presence of cognitive disorders, pyramidal signs, falls, pseudobulbar palsy, or urinary incontinence may also support its diagnosis (Kalra et al, 2010, for review).

There are a variety of neurodegenerative disorders that can cause parkinsonism, and a group of hereditary

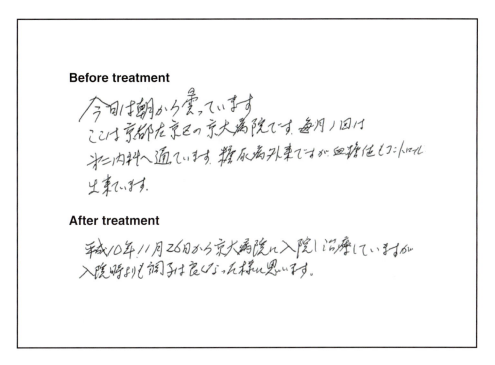

Figure 16-16 Micrographia seen in a Japanese patient with Parkinson disease. Before treatment, the hand-written letters become smaller toward the end of each line, which has improved after treatment.

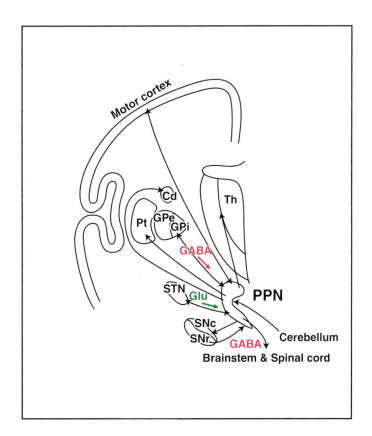

Figure 16-17 Schematic diagram showing the input and output of the pedunculopontine nucleus (PPN) in human. Cd: caudate nucleus, Pt: putamen. Otherwise the same abbreviations as in the Figures 16-9, 16-10 and 16-11. (Modified from Jenkinson et al, 2009, with permission)

diseases manifesting parkinsonism has drawn increas-ing attention (Table 16-1). In addition to the diseases listed in Table 16-1, some cases of **Gaucher disease** have been shown to develop parkinsonism and Lewy body dementia (see Chapter 22-2A) (Kraoua et al, 2009). In particular, those patients with heterozygous mutation of glucocerebrosidase gene develop parkinsonism at a younger age and commonly have nonmotor symptoms such as cognitive disorders and autonomic nervous dis-turbance (Brockmann et al, 2011; Seto-Salvia et al, 2012; Siebert et al, 2014, for review).

A syndrome characterized by parkinsonism of young onset and hypoventilation is known as **Perry syndrome**. In this condition, other various symptoms such as depression, behavioral abnormality, body weight loss, and vertical gaze palsy may be also seen. This is a rare autosomal dominant disease due to mutation of DCTN1 gene, and it responds to L-dopa (Newsway et al, 2010). Recently several condi-tions characterized by parkinsonism and brain iron accu-mulation have drawn increasing attention (Figure 16-18, Box 28).

L-3,4 dihydroxyphenylalanine (L-dopa) is known to be effective almost specifically for Parkinson disease, but L-dopa may improve the parkinsonian symptoms in other conditions as well, at least at a certain stage of the clinical course (Box 29).

Disability Rating Score of Parkinson Disease

On neurologic examination, it is quite important to rate the disability state objectively, which will serve as the basis for evaluating the effect of treatment. A commonly used disability scale for Parkinson disease is that of Hoehn and Yahr (Table 16-2). As the symptoms and signs of parkin-sonism tend to fluctuate especially over a course of L-dopa treatment (Box 41), the disability also varies according to the time when it is evaluated. For reporting the results of research or treatment of Parkinson disease internationally, the Unified Parkinson's Disease Rating Scale (UPDRS) is commonly used. The revised version of this scale (MDS-UPDRS) is made up of evaluation of mentation; beha-vior and mood; self-evaluation of the activities of daily life (ADLs) including speech, swallowing, handwriting, dress-ing, hygiene, falling, salivating, turning in bed, walking, and cutting food; clinician-scored monitored motor evalu-ation; Hoehn and Yahr staging of severity of Parkinson dis-ease; Schwab and England ADL scale; and complications of treatment (Goetz et al, 2008). The UPDRS has been recently revised.

TABLE 16-1 NEURODEGENERATIVE DISEASES PRESENTING WITH PARKINSONISM

Classical parkinsonism
Sporadic: idiopathic Parkinson disease
Hereditary: mutation of LRRK2, SNCA, Parkin, PINK1 and DJ-1 gene, and SCA2, etc.
Atypical parkinsonism
Sporadic: Lewy body disease, multiple system atrophy, progressive supranuclear palsy, corticobasal degeneration, etc.
Hereditary: mutation of FTDP-17 and SNCA, etc.
(from Galpern & Lang, 2006)

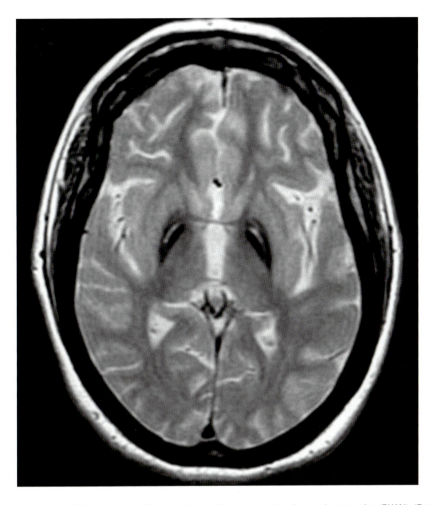

Figure 16-18 "The eye-of-the-tiger sign" on MRI in a patient with pantothenate kinase-associated neurodegeneration (PKAN). (Reproduced from Valentino et al, 2006, with permission)

C. CEREBELLUM

The cerebellum is a relatively large symmetric structure located in the posterior cranial fossa, and plays an important role in regulating the activity of motor cortices through the circuit with the cerebral cortex (Figure 16-7).

Cytoarchitecture of Cerebellum

The cerebellum receives cerebral input mainly from the frontal cortex through the **corticopontine tract**, which descends through the medial and lateral borders of the cerebral peduncle to project to the ipsilateral **pontine nucleus** (see Figure 5-2). The output projection from the pontine nucleus crosses at that level and reaches the contralateral cerebellar cortex through the **middle cerebellar peduncle** (brachium conjuntivum) (Figure 16-19).

In the cerebellar cortex, the middle cerebellar peduncle projects to the **granule cells** of the **granular layer** as **mossy fibers**, and axons of the granule cells project to the **molecular layer**, where they form the **parallel fibers**. Cerebellar granule cells are the most numerous cells in the brain. The parallel fibers make synaptic contact with the dendrites of **Purkinje cells** (Figure 16-20). Axons of Purkinje cells project to the deep cerebellar (intracerebellar) nuclei. The main output from the cerebellum to the cerebral cortex originates in the dentate nucleus and ascends as the **dentatothalamic tract (superior cerebellar peduncle)**, which crosses at the lower midbrain to pass through the red nucleus and projects to the **ventral lateral nucleus (VL)** of the contralateral thalamus (Figures 16-7 and 16-19). This area of the thalamus corresponds to the **ventral intermediate nucleus (Vim)** of Hassler's nomenclature (Krack et al, 2002, for review; Molnar et al, 2005). The dentato-thalamo-cortical pathway projects primarily to the lateral premotor area and the MI.

Cerebellar Circuit and Clinical Symptomatology

As the input from the cerebral cortex to the cerebellum
crosses at the pons as the middle cerebellar peduncle, and as
the output from the cerebellum to the motor cortex crosses
at the midbrain as the superior cerebellar peduncle, the cerebellar hemisphere is functionally connected to the contralateral cerebral hemisphere (Figure 16-7). Therefore, if
a cerebellar hemisphere is unilaterally involved by a lesion,
the motor disturbance is expected to occur in the ipsilateral extremities. This circuit is considered to regulate the
motor cortex so that the limb movement can be executed
skillfully, and its impairment will result in clumsy execution of voluntary movement (**ataxia**). Namely, all voluntary movements including eye movements, speaking, and
limb movements are executed with large variability in size
and time interval and with unstable rhythm. For speech,
the sounds become suddenly loud (**explosive speech**), and
the intervals among syllables become slurred and variable
(**scanning speech**, **slurred speech**). Limb movements
become clumsy because the related muscles cannot contract appropriately (**incoordination**, decomposition of
movement), and they often overshoot the target (**dysmetria**, **hypermetria**). Furthermore, repetitive alternating
movements (diadochokinesis) such as pronation and supi-
nation of hands are poorly executed (**adiadochokinesis**,
dysdiadochokinesis).

For cerebellar control of limb movement, the neocer-
ebellum (embryologically new cerebellum) which corresponds to the cerebellar hemispheres plays an important
role (Figure 16-21). In the cerebellar cortex, there is some
somatotopic organization.

TABLE 16-2 THE HOEHN AND YAHR SCALE FOR THE LEVEL OF DISABILITY IN PARKINSON DISEASE

Stage 0—no signs of disease
Stage 1—symptoms on one side only (unilateral)
Stage 1.5—symptoms unilateral and also involving the neck and spine
Stage 2—symptoms on both sides (bilateral) but no impairment of balance
Stage 2.5—mild bilateral symptoms with recovery when the "pull" test is given (the doctor stands behind the person and asks them to maintain their balance when pulled backward)
Stage 3—balance impairment. Mild to moderate disease. Physically independent
Stage 4—severe disability, but still able to walk or stand unassisted
Stage 5—needing a wheelchair or bedridden unless assisted

The outputs from the vestibular nerve and the medial and inferior vestibular nuclei are projected through the inferior cerebellar peduncle to the vermis, flocculus, and nodulus of the cerebellum, which corresponds to the archicerebellum (Figure 16-21). If this region is involved by a lesion, equilibrium of trunk is impaired (**truncal ataxia**). As was described in Chapter 13-1, a localized lesion in the cerebellum could cause vertigo in relation to this connection.

A large part of the cerebellar vermis and the medial part of the cerebellar hemisphere belong to the paleocerebellum (Figure 16-21). The anterior lobe of the cerebellum receives projection from the proprioceptive receptors of muscles through the spinocerebellar tracts (Figure 16-19). The spinocerebellar tracts ascend through the most lateral part of the spinal cord as the dorsal and ventral spinocerebellar tracts. The **dorsal spinocerebellar tract**

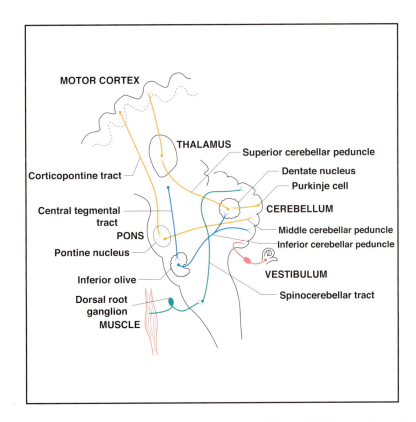

Figure 16-19 Input and output circuits of cerebellum. In this figure, the input from the vestibular nuclei of brainstem is not shown, and only the direct input from vestibulum is shown (see Chapter 13-1).

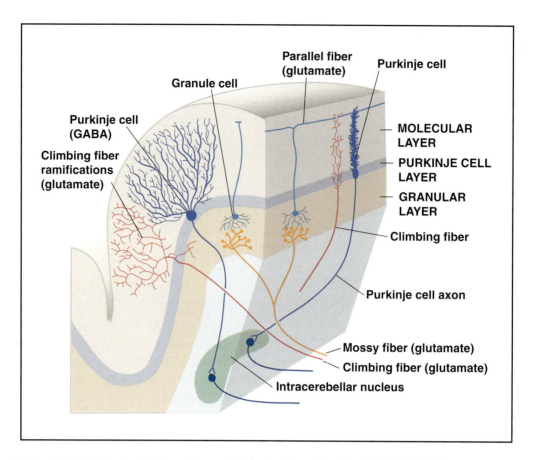

Figure 16-20 Schematic diagram showing cytoarchitecture of the cerebellar cortex. (Reproduced from Brodal, 2010, with permission)

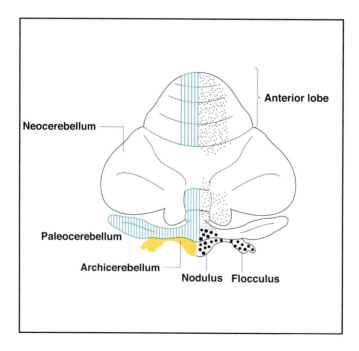

Figure 16-21 Embryological division of cerebellum.

originates in the column of Clarke in the posterior horn and ascends through the dorsal lateral cord to project to the ipsilateral cerebellum. The **ventral spinocerebellar tract** originates in the interneurons of layer 7 in the posterior horn caudal to the midthoracic level, and crosses and ascends through the contralateral lateral column to project to the cerebellum through the superior cerebellar peduncle, and most fibers cross again in the cerebellum. The function of the spinocerebellar tracts has not been fully elucidated, but it is believed that the dorsal tract sends information about complex joint movements to the cerebellum while the ventral tract sends information about the activity of inhibitory interneurons (Brodal, 2010, for review). Clinically, it is also believed to control muscle tone. In an acute cerebellar lesion, muscle tone is said to be decreased, but this is not always the case, and its underlying mechanism has not been fully clarified. It is known that section of the spinocerebellar tract at the time of spinal surgery does not cause any ataxia.

Another input to the cerebellum comes from the inferior olive (Figure 16-19). The inferior olive receives input from the ipsilateral red nucleus and probably also from the hypothalamus through the central tegmental tract. There may be also a direct pathway from the dentate nucleus of the contralateral cerebellum through the superior cerebellar peduncle and the central tegmental tract, forming the Guillain-Mollaret triangle (see Box 60). Fibers from the inferior olive cross at that level and project through the inferior cerebellar peduncle directly to the contralateral deep cerebellar nuclei as the climbing fibers. The function of this circuit has not been clearly elucidated, but the inferior olive may be related to adaptation learning that is an important function of cerebellum.

Spinocerebellar Degeneration

A number of neurodegenerative disorders primarily involving the cerebellum are known, and recently genetic abnormalities have been identified in many of them. Among those disorders, a group of diseases of autosomal dominant inheritance is categorized into **spinocerebellar ataxia (SCA)**, and now more than 35 diseases have been reported in the category (Durr, 2010, for review; Ikeda et al, 2012; Sugihara et al, 2012; Guo et al, 2014; Smets et al, 2014). Genetically SCA is classified into three groups. The first group is characterized by polyglutamine deposit in neurons due to CAG repeat expansion (**triplet repeat disease**) and is known as **polyglutamine disease**. To this group belong **SCA1, SCA2, SCA3, SCA6, SCA7, SCA17** and

dentato-rubro-pallido-luysian atrophy (DRPLA). Besides SCA, Huntington disease (see Box 51) and bulbospinal muscular atrophy (Box 33) also belong to the triplet repeat disease.

The second group of SCA also belongs to the triplet repeat disease, but in this group the repeat is in the intron rather than the exon. The mechanism of damage of such mutations is not clear, but is believed by some to be mediated by RNA (Todd & Paulson, 2010, for review). To this group **SCA10** and **SCA12** and probably **SCA8** belong. Other diseases like myotonic dystrophy and **fragile X-associated tremor/ataxia syndrome** also belong to the same genetic category. The third group of SCA is due to the ordinary single base pair mutation, and **SCA5, SCA13, SCA14,** and **SCA27** belong to this group.

Prevalence of SCAs is different among ethnic groups. In Japan, for example, SCA3 (Machado-Joseph disease), SCA6, chromosome 16q-linked dominant cerebellar ataxia, and DRPLA are common. Among others, SCA6 is characterized by pure cerebellar ataxia of late onset and sporadic occurrence. Some types of SCA are associated with unique clinical features. **Machado-Joseph disease** typically begins between the ages of 20 and 50 years, and is characterized by cerebellar ataxia, progressive external ophthalmoplegia, fasciculation in facial muscles, dysarthria, dysphagia, pyramidal signs, dystonia, rigidity, and distal muscle atrophy. SCA36 is characterized by cerebellar ataxia of late onset associated with motor neuron involvement (Ikeda et al, 2012).

In many triplet repeat diseases, it is known that the longer the repeat expansion, the greater is the disease severity. Furthermore, the repeat expansion tends to be longer in the offspring so that the onset age becomes younger in succeeding generations (**anticipation**).

There is also a group of cerebellar degenerative disorders of autosomal recessive inheritance. **Friedreich ataxia** is its representative form, and in fact it is the most common cause of hereditary cerebellar ataxia in the world (Fogel & Perlman, 2007, for review). This is due to a GAA expansion in the first intron of the frataxin gene on the chromosome 9q13. Clinically, ataxia of gait and limb movement, dysarthria, loss of vibration and joint position sense, loss of tendon reflexes, and pyramidal signs start at age 5 ~ 25 years (Koeppen, 2011, for review). Pathologically, it is characterized by degeneration of large sensory neurons in the dorsal root ganglion, dentate nucleus of the cerebellum, and upper motor neurons. Friedreich ataxia is conventionally classified into spinal ataxia, but diagnostically it is important to note that there are also abnormalities in eye movements such as square-wave jerks and ocular flutter, although the saccadic speed has been reported to be normal (Fahey et al, 2008). Furthermore, systemic abnormalities such as cardiomyopathy, diabetes mellitus, scoliosis, and pes cavus are common, and in fact cardiomyopathy is the most common cause of death in this disease.

A variety of conditions may manifest clinical symptomatology similar to Freidreich ataxia. Those include vitamin E deficiency, abetalipoproteinemia (Bassen-Kornzweig disease) (Box 30), Refsum disease, cerebrotendinous xanthomatosis (Box 31), mitochondrial encephalomyopathy (see Box 57), ataxia-telangiectasia (Louis-Bar syndrome), early-onset ataxia with ocular motor apraxia and hypoalbuminemia (Yokoseki et al, 2011), Charlevoix-Saquenay syndrome (Box 37), and Marinesco-Sjögren syndrome (Box 31). **Ataxia telangiectasia** is an autosomal recessive hereditary disease due to mutation of the ATM gene. The disease exhibits progressive cerebellar ataxia in early childhood associated with conjunctival telangiectasia, immunoglobulin deficiency leading to recurrent infections, endocrine abnormalities, and increased risk of cancer. When children with this condition grow up, they may show a wide spectrum of movement disorders.

Acquired Cerebellar Ataxia

A number of acquired conditions due to toxic, inflammatory, metabolic, and autoimmune disorders may present with ataxia, and some of them may show clinical pictures similar to the neurodegenerative disorders. As many of

---

BOX 30 BASSEN-KORNZWEIG DISEASE

The authors saw a 36-year-old man with genetically proved Bassen-Kornzweig disease at NINDS, NIH. The patient was noted to have clumsy hand movement at age 5 years, and difficulty in writing and walking and tremor in head and voice at age 14. At age 16, loss of tendon reflexes, decrease in joint position sense and vibration sense, abetalipoproteinemia, hypocholesterolemia, acanthocytosis, decreased vitamin E level in serum, and steatorrhea were found. There was no similar disease in his family except for hand tremor. Neurologically, there were postural and action tremors in the head, limb, and truncal ataxia, hypotonia of limbs and ataxic-spastic gait. There was no pseudoathetosis, and Romberg sign was negative. This disease was reported by Bassen and Kornzweig of New York in 1950 as a case of atypical retinal pigment degeneration and acanthocytosis (Bassen & Kornzweig, 1950). This is inherited in an autosomal recessive trait, and mutation of microsomal triglyceride transfer protein (MTP) gene has been reported (Zamel et al, 2008).

BOX 31 HEREDITARY DISORDERS CHARACTERIZED BY CEREBELLAR ATAXIA, SPASTIC PARALYSIS, AND CATARACT

Cerebrotendinous xanthomatosis and Marinesco-Sjögren syndrome are clinically similar in that both are inherited in autosomal recessive trait and both manifest cataracts and cerebellar ataxia from childhood. **Cerebrotendinous xanthomatosis** is caused by mutation of the CYP27A1 gene and is characterized by deposit of cholestanol in the brain, lens, and tendon due to lack of sterol-27-hydroxylase, which interferes with the synthesis of chenodeoxycholic acid (CDCA). Clinically, cataract and xanthoma in the tendon appear in the school age child or young adult, and psychomotor retardation, cognitive decline, cerebellar ataxia, and pyramidal signs are seen. In addition, epileptic attacks, parkinsonism, psychiatric symptoms, and polyneuropathy may be also seen. The diagnosis is made by documenting enlargement of the Achilles tendon by visual inspection and MRI, and elevated cholestanol in the serum. It has been reported that supplementation of CDCA ameliorates the cholestanol deposit (Pilo-de-la-Fuente et al, 2011). By contrast, **Marinesco-Sjögren syndrome** is characterized by appearance of cataracts, cerebellar ataxia, psychomotor retardation, chronic myopathy, small stature, hypogonadotropic hypogonadism and skeletal abnormalities in infancy, thus clinically resembling cerebrotendinous xanthomatosis. In a large proportion of cases with this condition, mutation of SILI gene on chromosome 5q31 has been detected (Yis et al, 2011; Krieger et al, 2013).

---

them are treatable if diagnosed in the early stage of illness, the diagnosis of those conditions is important (Ramirez-Zamora et al, 2015, for review).

The cerebellum is especially vulnerable to ethanol, pharmaceutical drugs such as diphenylhydantoin and lithium, and some heavy metals (**toxic cerebellar diseases**). **Hunter-Russell syndrome (Minamata disease)** is a typical example of organic mercury poisoning (see Chapter 1-1). The cerebellum is also a predilection for the demyelinating plaques in **multiple sclerosis**.

Purkinje cells are vulnerable to autoimmune pathology in relation to either viral infection or neoplasm of other organs. The latter condition is called **subacute cerebellar degeneration**, which is associated with elevated anti-Yo antibody in association with cancer of the uterus, ovary, or breast or with elevated antibody against voltage-gated calcium channel (VGCC) in association with pulmonary small cell carcinoma (see Chapter 25-2). Other antibodies such as anti-Hu, anti-Ri, anti-CV2, anti-Tr, anti-Ma, anti-Ta, anti-zic 4, and anti-mGluR1 might also be detected in paraneoplastic cerebellar degeneration.

Subacute combined degeneration of the spinal cord due to vitamin B12 deficiency, although it does not directly involve the cerebellum, may manifest as an ataxic-like gait due to proprioceptive loss in the lower extremities in addition to hyperactive tendon reflexes (other than at the ankle) and Babinski signs. The ankle jerk may be lost because of the coexistence of polyneuropathy (see Chapter 19-2C). Its most common cause is pernicious anemia, but it may be also caused by gastric resection and other forms of malnutrition. Pathologically, it is characterized by myelin loss of the posterior column and the lateral column of the spinal cord. When it is severe, it may also damage cerebral white matter and cause cognitive impairment. Therefore, this condition is an important differential diagnosis for spinocerebellar degeneration.

Since Hadjivassiliou et al. of Sheffield reported 28 patients with **gluten-sensitive ataxia** in 1998, this condition has drawn the attention of many investigators (Hadjivassiliou et al, 1998; Hernandez-Lahoz et al, 2014). Gluten ataxia is characterized by sporadic, progressive cerebellar ataxia of late onset and elevated antigliadin antibodies in the serum. The entity is highly controversial, but is now considered by some to be a gluten-induced autoimmune disease. A gluten-free diet is recommended for treatment although no controlled studies have been done (Hernandez-Lahoz et al, 2014).

Tumors of the Cerebellum

Tumors of the cerebellum are more common in children than in adults, and most of them are **astrocytomas** or **medulloblastomas**. In adults, **hemangioblastoma** is the most common tumor of the cerebellum. Familial hemangioblastoma is known as **von Hippel-Lindau disease**, which, in addition to hemangioblastoma in the central nervous system and retina, is often complicated by pheochromocytoma and tumors in other visceral organs (Frantzen et al, 2012; Binderup et al, 2015). **Lhermitte-Duclos disease** is cerebellar dysplastic gangliocytoma, which is characterized by a striated appearance on MRI (Figure 16-22), and this tumor is commonly associated with an autosomal dominant hereditary cancer syndrome called Cowden syndrome (Abi Lahoud et al, 2014; Mester & Eng, 2015, for review).

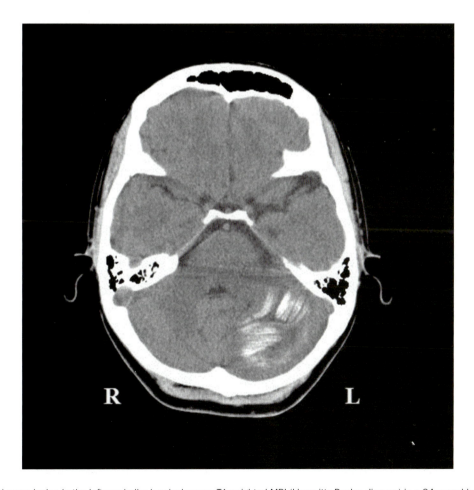

Figure 16-22 A striated mass lesion in the left cerebellar hemisphere on T1-weighted MRI (Lhermitte-Duclos disease) in a 24-year-old patient with Cowden syndrome. (Courtesy of Dr. Hidefumi Suzuki, Ijinkai Takeda General Hospital, Kyoto)

3. EXAMINATION OF MOTOR FUNCTIONS

Motor system can be examined in the following order. In general, the examination may start with observation of visible findings, followed by manual examination of objective findings, and finally observation of the execution of the patient's voluntary movements; namely posture, the presence or absence of muscle atrophy and fasciculation, muscle power (muscle strength), muscle tone, the presence or absence of muscle spasm and myotonia, and coordination.

A. POSTURE

First it is useful to observe the **posture** of upper limbs while they are kept in the natural **position** or in the forward-extended position. Any abnormal posture, especially of twisted nature, suggests a possibility of **dystonia**. If it is simply an abnormal posture of either flexion or extension, the range of joint motion should be tested in order to exclude joint pathology. Generally speaking, postural abnormality due to central nervous system pathology tends to disappear during sleep, whereas abnormality of the joint itself is unchanged during sleep. Patients with spastic hemiplegia show a characteristic posture with the upper limb flexed and with the lower limb extended and externally rotated (**Wernicke-Mann posture**). Postural abnormality of basal ganglia disorders, especially of Parkinson disease, has been described in Chapter 15-1.

B. MUSCLE ATROPHY AND FASCICULATION

If the history suggests a possibility of neuromuscular diseases, muscles should be carefully examined by visual inspection and palpation.

Muscle Atrophy

First of all, muscle volume should be carefully observed or palpated. If there is muscle atrophy, its distribution should be evaluated in detail. Generally speaking, in myopathy like **progressive muscular dystrophy**, atrophy is seen mainly in the muscles of shoulder and pelvic girdles, and of proximal limbs. A typical form is **limb-girdle muscular dystrophy** (Narayanaswami et al, 2014), but **facioscapulohumeral muscular dystrophy** (FSMD) is not rare (Deenen et al, 2014). There are two types in FSMD, and FSMD type 1 results from deletion of a critical number of D4Z4 repeats on the A allele (Tawil et al, 2015). In these conditions, the scapula may look protruded backward because of atrophy of the adjacent muscles (**scapula alata**, **winged scapula**) (Figure 16-23). **Oculopharyngeal muscular dystrophy** shows an unusual distribution of muscle atrophy for myopathy. It is an autosomal dominant hereditary myopathy due to GCN repeat expansion of the PABPN1 gene and it is associated with cognitive decline in some cases (Mizoi et al, 2011). The distribution of muscle atrophy in **Emery-Dreifuss syndrome** is the same as that of ordinary limb-girdle muscular dystrophy, but it is

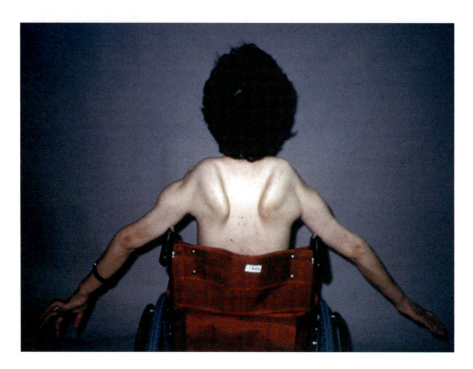

Figure 16-23 Scapular winging (scapula alata) seen in a patient with facioscapulohumeral muscular dystrophy. (Courtesy of Dr. Akio Ikeda of Kyoto University)

characterized by joint contracture and cardiomyopathy with conduction block (Liang et al, 2011).

The distal predominance of muscle atrophy usually suggests **neurogenic muscle atrophy**, but exceptions are not rare, like **distal myopathy** and **myotonic dystrophy**. Three groups of **distal muscular dystrophy** are known; Welander type of autosomal dominant inheritance, and Nonaka type and Miyoshi type of autosomal recessive inheritance. In the Miyoshi type, the calf muscle is predominantly affected and the serum creatine kinase is elevated, whereas in the Nonaka type the atrophy of the calf muscle is little if any. In **inclusion body myositis** (Box 32), the quadriceps femoris muscle is mainly involved in the lower limb whereas, in the upper limb, the finger flexor and extensor muscles are primarily affected.

By contrast, **Kugelberg-Welander disease** is a progressive spinal muscular atrophy of juvenile onset and of autosomal recessive inheritance, but in this case atrophy is primarily seen in the proximal muscles in spite of the fact that it is a typical neurogenic muscle atrophy associated with fasciculation. In **bulbospinal muscular atrophy**, neurogenic muscle atrophy is seen in the bulbar muscles and proximal limb muscles (Box 33) (see Figure 14-7).

Amyotrophic lateral sclerosis (ALS) is one of the most incurable neurological diseases, characterized by rapidly progressive neurogenic muscle atrophy occurring in adults above middle age. Muscle atrophy and weakness of the limbs usually start distally, but they may also start from the proximal upper limb (Figure 16-24) or bulbar muscles. It is usually sporadic, but about 10% of cases are familial. In 1993, the superoxide dismutase 1 (SOD1) gene was reported as a responsible cause of familial cases, and it is found in about 20% of the familial cases, but more recently, mutation of other genes including TARDBP, FUS, optineurin, and VCP has been discovered (Yamashita & Ando, 2015, for review). Some of these gene mutations have been found also in other neurodegenerative diseases (Renton et al, 2011) (see Chapter 22-2B). C9orf72 hexanucleotide repeat expansions are the most common cause of familial frontotemporal dementia and ALS, although patients with ALS with these expansions more frequently show behavioral and cognitive symptoms than those with classical ALS (Rohrer et al, 2015, for review).

In muscle atrophy following a nerve lesion, the speed of development of muscle atrophy and its severity heavily depend on etiology (whether trauma or inflammation), speed and severity of the nerve damage, and especially which of the two pathologies, axonal damage versus demyelination, is predominant (see Chapter 30-1).

BOX 32 INCLUSION BODY MYOSITIS

This myopathy used to be considered as a kind of chronic myositis because of the presence of unique inclusion body in the cytoplasm as well as in the nucleus of muscle cells. It may be hereditary but most cases are sporadic. The sporadic form mainly affects males older than 50 years. Muscle atrophy and weakness are mainly seen in the quadriceps femoris muscle and the finger flexors and extensors (Lloyd et al, 2014). The clinical course is slowly progressive, and there is no effect of immunosuppressive treatments (Mastaglia & Needham, 2015, for review). As a result of long-term follow-up study of many sporadic cases, it was shown that daily activity is significantly impaired due to progressive muscle weakness (Benveniste et al, 2011; Cox et al, 2011). Recently the deposit of β amyloid has been demonstrated in the muscle fibers of patients with this condition, and it has drawn special attention in relation to the mixture of an aging effect and inflammation. In relation to this, it should be noted that a similar term "hereditary inclusion body myopathy" is applied to the condition histologically characterized by "distal myopathy with rimmed vacuoles."

BOX 33 BULBOSPINAL MUSCULAR ATROPHY

This is characterized by slowly progressive bulbar palsy and neurogenic muscle atrophy predominantly involving the proximal limbs in males over middle age and is often associated with gynecomastia and testicular atrophy. This clinical picture was initially described by Kawahara of Nagoya University at the end of the 19th century, and Kennedy, Alter, & Sung of Minnesota University in 1968 coined the term "progressive proximal spinal and bulbar muscular atrophy of late onset" for this condition. This is a polyglutamine disease due to a CAG repeat in the androgen receptor gene on chromosome Xq11-12. Extraocular muscles are not involved, but unlike amyotrophic lateral sclerosis, the upper motor neuron is not affected and its clinical course is much slower (Chahin et al, 2008). There is a deposit of pathogenic androgen receptors in the nucleus of the remaining neurons, and the effect of androgen deprivation therapy has been experimentally shown by Sobue and his group (Adachi et al, 2007). Recently, in a double blind, long-standing follow-up study in patients who were treated with subcutaneous injection of anti-androgen leuprorelin, it was shown to be effective for slowing progression of motor disabilities.

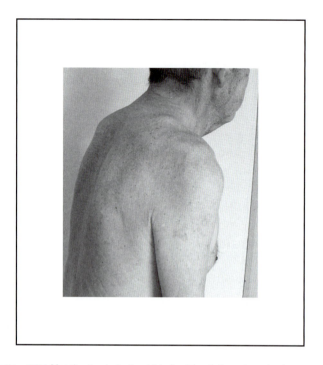

Figure 16-24 Muscle atrophy in the right shoulder girdle and proximal upper limb seen in a patient with clinical diagnosis of amyotrophic lateral sclerosis and progressive supranuclear palsy. (Courtesy of Dr. Manabu Inoue, Ijinkai Takeda General Hospital, Kyoto)

Fasciculation

Irregular twitches observed in the resting muscle are called fasciculations and are pathognomonic of neurogenic muscle disease. Therefore, if muscle atrophy is found, the presence or absence of fasciculation should be carefully examined. This phenomenon is caused by an increased spontaneous discharge of an enlarged motor unit as a result of reinnervation following chronic denervation. If fasciculation occurs in small muscles like the hand intrinsic muscles, it manifests as small finger movements resembling tremor. In this case, twitches may be palpable in individual interosseous muscles, which will exclude a possibility of tremor. Occasionally, fasciculation might be seen in healthy subjects with no muscle atrophy (benign fasciculation).

In active degeneration of anterior horn cells, the needle EMG of the completely resting muscle might delineate small muscle discharges (**fibrillation**) and **positive sharp waves**, both of which are called **denervation potentials**. This represents the spontaneous activity of single muscle fibers.

Myokymia is a continuous, relatively slow undulation seen in the surface of muscle, and it is thought to be generated by an abnormal excitability of anterior horn cells like fasciculation. The needle EMG will show repetitive bursts of rhythmic discharges of a single motor unit potential associated with this phenomenon.

Muscle Hypertrophy

Muscle can be hypertrophic in some conditions. Calf muscle may look enlarged in patients with **Duchenne muscular dystrophy** and those with **Becker muscular dystrophy** of late onset, but this phenomenon is considered to be **pseudohypertrophy** because it is not real hypertrophy of the muscle fiber. In some patients with muscular dystrophy, a part of the biceps brachii muscle may look swollen like a ball (**boule musculaire**). Muscle hypertrophy may appear in patients with hypothyroid myopathy. This condition is called **Hoffmann syndrome** in the adults and **Kocher-Debre-Semelaigne syndrome** in infants.

Firmness and tenderness of muscle can be checked by palpation and pressing with the examiner's fingers. In polymyositis, muscle is often painful spontaneously as well as on pressure and may feel firm likely due to inflammatory changes.

C. MUSCLE STRENGTH

As muscle strength varies even among healthy subjects depending on sex, age, and body build, it is important to evaluate strength of the muscle in question in comparison with normal muscles in each individual. How much in detail the muscle strength should be evaluated depends on the tentative clinical diagnosis derived from the history taking. If detailed information about the muscle strength was judged to be unnecessary from the history, it is practical to test a few representative muscles from the proximal and distal limbs. It is important to pay attention to the symmetry between two sides, but there may be significant asymmetry even in healthy subjects depending on the handedness, occupation, and sports of the subject. In patients with mild hemiparesis, if both upper limbs are held in extension straight forward at the shoulder level with the palm up, the weaker arm might fall depending on the degree of weakness. This phenomenon is called **Barré sign**. This phenomenon becomes manifest especially when the eyes are closed, but in this case it has to be judged whether it is due to weakness or pseudoathetosis as a result of proprioceptive loss (see Chapter 19-2B). A similar phenomenon can be observed in the lower limbs if the lower legs are kept raised by flexing the knees with the patient placed in the prone position.

Manual Muscle Testing

In order to express the degree of weakness quantitatively, manual muscle testing or manual strength testing is used. In the MRC scale shown below, the degree of weakness can be rated into 5 categories (0 to 4) while normal strength is rated 5.

5: normal

4: good (weaker than normal, but the patient can move against the examiner's moderate resistance)

3: fair (can move well against gravity)

2: poor (can move well if gravity is removed)

1: trace (can contract the muscle but no joint movement)

0: zero (complete paralysis)

In the above manual muscle testing, if scale 4 is judged insufficiently precise, intermediate ratings of 4- or 4+ can be used.

Muscle Pain

In patients with severe muscle pain (**myalgia**), it may be difficult to evaluate the muscle strength precisely. Although myalgia is common in **polymyositis** and **dermatomyositis** (see Chapter 3-1), myalgia is more severe in the condition called **polymyalgia rheumatica**. This is a systemic angitis seen in aged subjects and shares pathogenesis with **temporal arteritis** (see Chapter 7-1A). In fact, these two conditions commonly coincide or occur independently in the same patient. It is characterized by marked elevation of erythrocyte sedimentation rate and good response to corticosteroid treatment. By contrast, polymyositis is characterized by predominant muscle weakness with relatively mild myalgia, myogenic abnormality on the needle EMG, and elevated creatine kinase level in the serum. Regarding the needle EMG, it should be kept in mind that, in polymyositis, the so-called active denervation potentials like fibrillation and positive sharp waves can be observed especially upon needle insertion. This is considered to be due to denervation which could result either from segmental necrosis of muscle fibers separated from the end-plate region or from involvement of the terminal nerve endings (Kimura, 2013, for review). It is important to keep in mind that dermatomyositis in aged subjects is often a manifestation of paraneoplastic syndrome (see Box 5).

A condition similar to polymyalgia rheumatica, but more often associated with widespread musculoskeletal pain accompanied by fatigue, but no objective findings, is sometimes diagnosed as **fibromyalgia**. It is more common in females than in males, and there are often tender spots on the shoulder, low back, and proximal lower limbs. As there is no specific laboratory abnormality in this condition, and as the clinical course varies among patients, the diagnostic criteria are still controversial. Depression is common in these patients and some cases are thought to be psychogenic. There is a controversy as to its relationship with chronic fatigue syndrome.

Sites of Lesion for Monoplegia

When one finds muscle weakness in one hand or foot (**monoplegia**), it has to be distinguished whether it is due to disturbance of the central nervous system or the peripheral nervous system, and if it is peripheral, what part of the motor nerve is affected. In general, flaccid paralysis suggests a peripheral cause while hypertonia or enhanced tendon reflex supports the diagnosis of central paralysis. The presence of muscle atrophy in the hand or foot suggests a peripheral pathology, but cases with no muscle atrophy are more often difficult. That is because muscle atrophy does not appear until several days after the onset of weakness of peripheral origin. Even in this case, however, muscle tone and tendon reflexes might give a clue to the diagnosis.

In a case with monoplegia of peripheral origin, it can be judged clinically whether the lesion is in the anterior spinal root, brachial plexus, or lumbar plexus, or a single nerve or multiple nerves. In a case with monoplegia of the hand, for example, it is useful to start evaluating whether the muscle atrophy or weakness is localized to those muscles innervated by any one of the median nerve, ulnar nerve, and radial nerve, or more than one of them. For this purpose, the information about nerve innervation and segment of each representative muscle is helpful (Table 16-3). **Juvenile muscular atrophy of unilateral upper extremity (Hirayama disease)** is an example of segmental muscle atrophy (Box 34) (Figure 16-25).

A lesion of each nerve innervating hand muscles shows characteristic posture of the hand. In an ulnar nerve palsy, atrophy is seen in the interosseous and hypothenar muscles, and the metacarpal-phalangeal joints of the fourth and fifth fingers are hyperextended (**claw hand**) (Figure 16-26a). In a median nerve palsy, marked atrophy is seen in the thenar muscles, and the thumb is unopposed at the same plane as the palm (**ape hand**) (Figure 16-26b). In a radial nerve palsy,

TABLE 16-3 NERVE INNERVATION AND FUNCTION OF REPRESENTATIVE LIMB MUSCLES

Muscle	Nerve	Segment	Function
Upper limbs			
Supraspinatus	Suprascapular	C5	Initial abduction of arm from side of body
Infraspinatus	Suprascapular	C5	External rotation of arm at shoulder
Deltoideus	Axillary	C5	Abduction of arm
Biceps brachii	Musculocutaneous	C6	Flexion of forearm at elbow
Triceps brachii	Radial	C7	Extension of forearm at elbow
Pronator teres	Median	C6	Pronation of forearm
Supinator	Posterior inerosseus	C6	Supination of forearm
Flexor carpi radialis	Median	C7	Flexion of hand at wrist
Flexor carpi ulnaris	Ulnar	C8	Flexion and ulnar deviation of hand at wrist
Extensor carpi radialis	Radial	C7	Extension of hand at wrist
Extensor carpi ulnaris	Radial	C7	Extension and ulnar deviation of hand at wrist
Extensor digitorum	Radial	C7	Extension of fingers at MP joints
Flexor digitorum sublimis	Median	C8	Flexion of middle phalanges at proximal IP joints
Abductor pollicis brevis	Median	C8	Palmar abduction of thumb
Opponens pollicis brevis	Median	T1	Opposition of first metacarpal across palm
Interossei	Ulnar	T1	Abduction and adduction of fingers
Lower limbs			
Iliopsoas	Lumbar plexus	L2	Flexion of thigh at hip
Quadriceps femoris	Femoral	L3	Extension of leg at knee
Hamstrings	Sciatic	L5	Flexion of leg at knee
Tibialis anterior	Deep peroneal	L4	Dorsiflextion of foot
Gastrocnemius-soleus	Tibial	S2	Plantar flexion of foot
Peroneus longus, brevis	Superficial peroneal	L5S1	Eversion of foot
Tibialis posterior	Posterior tibial	L5S1	Inversion of foot
Extensor hallucis longus	Deep peroneal	S1	Extension of big toe
Flexor digitorum longus	Posterior tibial	L5S1	Plantar flexion of toes at distal IP joints

MP: metacarpophalangeal, IP: interphalangeal, C: cervical, T: thoracic, L: lumbar, S: sacral

wrist drop is seen due to weakness of wrist extensors (Figure 16-26c). Furthermore, in an ulnar nerve palsy, a maneuver of firm grasping of a piece of paper with the thumb and index finger of each hand and of strong lateral pulling causes flexion of the distal phalanx of the thumb on the affected side because of inability to adduct the thumb, which is compensated by the flexor pollicis longus muscle innervated by the intact median nerve (**Froment sign**) (Figure 16-27). In the lower limbs, **foot drop** occurs in a peroneal nerve palsy.

If a single nerve is severely damaged, muscles innervated by other nerves may also appear weak to some extent on manual muscle testing. That is because, in order to fully contract a particular muscle, that muscle has to be set ready in the most appropriate posture, which can only be done by other related muscles. For example, if the median nerve is markedly impaired due to **carpal tunnel syndrome** (see Box 64), the muscles innervated by the ulnar nerve might be also judged slightly weak.

Root Lesions

A lesion of the anterior spinal root causes atrophy in the muscles innervated by the corresponding segment (Table 16-3). It is often associated with radicular pain and sensory symptoms in the segmental distribution due to a simultaneous involvement of the posterior spinal root. A spread of metastatic carcinoma selectively involving anterior roots might cause rapidly expanding neurogenic muscle atrophy across multiple segments.

Plexus Lesions

By contrast with a segmental lesion or a peripheral nerve lesion, lesions of the **brachial plexus** (Figure 16-28) and **lumbosacral plexus** (Figure 16-29) may involve multiple nerve roots or multiple peripheral nerves. Thus, if muscle weakness cannot be explained by a lesion of either a nerve root or of a peripheral nerve or nerves, it is advisable to consider a possibility of plexus lesion. Idiopathic inflammation of the brachial plexus can cause neuralgic pain and muscle atrophy in a unilateral upper limb. This condition is called **neuralgic amyotrophy** and is considered to be of autoimmune pathogenesis. In this condition, even though the clinical manifestation is limited to a unilateral upper limb, the EMG study might disclose abnormality also in the opposite upper limb.

Compression of the lower part of brachial plexus at the thoracic outlet will cause pain and numbness in the upper limb. This condition is called **thoracic outlet syndrome** and is most commonly caused by a cervical rib which is the rib coming out from the eighth cervical spine. Clinically, it is characterized by sensory loss on the ulnar side of the hand with atrophy of the thenar muscle due to a lesion of the lower trunk. The maneuver called the **Adson test** is often applied. In this test, with the patient placed in the sitting position, the examiner palpates the radial pulse bilaterally, and the patient is asked to take a rapid deep breath and rotate the extended neck to either side. If the pulsation diminishes on either side, the test is judged positive. In

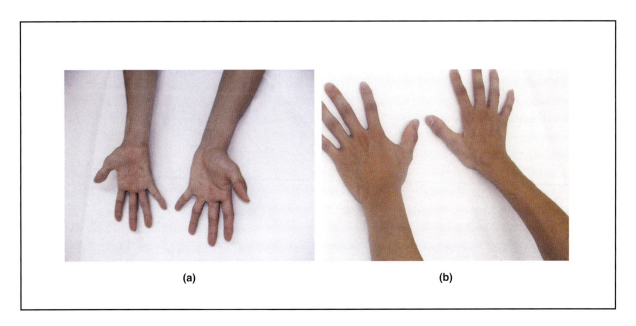

(a)   (b)

Figure 16-25 Juvenile muscular atrophy of unilateral upper extremity seen in a 23-year-old Japanese male with clinical diagnosis of Hirayama disease: (a) palmar view, (b) dorsal view.

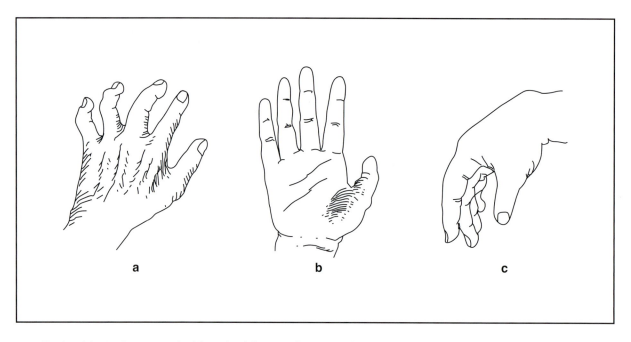

Figure 16-26 Claw hand due to ulnar nerve palsy (a), ape hand due to median nerve palsy (b), and wrist drop due to radial nerve palsy (c). (Modified from Chusid & McDonald, 1964)

this case, a vascular bruit may be audible in the subclavian artery. However, the sensitivity and specificity of this test may not be very high.

In patients with diabetes mellitus, **painful sensory polyneuropathy** is common (see Chapter 19-2B), but painless motor neuropathy may also appear in the territory of lumbosacral plexus (**painless diabetic motor neuropathy**) (Garces-Sanchez et al, 2011).

Acute Polyneuritis

Diffuse inflammatory involvement of peripheral nerves of acute onset is called **acute polyneuritis** or **acute polyradiculoneuritis**. This condition is generally called **Guillain-Barré syndrome** and is important because it is relatively common and mostly curable if appropriately treated in the early phase. In most cases, it is preceded by symptoms of upper respiratory or gastrointestinal infection either immediately or by a week or two. The common initial symptoms are weakness and numbness of hands or feet, which is followed by rapid progression in degree and distribution. Rapid ascending of the symptoms from the feet to respiratory muscles is not infrequent. Occasionally cranial nerves may also be involved. Tendon reflexes are diffusely lost from the acute phase. The signs are usually symmetric, but there may be asymmetry. An autoimmune pathogenesis is considered in most cases. After the acute phase, electrophysiological studies will disclose its demyelinating nature, but in some cases axonal impairment may be a main feature. In the axonal type, muscle weakness

tends to be severe, and muscle atrophy will become apparent from about a week after the onset, and the functional recovery is worse than the demyelinating type (Figure 16-30). In those cases of acute axonal polyneuritis who manifest gastrointestinal symptoms before the clinical onset, infection with *Campylobacter jejuni* may be found for its pathogenesis (Huizinga et al, 2015).

Guillain-Barré syndrome has to be differentiated from other conditions characterized by acute or subacute motor weakness, such as botulism (see Box 97), acute anterior poliomyelitis, tic paralysis including Lyme disease, AIDS-related polyneuropathy, diphtheritic neuropathy, porphyric polyneuropathy, and polyneuropathies caused by toxins such as lead, hexane, thallium, acrylamide, and vincristine. These conditions usually show characteristic patterns of weakness

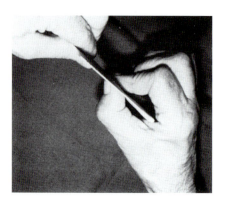

Figure 16-27 Froment sign in the right hand seen in ulnar nerve palsy. (Reproduced from Dawson et al, 1999, with permission)

THE NEUROLOGIC EXAMINATION

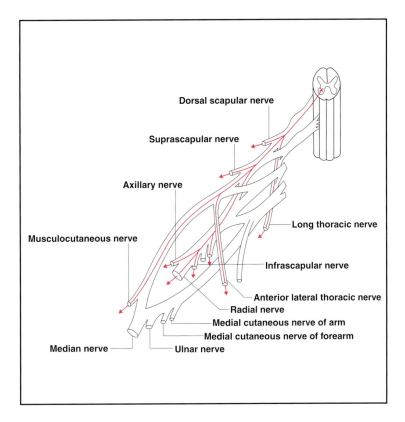

Figure 16-28 Schematic diagram of the brachial plexus.

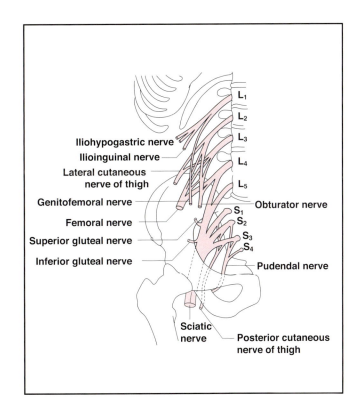

Figure 16-29 Schematic diagram of the lumbosacral plexus. (Modified from Mayo Clinic and Mayo Foundation, 1998)

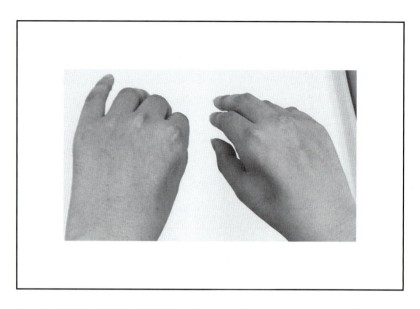

Figure 16-30 Muscle atrophy of hands seen 6 months after acute axonal polyneuritis.

and associated systemic findings, and the mode of onset is usually different from typical Guillain-Barré syndrome.

In typical Guillain-Barré syndrome, motor paralysis predominates whereas sensory impairment is mild, if any. Furthermore, as motor paralysis is commonly seen in proximal muscles, differentiation from polymyositis of subacute onset may be even necessary in the acute phase. Even in cases with no sensory symptoms, if the straight leg-raising test induces radiating pain over the posterior aspect of lower limb (positive Lasègue sign), it may suggest inflammatory involvement of the posterior roots.

In some patients with acute polyneuritis, only sensory symptoms may be present. In these cases, unlike typical Guillain-Barré syndrome, the posterior root ganglion cells are considered to be affected by an autoimmune pathogenesis (**polyganglionitis**). Moreover, impairment of the autonomic nervous system might predominate, suggesting involvement of autonomic ganglion cells or autonomic nerve fibers. As the postganglionic fibers are either A-δ fibers or unmyelinated C fibers (see Chapter 20), axons are primarily involved in these cases, resulting in greater resistance to treatment. In autoimmune polyneuritis, antibodies against various gangliosides have been demonstrated (Kusunoki & Kaida, 2011, for review).

Atypical Acute Polyneuritis

If acute polyneuritis is preceded by symptoms of systemic infection and is associated with an atypical clinical picture, a possibility of infection with a variety of microorganisms has to be taken into account. Those include **Epstein-Barr virus**, **mycoplasma pneumoniae** and *Borrelia burgdorferi*, a spirochete causing Lyme disease.

Collagen diseases like **systemic lupus erythematosus (SLE)** and Sjögren syndrome may present with polyneuritis based on autoimmune angitis. In **Sjögren syndrome**, sensory symptoms are especially common in the trigeminal nerve territory. By contrast, in **polyarteritis nodosa**, **multiple mononeuritis (mononeuritis multiplex)** is especially common. Multiple mononeuritis associated with severe pain and marked eosinophilia characterizes **Churg-Strauss syndrome**.

Acute anterior poliomyelitis (polio, Heine-Medin disease) and **diphtheria** used to be known as common causes of acute focal motor paralysis, and may be still prevalent in some regions of the world. Polio paralyzes predominantly unilateral upper or lower limb or respiratory muscles, but other limbs may also be affected to a certain extent, and sensory impairment may also be present. By contrast, diphtheria is known to cause especially bulbar palsy. There have been some reports of vaccine-associated paralytic poliomyelitis following oral administration of live polio vaccine. Nowadays, therefore, subcutaneous injection of inactivated polio vaccine is being used in many parts of the world. Recently in the United States, a possible link between an outbreak of enterovirus D68 infection and acute flaccid myelitis has drawn attention (Greninger et al, 2015), although their causative relationship has not been confirmed.

Chronic Inflammatory Demyelinating Polyneuropathy

A chronic form of polyneuritis is not uncommon. There are three groups: **chronic inflammatory demyelinating** polyneuropathy (CIDP), chronic inflammatory axonal polyneuropathy (CIAP), and multifocal motor neuropathy with conduction block. In the latter condition, multiple nerves may not necessarily be affected all at one time, but it may be just mononeuritis at a certain stage of illness which is later followed by involvement of other nerves. This condition is occasionally called Lewis-Sumner syndrome, but in their original report of five cases published in 1982, there was also sensory impairment (Lewis et al, 1982). In many cases of this disease, IgM antibody against GM1 is elevated in the serum, and it is especially so in the severe cases (Cats et al, 2010). For these kinds of chronic polyneuritis, intravenous injection of immunoglobulin (IVIg) is used for the treatment. There might be some improvement, but it tends to show remissions and relapses just as in multiple sclerosis of the central nervous system.

Misdiagnosis of CIDP is common (Allen & Lewis, 2015). The initial symptoms of CIDP might appear acutely, and some cases of Guillain-Barré syndrome might show worsening of the symptoms after the acute phase, thus creating some diagnostic difficulty in the acute phase. It has been reported that, if patients with initial diagnosis of Guillain-Barré syndrome show worsening of the symptoms more than 8 weeks after the onset or if they repeat more than three times, it is more likely CIDP (Ruts et al, 2010).

Toxic Polyneuropathy

As the peripheral nerves, like the cerebellum, are vulnerable to heavy metals and drugs, a possibility of toxic polyneuropathy should be considered in any polyneuropathy of subacute onset. Intoxication with lead, vincristine, and acrylamide presents primarily with motor paralysis. Toxins like arsenic, organic mercury, cisplatin, and n-hexane tend to affect the sensory ganglion, and those including organophosphate and thallium are known to affect the autonomic nervous system.

Metabolic Polyneuropathy

Metabolic diseases such as diabetes mellitus, malnutrition, vitamin deficiency due to ethanol abuse, and porphyria are known to cause chronic polyneuropathy. Among others, diabetic polyneuropathy and alcohol vitamin deficiency polyneuropathy are notorious for causing severe dysesthesia with burning pain (see Chapter 19-2B).

Hereditary Polyneuropathy

There are a number of diseases in this category, but its most representative form is hereditary motor sensory neuropathy (HMSN). HMSN is classified into three groups: type I (Charcot-Marie-Tooth disease type I) is characterized by a decrease in the motor nerve conduction velocity, type II (Charcot-Marie-Tooth disease type II) is characterized by axonal damage, and type III is characterized by nerve hypertrophy due to demyelination (Dejerine-Sottas disease). The mode of inheritance is autosomal dominant for type I, but not consistent for type II and type III. In HSMN type I and type III, the myelin sheath is primarily affected and they are characterized by the presence of onion bulb formation in the histology of the peripheral nerve. In type III, there is prominent enlargement of the peripheral nerves, and the hypertrophy can be observed or palpated in the greater auricular nerve and peroneal nerve. An autosomal dominant hereditary polyneuropathy initially presenting with ataxic gait, pes cavus, and loss of tendon reflexes, and later manifesting distal muscle atrophy, postural tremor, and sensory loss used to be called Roussy-Lévy syndrome, but this form is now considered to be a subtype of Charcot-Marie-Tooth disease type I (Planté-Bordeneuve et al, 1999). Genetic abnormalities have been elucidated for many subtypes of HMSN (Gutmann & Shy, 2015, for review).

Other autosomal dominant forms of hereditary neuropathy include hereditary sensory neuropathy, hereditary sensory and autonomic neuropathy, familial amyloid polyneuropathy (see Box 68), and hereditary neuropathy with liability to pressure palsy (pressure sensitive neuropathy). Pressure sensitive neuropathy is characterized by occurrence of motor paralysis following mechanical compression of the corresponding nerve and the histological appearance of sausage due to beads-shaped hypertrophy of nerve (tomaculous neuropathy). Clinically, this neuropathy is manifested as multiple mononeuropathy, but the tendon reflexes are lost not only in the compressed nerve but also diffusely. Another autosomal recessive form of hereditary polyneuropathy is giant axonal neuropathy, which is histologically characterized by deposits of neurofilaments in the axon. Generally speaking, in these hereditary neuropathies, it is rare for the patients to be aware of numbness or pain even if the sensory nerves are involved.

Spastic Paralysis

Motor paralysis due to a lesion of the pyramidal tract is associated with increased muscle tone (spasticity) and is thus called spastic paralysis (Boxes 35, 36, 37, 38 and 39).

As there is a clear somatotopic organization in the motor cortex (Figure 16-1, see also Figure 11-2), a localized lesion in the motor cortex causes monoplegia in the contralateral upper or lower limb. By contrast, a lesion in the internal capsule causes contralateral hemiplegia because all fibers of the corticospinal tract converge there. In this case, the paralysis also involves the contralateral orbicularis oris muscle and the tongue, which will deviate to the hemiplegic side upon protrusion (see Box 22).

In a transverse lesion of the spinal cord, spastic paralysis is seen bilaterally below the level of the lesion, namely paraplegia in a thoracic cord lesion and quadriplegia in a cervical cord lesion. If there is marked paraplegia while the upper limbs are intact or only mildly weak if at all, the main lesion is usually in the thoracic cord. If a transverse lesion is just at the level of the Th10 segment, voluntary flexion of the neck in the supine position will shift the umbilicus rostrally (**Beevor sign**). This phenomenon occurs because the rostral half of the rectus abdominis muscle above the Th10 segments contracts normally whereas the caudal half is paralyzed.

Gowers Sign

Patients who have marked weakness in the pelvic girdle and muscles of the proximal lower limb have great difficulty in standing up from a squatting position, and they can barely climb themselves up with legs widely placed and by holding on to the near objects like a chair. This phenomenon is called **Gowers sign**. Furthermore, they tend to swing the waist when walking (**waddling gait**). This condition is commonly seen in myopathy, but may be also seen in patients with proximal neurogenic muscular atrophy like Kugelberg-Welander disease.

Disuse Atrophy

In patients who have remained in bed for a long time for nonneurologic diseases or in patients with neurologic diseases without direct involvement of the neuromuscular system, muscles may lose their volume. This kind of muscle wasting is called **disuse atrophy**, and sometimes its distinction from real muscle disease becomes a practical problem. In disuse atrophy, muscle strength is relatively well preserved in spite of small muscle volume, and tendon reflexes are preserved. Needle EMG study does not show any primary abnormality in this case.

Psychogenic motor paralysis is not rare, and is described in the chapter of psychogenic disorders (Chapter 26).

D. MUSCLE TONE

Muscle tone is tested by passively stretching the relaxed muscle and is judged by the degree of resistance against passive stretch. Therefore, it is important to place the corresponding muscle in complete relaxation. In order to distinguish between **spasticity** and **rigidity**, the passive stretch has to be given with two different speeds. Spasticity is speed-dependent and can be elicited only by quick stretch, whereas rigidity is independent of the stretch speed. Stretch of intermediate speed may not help to distinguish one from the other.

Spasticity

Spasticity is characterized by a sudden increase in the resistance during passive stretch, and if a flexor stretch

is maintained, the resistance may suddenly disappear leading to an extension movement. This phenomenon is called **clasp-knife phenomenon** and is explained based on the physiological principle of **lengthening reaction**. Spasticity is commonly tested in the forearm flexor (biceps brachii muscle) for the upper limb and in the quadriceps femoris muscle for the lower limb. If we take passive stretch of the biceps brachii muscle as an example (Figure 16-31), an impulse produced by stretch of the stretch receptor (muscle spindle) is conducted through the Ia fibers to the anterior horn of the corresponding cervical cord segment where the α motor neurons are monosynaptically activated, causing the reflex contraction of the muscle. This muscle contraction is excessively enhanced because the anterior horn cells are hyperexcitable due to a lesion of the pyramidal tract. Then the α motor neurons are inhibited by the inhibitory interneurons postsynaptically, causing the clasp-knife phenomenon. Regarding the afferent input for this phenomenon, it used to be believed that the Ib afferent fibers originating from the tension receptor (tendon organ) play

HTLV-I-ASSOCIATED MYELOPATHY/TROPICAL SPASTIC PARALYSIS (HAM/TSP) AND SUBACUTE MYELO-OPTICO-NEUROPATHY (SMON)

HAM/TSP and SMON, characterized predominantly by spastic paraparesis, are noteworthy because there has been a dramatic drop in the number of new cases after discovery of the etiology in both diseases. HAM/TSP used to be prevalent especially in Martinique and Japan. It was shown to be associated with chronic infection with the human T-lymphotropic virus type I (HTLV-I), the virus known to cause adult T-cell leukemia, and its pathomechanism was clarified by Osame et al. (Osame, 2002, for review). It manifests symmetric spastic paraparesis associated with only mild hyperreflexia in the arms, clinical and electrophysiological evidence of moderate posterior column involvement at the thoracic level, and urinary frequency and urgency associated with the detrusor-urethral sphincter dyssynergia, suggesting a diffuse white matter lesion predominantly involving the thoracic cord (Shibasaki et al, 1988). SMON has been endemic in Japan since 1955 and was proven to be due to the chronic use of clioquinol, the drug used for diarrhea (Igata, 2010, for review). It manifests severe painful dysesthesia in the distal portion of the legs and perineum, and spastic paraparesis with or without visual loss. The central distal axonopathy of the dorsal root ganglion was shown to cause the severe sensory symptoms pathologically and electrophysiologically (Shibasaki et al, 1982).

a major role, but its precise mechanism in humans still remains controversial (Cleland et al, 1990; Burke et al, 2013, for review).

Clonus

When testing muscle tone in patients with marked spasticity, a single muscle stretch might induce repetitive brisk contractions in the same muscle, which is called clonus. Clonus is interpreted as a repetition of the excessively enhanced stretch reflexes. Clonus is most easily demonstrated in the calf muscle (**ankle clonus**), but it can be also seen in the quadriceps femoris, wrist flexor, and masseter muscles. Clonus may occur spontaneously, and when it is vigorous, it may look like convulsions.

Rigidity

Rigidity is one of the most representative signs of parkinsonism. In rigidity, resistance against the passive muscle stretch appears independent of the speed of stretch, and typically it continues throughout the passive stretch in a cogwheel fashion (**cogwheel phenomenon**), which is due to action tremor superimposed upon the increased tone (Lance et al, 1963). Rigidity sometimes may continue throughout the passive stretch smoothly without cogwheel. In contrast

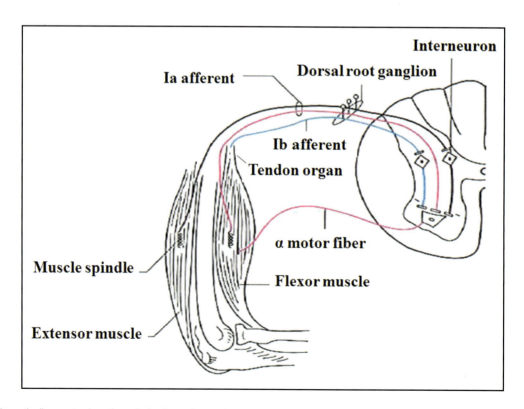

Figure 16-31 Schematic diagram to show the spinal reflex pathways. Interneurons are shown much posterior from the real location for the sake of clarity.

with rigidity, **Gegenhalten** (paratonia) appears as a continuous resistance against the passive movement of joint and is proportional to the effort with which the examiner tries to move. It is usually seen in association with diffuse cerebral lesion (Boxes 40 and 41).

Hypotonia

Decreased muscle tone is commonly seen in disorders of the peripheral nervous system or muscles. Among others, **tabes dorsalis** is known to cause marked hypotonia so that the toes may even touch the face upon the straight leg-raising test. Tabes dorsalis is a representative form of neurosyphilis with main involvement of the dorsal roots.

Hypotonia may be also seen in disorders of the central nervous system. In the acute stage of severe cerebral apoplexy, flaccid paralysis may be seen. This condition is called **spinal shock** even if the paralysis is caused by cerebral lesions. In newborns and infants with chronic diffuse cerebral lesions, flaccid paralysis is often seen (**floppy infant**).

BOX 40 MALIGNANT SYNDROME AND MALIGNANT HYPERTHERMIA

Rigidity of acute or subacute onset can be seen in **malignant syndrome (syndrome malin)**. This condition commonly occurs during chronic medication of neuroleptics or after the patient suddenly stops taking antiparkinsonian medications (**neuroleptic malignant syndrome**). This is especially common for the antipsychotic drugs blocking the dopamine D2 receptor, but may be also seen with other neuroleptics (Nisijima et al, 2007, for review). Clinically, in addition to marked rigidity, it is characterized by hyperthermia, consciousness disturbance, various autonomic symptoms, elevated serum creatine kinase and leukocytosis in the peripheral blood. It is treated by water, physical cooling, and administration of dantrolene sodium. In terms of hyperthermia, it is similar to serotonin syndrome (see Chapter 4-4) and malignant hyperthermia. **Malignant hyperthermia** is induced by inhalation anesthesia, and presents with muscle rigidity and respiratory as well as metabolic acidosis in addition to hyperthermia. It is commonly encountered in patients with various kinds of myopathy, among others, central core disease. For its pathogenesis, it is considered that the inhalation anesthetics act on muscles to cause excessive muscle contraction and hyperthermia. The mechanism of the malignant syndrome has not been fully elucidated, but a decrease in the central dopaminergic function, block of the dopamine receptors, and abnormal transmission of other catecholamines are considered (Nisijima et al, 2007, for review).

BOX 41 WHAT CAN OCCUR IN PARKINSON PATIENTS DURING L-DOPA TREATMENT?

A variety of untoward symptoms can occur in patients with Parkinson disease over a period of long-term treatment with L-dopa or dopa agonists (Aquino & Fox, 2015, for review). The most common phenomenon is the **wearing-off phenomenon**, in which the symptoms show diurnal fluctuation as a result of shortened duration of the drug effect (Antonini et al, 2011). By contrast, bradykinesia and rigidity might suddenly worsen and suddenly improve with no relation to the time of drug administration (**on-off phenomenon**). **Dyskinesia** (see Chapter 18-7) is seen in about a half of patients at 5 years after the initiation of L-dopa treatment (Gottwald & Aminoff, 2011, for review). Dyskinesia and wearing-off occur earlier after the treatment onset especially in patients with higher L-dopa dose and younger age at onset (Olanow et al, 2013). In addition, a variety of behavioral abnormalities may appear. In particular, the patients cannot control their impulses for gambling, shopping, sexual behavior, and appetite (**impulse control disorders**) (Voon et al, 2011; Weintraub et al, 2015, for review). These disorders are mediated by the nigrostriatal dopaminergic system and another dopaminergic pathway from the ventral tegmental area to the ventral pallidum and nucleus accumbens, which are both related to reward and addiction (Wise, 2009, for review). **Pathological gambling** is related to functional abnormality of the ventral pallidum, nucleus accumbens, hippocampus, amygdala, insula, and orbitofrontal cortex, and it is more common with the treatment with dopa agonists than with L-dopa (Djamshidian et al, 2011, for review). As for the tendency to repeat the same behavior (**punding**) and **compulsive behavior**, it has not been solved whether those are related to L-dopa treatment or the pathology of Parkinson disease itself (Spencer et al, 2011). For dopa-induced dyskinesia and punding, a favorable effect of amantadine has been reported (Kashihara & Imamura, 2008).

Hypotonia is also seen in acute cerebellar lesions, although its mechanism has not completely been elucidated. In relation to this, the cerebellar form of multiple system atrophy (MSA-C) may manifest hypotonia whereas its parkinsonian form (MSA-P) commonly shows rigidity (see Box 69).

E. MUSCLE SPASM AND CRAMP

A continuous or intermittent state of spontaneous abnormal muscle contraction is called **muscle spasm**. Muscle spasm associated with pain is called muscle cramp or just **cramp**. Spasm is caused by the occurrence of abnormal electrical discharge in the nervous system or muscles. For neurogenic spasm, any part of the motor system may be responsible, including motor cortex, corticospinal or corticobulbar tract, anterior horn cells or brainstem motor nuclei, α motor fibers, neuromuscular junction, and muscles. Therefore, the distribution of spasm is variable depending on its responsible source. A phasic repetitive form of spasm originating in the motor cortex may present with **epilepsia partialis continua (Kojevnikoff epilepsy)**.

Convulsion rarely originates in the white matter, but **painful tonic spasm** can occur in multiple sclerosis including neuromyelitis optica as a result of abnormal discharge and abnormal conduction of electrical discharges following demyelination (Shibasaki & Kuroiwa, 1974). In this case, pain is induced by a somatic stimulus applied to the skin and it spreads rostrally as well as caudally along with painful spasm.

Hemifacial Spasm

Hemifacial spasm is manifested as repetitive twitches or continuous spasm of the orbicularis oculi and oris muscles or either one of the two muscles. This is due to abnormal electrical discharge of the facial nucleus or facial nerve. The underlying cause is, like trigeminal neuralgia, considered to be demyelination of the facial nerve secondary to its compression by tortuous arteries in the posterior cranial fossa, but it has also been shown that excitability of the facial motor nucleus is increased (see Chapter 11-1A). Decompression surgery can be done and can be curative, but nowadays the local injection of botulinum toxin has been effectively used and may be more common.

Tetanus

The α motor neuron is particularly vulnerable to **tetanus toxin** produced by an anaerobic bacterium *Clostridium tetani*. **Tetanus** is caused by infection of injured skin with the bacteria, and the toxin produced there is transported retrogradely through the α motor fibers to reach the anterior horn or brainstem motor nuclei. At the synaptic terminal, the inhibitory neurotransmitters glycine and GABA are blocked by the toxin, causing massive vigorous spasm. As the toxin has special affinity to the motor nucleus of the trigeminal nerve, the most common initial symptom is inability to open the mouth due to marked spasm of the masseter (**trismus**) (see Chapter 10-2A and Chapter 29-3).

Stiff-person Syndrome and Progressive Encephalomyelitis with Rigidity and Myoclonus

Stiff-person syndrome, previously called stiff-man syndrome, is characterized by continuous painful spasms involving the trunk and limb muscles which is dramatically aggravated by movement or various kinds of stimuli. This condition is considered to be caused by excessive excitability of anterior horn cells through an autoimmune mechanism. In many cases, antibodies against glutamic acid decarboxylase (GAD) are elevated in the serum and cerebrospinal fluid, which is expected to cause deficiency of GABA, thus impairing the inhibitory transmissions. In some cases of this condition, antibodies against GABAA-receptor-associated protein (GABARAP) are elevated instead of anti-GAD antibody (Raju et al, 2006). Furthermore, stiff-person syndrome can occur as a paraneoplastic syndrome in association with breast cancer and small cell carcinoma of the lung, and in these cases, antibody against amphiphysin might be elevated (Murinson & Guarnaccia, 2008).

Progressive encephalomyelitis with rigidity and myoclonus (PERM) is similar to stiff-person syndrome but more severe than stiff-person syndrome with additional brainstem or other neurological defects (Balint et al, 2014). Recently a relationship of this syndrome with glycine receptor antibodies has drawn special attention (Carvajal-Gonzalez et al, 2014).

Isaacs syndrome is also characterized by muscle spasm, but in contrast with stiff-person syndrome, the spasm in this condition is more pronounced in the distal limb muscles. Isaacs syndrome is caused by an autoimmune abnormality of the voltage-gated potassium channel (VGKC) of α motor fibers (see Chapter 25-2).

It is important to note that spasm or cramp is not infrequently seen in patients with motor neuron diseases, especially in their early clinical stage, probably due to increased excitability of lower motor neurons.

Painful Muscle Spasm (Cramp)

The most common form of cramp is **idiopathic cramp**, of which a cause is unidentified. **Tetany** is caused by hypocalcemia in association with hypoparathyroidism, metabolic alkalosis, and hyperventilation syndrome. In tetany, the needle EMG shows repetitive discharges of doublets or triplets. In this case, excitability of motor nerves is increased so that tapping of the facial nerve will cause spasm in the facial muscles (**Chvostek sign**), and tapping of the median nerve will cause spasm in the hand muscles (**Trousseau sign**). In practice, the Trousseau sign can be noted while a tourniquet is tied around the arm for the purpose of blood pressure measurement.

In **glycogen storage disease**, among others McArdle disease (muscle phosphorylase deficiency), painful spasms are induced by vigorous physical exercise, and in fact this is the most common chief complaint in this condition. **McArdle disease** is an autosomal recessive hereditary disease, but it is more common in males. Vigorous physical exercise mobilizes anaerobic glycolysis, which produces a large amount of lactic acid. In this disease, as the aerobic glycolysis is impaired due to phosphorylase deficiency, lactic acid cannot be metabolized and accumulates in the muscle, which then causes painful spasm.

F. MYOTONIA

Myotonia is manifested as stiffness of muscles and difficulty in muscle relaxation due to repetitive depolarization of sarcolemma. The main feature of myotonia is difficulty in relaxing the contracted muscle, and in the resting state of muscles, stiffness may or may not be present (Figure 16-32a). Furthermore, myotonia is induced by tapping the thenar muscle or tongue (**percussion myotonia**) (Figure 16-32b). The needle EMG of myotonia shows rhythmic discharges at 50 ~ 100 Hz, and its frequency fluctuates so that it sounds like motorbike, which is also called the dive bomber sound.

In ordinary myotonia, muscle relaxation becomes increasingly easier as the patient repeats voluntary muscle contraction (**warm-up phenomenon**), which is seen in patients with **myotonic dystrophy** and **myotonia congenita**. In special conditions like **paramyotonia congenita**, muscle relaxation becomes increasingly difficult as the patient repeats muscle contraction. This phenomenon is called **paramyotonia**, which becomes characteristically worse in a cold environment.

In myotonic dystrophy, the patient has muscle atrophy and weakness in addition to myotonia, but in some kinds of myotonic disorders, myotonia is the sole manifestation. Furthermore, myotonia is closely related to periodic paralysis. Especially in hyperkalemic periodic paralysis, the patient shows myotonia during the intervals of paralytic attacks. Recently, mutation of ion channel genes has been identified in many of these conditions (see Chapter 25-1C).

In myotonic dystrophy, myocardial conduction abnormality and arrhythmia are commonly present, and they may be a cause of sudden death (Groh et al, 2008). A question as to whether myotonia involves the extraocular muscles or not has not been solved. In some patients, the return from lateral saccade looks slow, but in other cases, saccades look relatively normal even when there is marked myotonia in hands.

G. COORDINATION

For testing coordination of upper extremities, the **nose-finger-nose test** (also called **finger-nose-finger test**) is used to detect **dysmetria** and **dyssynergia**. These tests can be done either in a sitting or supine position. If a patient has visual disturbance, it may be replaced by the **finger-to-nose test** without any visual target. Then **rapid alternating movement** is tested with shin tapping. For testing the distal upper limbs, finger tapping is useful. Patients are asked to tap the index finger rhythmically on the metacarpal-phalangeal joint of the thumb. Fisher described the test, but his name has not been attached to it. When these tasks are poorly performed, it is called **dysdiadochokinesis** or **adiadochokinesis**. For testing coordination of lower extremities, the **heel-knee test** is used to detect dysmetria and dyssynergia. For this test, the patient is placed in a supine position and asked to put a heel on the knee of the other leg and slide it down over the anterior aspect of the lower leg smoothly. The patient may be also asked to repeat tapping the middle of the shin with the heel to see rhythmic performance. These tests of lower extremities may be also done in a sitting position.

Cerebellar ataxia due to a unilateral cerebellar lesion is seen in the ipsilateral extremities, because the cerebellar hemisphere is functionally connected to the contralateral motor cortex (Figure 16-7). There is some somatotopic organization in the cerebellar hemisphere, because the degree of ataxia is not infrequently discrepant between the upper and lower extremities.

While testing strength of the forearm flexor muscles by manual muscle testing, if the examiner suddenly releases the resistance, some patients cannot stop the muscle contraction and may hit their own chest, which a healthy subject can avoid. This phenomenon is called **rebound phenomenon**. It is generally considered to be specific for cerebellar lesions, but if this is the only abnormality, it is not necessarily pathognomonic of cerebellar lesion.

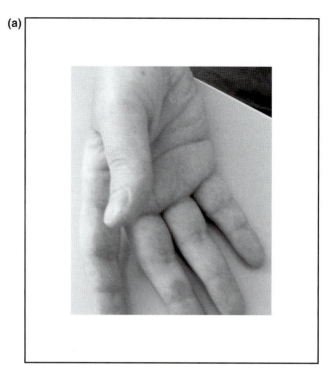

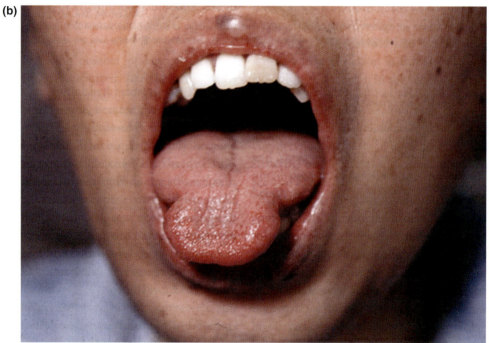

Figure 16-32 Myotonia seen in the thumb during an attempt to relax the grasped hand in a patient with myotonic dystrophy (a) and percussion myotonia elicited by tapping the tongue in another patient with myotonic dystrophy (b). [Figure (b) courtesy of Dr. Akio Ikeda, Kyoto University]

BIBLIOGRAPHY

Abi Lahoud G, Chalouhi N, Zanaty M, Rizk T, Jabbour P. Association of Lhermitte-Duclos disease and split cord malformation in a child. J Clin Neurosci 21:1999–2002, 2014.

Adachi H, Waza M, Katsuno M, Tanaka F, Doyu M, Sobue G. Pathogenesis and molecular targeted therapy of spinal and bulbar muscular atrophy. Neuropathol Appl Neurobiol 33:135–151, 2007.

Allen JA, Lewis RA. CIDP diagnostic pitfalls and perception of treatment benefit. Neurology 85:498–504, 2015.

Antonini A, Martinez-Martin P, Chaudhuri RK, Merello M, Hauser R, Katzenschlager R, et al. Wearing-off scales in Parkinson's disease: critique and recommendations. Mov Disord 26:2169–2175, 2011.

Aquino CC, Fox SH. Clinical spectrum of levodopa-induced complications. Mov Disord 30:80–89, 2015. (review)

Balint B, Jarius S, Nagel S, Haberkorn U, Probst C, Blöcker IM, et al. Progressive encephalomyelitis with rigidity and myoclonus: a new variant with DPPX antibodies. Neurology 82:1521–1528, 2014.

Bassen FA, Kornzweig AL. Malformation of the erythrocytes in a case of atypical retinitis pigmentosa. Blood 5:381–387, 1950.

Benveniste O, Guiguet M, Freebody J, Dubourg O, Squier W, Maisonobe T, et al. Long-term observational study of sporadic inclusion body myositis. Brain 134:3176–3184, 2011.

Binderup MLM, Budrz-Jørgensen E, Bisgaard ML. New von Hippel-Lindau manifestations develop at the same or decreased rates in pregnancy. Neurology 85:1500–1503, 2015.

Bohnen NI, Müller MLTM, Koeppe RA, Studenski SA, Kilbourn MA, Frey KA, et al. History of falls in Parkinson disease is associated with reduced cholinergic activity. Neurology 73:1670–1676, 2009.

Braak H, Del Tredici K. Invited article: nervous system pathology in sporadic Parkinson disease. Neurology 70:1916–1925, 2008. (review)

Brockmann K, Srulijes K, Hauser A-K, Schulte C, Csoti I, Gasser T, et al. GBA-associated PD presents with nonmotor characteristics. Neurology 77:276–280, 2011.

Brodal P. The Central Nervous System: Structure and Function. Oxford University Press, New York, 3rd ed. 2004, and 4th ed. 2010.

Burke D, Wissel J, Donnon GA. Pathophysiology of spasticity in stroke. Neurology 80 (Suppl 2): S20–S26, 2013. (review)

Carvajal-Gonzalez A, Leite MI, Waters P, Woodhall M, Coutinho E, Balint B, et al. Glycine receptor antibodies in PERM and related syndromes: characteristics, clinical features and outcomes. Brain 137:2178–2192, 2014.

Cats EA, Jacobs BC, Yuki N, Tio-Gillen AP, Piepers S, Franssen H, et al. Multifocal motor neuropathy: association of anti-GM1 IgM antibodies with clinical features. Neurology 75:1961–1967, 2010.

Chahin N, Klein C, Mandrekar J, Sorenson E. Natural history of spinal-bulbar muscular atrophy. Neurology 70:1967–1971, 2008.

Chahin S, Garwood MD, St Louis EK, Shivapour ET, Kelkar PM, Granner MA. Intramedullary Sjögren syndrome. Neurology 73:2041–2042, 2009.

Christopher L, Koshimori Y, Lang AE, Criaud M, Strafella AP. Uncovering the role of the insula in non-motor symptoms of Parkinson's disease. Brain 137:2143–2154, 2014. (review)

Chusid JG, McDonald JJ. Correlative Neuroanatomy and Functional Neurology. 12th ed. Lange, Maruzen Asian Edition, Tokyo, 1964.

Cleland CL, Hayward L, Rymer WZ. Neural mechanisms underlying the clasp-knife reflex in the cat. II. Stretch-sensitive muscular-free nerve endings. J Neurophysiol 64:1319–1330, 1990.

Cox FM, Titulaer MJ, Sont JK, Wintzen AR, Verschuuren JJ, Badrising UA. A 12-year follow-up in sporadic inclusion body myositis: an end stage with major disabilities. Brain 134:3167–3175, 2011.

Dawson DM, Hallett M, Wilbourn AJ. Entrapment Neuropathies. 3rd ed. Lippincott-Raven, Philadelphia, 1999.

de Beer M, Engelen M, van Giel BM. Frequent occurrence of cerebral demyelination in adrenomyeloneuropathy. Neurology 83:2227–2231, 2014.

Deenen JC, Arnts H, van der Maarel SM, Padberg GW, Verschuuren JJ, Bakker E, et al. Population-based incidence and prevalence of facioscapulohumeral dystrophy. Neurology 83:1056–1059, 2014.

Djamshidian A, Cardoso F, Grosset D, Bowden-Jones H, Lees AJ. Pathological gambling in Parkinson's disease—a review of the literature. Mov Disord 26:1976–1984, 2011. (review)

Duquette A, Brais B, Bouchard J-P, Mathieu J. Clinical presentation and early evolution of spastic ataxia of Charlevoix-Saguenay. Mov Disord 28:2011–2014, 2013.

Durr A. Autosomal dominant cerebellar ataxias: polyglutamine expansions and beyond. Lancet Neurol 9:885–894, 2010. (review)

El-Abassi R, Egnland JD, Carter GT. Charcot-Marie-Tooth disease: An overview of genotypes, phenotypes, and clinical management strategies. PM R 6:342–355, 2014. (review)

Etoh S, Noma T, Matsumoto S, Kamishita T, Shimodozono M, Ogata A, et al. Stroke patient with mirror movement of the affected hand due to an ipsilateral motor pathway confirmed by transcranial magnetic stimulation: a case report. Int J Neurosci 120:231–235, 2010.

Fahey MC, Cremer PD, Aw ST, Millist L, Todd MJ, White OB, et al. Vestibular, saccadic and fixation abnormalities in genetically confirmed Friedreich ataxia. Brain 131:1035–1045, 2008.

Fogel B, Perlman S. Clinical features and molecular genetics of autosomal recessive cerebellar ataxias. Lancet Neurol 6:245–257, 2007. (review)

Frantzen C, Kruizinga RC, van Asselt SJ, Zonnenberg BA, Lenders JW, de Herder WW, et al. Pregnancy-related hemangioblastoma progression and complications in von Hippel-Lindau disease. Neurology 79:793–796, 2012.

Galpern WR, Lang AE. Interface between tauopathies and synucleinopathies: a tale of two proteins. Ann Neurol 59:449–458, 2006. (review)

Garces-Sanchez M, Laughlin RS, Dyck PJ, Engelstad JK, Norell JE, Dyck PJ. Painless diabetic motor neuropathy: a variant of diabetic lumbosacral radiculoplexus neuropathy? Ann Neurol 69:1043–1054, 2011.

Girasole AE, Nelson AB. Probing striatal microcircuitry to understand the functional role of cholinergic interneurons. Mov Disord 30:1306–1318, 2015. (review)

Goedert M, Spillantini MG, Del Tredici K, Braak H. 100 years of Lewy pathology. Nat Rev Neurol 9:13–24, 2013. (review)

Goetz CG, Tilley BC, Shaftman ST, Stebbins GT, Fahn S, Martinez-Martin P, et al. Movement Disorder Society-sponsored revision of the Unified Parkinson's Disease Rating Scale (MDS-UPDRS): scale presentation and clinimetric testing results. Mov Disord 23:2129–2170, 2008.

Gottwald MD, Aminoff MJ. Therapies for dopaminergic-induced dyskinesias in Parkinson disease. Ann Neurol 69:919–927, 2011. (review)

Greninger AL, Naccache SN, Messacar K, Clayton A, Yu G, Somasekar S, et al. A novel outbreak enteriovirus D68 strain associated with acute flaccid myelitis cases in the USA (2012–14): a retrospective cohort study. Lancet Infect Dis 15:671–682, 2015.

Groh WJ, Groh MR, Saha C, Kincaid JC, Simmons Z, Ciafaloni E, et al. Electrocardiographic abnormalities and sudden death in myotonic dystrophy type 1. N Eng J Med 358:2688–2697, 2008.

Guo Y-C, Lin J-J, Liao Y-C, Tsai P-C, Lee Y-C, Soong B-W. Spinocerebellar ataxia 35. Novel mutations in TGM6 with clinical and genetic characterization. Neurology 83:1554–1561, 2014.

Gutmann L, Shy M. Update on Charcot-Marie-Tooth disease. Curr Opin Neurol 28:462–467, 2015. (review)

Hadjivassiliou M, Grunewald RA, Chattopadhyay AK, Davies-Jones GA, Gibson A, Jarratt JA, et al. Clinical, radiological, neurophysiological, and neuropathological characteristics of gluten ataxia. Lancet 352:1582–1585, 1998.

Hammond C, Bergman H, Brown P. Pathological synchronization in Parkinson's disease: networks, models and treatments. Trends Neurosci 30:357–364, 2007. (review)

Hattori N, Shibasaki H, Wheaton L, Wu T, Matsuhashi M, Hallett M. Discrete parieto-frontal functional connectivity related to grasping. J Neurophysiol 101:1267–1282, 2009.

Haymaker W. Bing's Local Diagnosis in Neurological Diseases. 5th ed. Mosby, St Louis, 1969.

Hernandez-Lahoz C, Rodrigo-Saez L, Vega-Villar J, Mauri-Capdevila G, Mier-Juanes J. Familial gluten ataxia. Mov Disord 29:308–310, 2014.

Hida A, Kowa H, Iwata A, Tanaka M, Kwak S, Tsuji S. Aceruloplasminemia in a Japanese woman with a novel mutation of CP gene: clinical presentations and analysis of genetic and molecular pathogenesis. J Neurol Sci 298:136–139, 2010.

Hilker R, Voges J, Weber T, Kracht LW, Roggendorf J, Baudrexel S, et al. STN-DBS activates the target area in Parkinson disease: an FDG-PET study. Neurology 71:708–713, 2008.

Hirayama K. Juvenile muscular atrophy of unilateral upper extremity (Hirayama disease)—half-century progress and establishment since its discovery. Brain Nerve 60:17–29, 2008. (review) (abstract in English)

Hitomi T, Mezaki T, Tsujii T, Kinoshita M, Tomimoto H, Ikeda A, et al. Improvement of central motor conduction after bone marrow transplantation in adrenoleukodystrophy. J Neurol Neurosurg Psychiatry 74:373–375, 2003.

Huizinga R, van den Berg B, van Rijs W, Tio-Gillen AP, Fokkink WJR, Bakker-Jonges LE, et al. Innate immunity to *Campylobacter jejuni* in Guillain-Barré syndrome. Ann Neurol 78:343–354, 2015.

Igata A. Clinical studies on rising and re-rising neurological diseases in Japan. A personal contribution. Proc Jpn Acad Ser B Phys Biol Sci 86:366–377, 2010. (review)

Ikeda Y, Ohta Y, Kobayashi H, Okamoto M, Takamatsu K, Ota T, et al. Clinical features of SCA36: a novel spinocerebellar ataxia with motor neuron involvement (Asidan). Neurology 79:333–341, 2012.

Jenkinson N, Nandi D, Muthusamy K, Ray NJ, Gregory R, Stein JF, et al. Anatomy, physiology, and pathophysiology of the pedunculopontine nucleus. Mov Disord 24:319–328, 2009. (review)

Kalra S, Grosset DG, Benamer HTS. Differentiating vascular parkinsonism from idiopathic Parkinson's disease: a systematic review. Mov Disord 25:149–156, 2010. (review)

Kashihara K, Imamura T. Amantadine may reverse punding in Parkinson's disease—observation in a patient. Mov Disord 23:129–130, 2008.

Katz M, Luciano MS, Carlson K, Luo P, Marks WJ, Larson PS, et al. Differential effects of deep brain stimulation target on motor subtypes in Parkinson's disease. Ann Neurol 77:710–719, 2015.

Kimura J. Electrodiagnosis in Diseases of Nerve and Muscle: Principles and Practice. 4th ed. Oxford University Press, New York, 2013.

Kitamura J, Shibasaki H, Kondo T. A cortical slow potential is larger before an isolated movement of a single finger than simultaneous movement of two fingers. Electroenceph Clin Neurophysiol 86:252–258, 1993a.

Kitamura J, Shibasaki H, Takagi A, Nabeshima H, Yamaguchi A. Enhanced negative slope of cortical potentials before sequential as compared with simultaneous extensions of two fingers. Electroencephalogr Clin Neurophysiol 86:176–182, 1993b.

Koeppen AH. Friedreich's ataxia: pathology, pathogenesis, and molecular genetics. J Neurol Sci 303:1–12, 2011. (review)

Krack P, Dostrovsky J, Ilinsky I, Kultas-Ilinsky K, Lenz F, Lozano A, et al. Surgery of the motor thalamus: problems with the present nomenclatures. Mov Disord 17 (Suppl 3): S2–S8, 2002. (review)

Kraoua I, Stirnemann J, Ribeiro MJ, Rouaud T, Verin M, Annic A, et al. Parkinsonism in Gaucher's disease type 1: ten new cases and a review of the literature. Mov Disord 24:1524–1530, 2009.

Krieger M, Roos A, Stendel C, Claeys KG, Sonmez FM, Baudis M, et al. SIL1 mutations and clinical spectrum in patients with Marinesco-Sjögren syndrome. Brain 136:3634–3644, 2013.

Kruer MC, Hiken M, Gregory A, Malandrini A, Clark D, Hogarth P, et al. Novel histopathologic findings in molecularly-confirmed pantothenate kinase-associated neurodegeneration. Brain 134:947–958, 2011.

Kusunoki S, Kaida K, Ueda M. Antibodies against gangliosides and ganglioside complexes in Guillain-Barré syndrome: new aspects of research. Biochim Biophys Acta 1780:441–444, 2008.

Kwon DH, Lee S-H, Kim E-S, Eoh W. Intramedullary sarcoidosis presenting with delayed spinal cord swelling after cervical laminoplasty for compressive cervical myelopathy. J Kor Neurosurg Soc 56:436–440, 2014.

Lance JW, Schwab RS, Peterson EA. Action tremor and the cogwheel phenomenon in Parkinson's disease. Brain 86:95–110, 1963.

Lewis RA, Sumner AJ, Brown MJ, Asbury AK. Multifocal demyelinating neuropathy with persistent conduction block. Neurology 32:958–964, 1982.

Liang W-C, Mitsuhashi H, Keduka E, Nonaka I, Noguchi S, Nishino I, et al. TMEM43 mutations in Emery-Dreifuss muscular dystrophy-related myopathy. Ann Neurol 69:1005–1013, 2011.

Lloyd TE, Mammen AL, Amato AA, Weiss MD, Needham M, Greenberg SA. Evaluation and construction of diagnostic criteria for inclusion body myositis. Neurology 83:426–433, 2014.

Lo Giudice T, Lombardi F, Santorelli FM, Kawarai T, Orlacchio A. Hereditary spastic paraplegia: clinical-genetic characteristics and evolving molecular mechanisms. Exp Neurol 261:518–539, 2014. (review)

Lossos A, Klein CJ, McEvoy KM, Keegan BM. A 63-year-old woman with urinary incontinence and progressive gait disorder. Neurology 72:1607–1613, 2009.

Mastaglia FL, Needham M. Inclusion body myositis: a review of clinical and genetic aspects, diagnostic criteria and therapeutic approaches. J Clin Neurosci 22:6–13, 2015. (review)

Matiello M, Lennon VA, Jacob A, Pittock SJ, Lucchinetti CF, Wingerchuk DM, et al. NMO-IgG predicts the outcome of recurrent optic neuritis. Neurology 70:2197–2200, 2008.

Mayo Clinic and Mayo Foundation. Mayo Clinic Examinations in Neurology, 7th ed. Mosby, St. Louis, 1998.

Mester J, Eng C. Cowden syndrome: recognizing and managing a not-so-rare hereditary cancer syndrome. J Surg Oncol 111:125–130, 2015. (review)

Mink JW. Functional organization of the basal ganglia. In Jankovic J and Tolosa E (eds), Parkinson's Disease and Movement Disorders. 5th ed. Lippincott Williams & Wilkins, Philadelphia, 2007, pp. 1–6. (review)

Mizoi Y, Yamamoto T, Minami N, Ohkuma A, Nonaka I, Nishino I, et al. Oculopharyngeal muscular dystrophy associated with dementia. Intern Med 50:2409–2412, 2011.

Molnar GF, Pilliar A, Lozano AM, Dostrovsky JO. Differences in neuronal firing rates in pallidal and cerebellar receiving areas of thalamus in patients with Parkinson's disease, essential tremor, and pain. J Neurophysiol 93:3094–3101, 2005.

Moreau C, Ozsancak C, Blatt JL, Derambure P, Destee A, Defebvre L. Oral festination in Parkinson's disease: biomechanical analysis and correlation with festination and freezing of gait. Mov Disord 22:1503–1506, 2007.

Moriya A, Kadowaki S, Kikuchi S, Nakatani-Enomoto S, Mochizuki H, Ugawa Y. Two cases of posterior spinal artery syndrome (PSAS). Clin Neurol 51:699–702, 2011. (abstract in English)

Murinson BB, Guarnaccia JB. Stiff-person syndrome with amphiphysin antibodies. Distinctive features of a rare disease. Neurology 71:1955–1958, 2008.

Nakamura A, Izumi K, Umehara F, Kuriyama M, Hokezu Y, Nakagawa M, et al. Familial spastic paraplegia with mental impairment and thin corpus callosum. J Neurol Sci 131:35–42, 1995.

Nakamura S, Kitami M, Furukawa Y. Opalski syndrome: ipsilateral hemiplegia due to a lateral-medullary infarction. Neurology 75:1658, 2010.

Narayanaswami P, Weiss M, Selcen D, David W, Raynor E, Carter G, et al. Evidence-based guideline summary: diagnosis and treatment of limb-girdle and distal dystrophies: report of the guideline development subcommittee of the American Academy of Neurology and the practice issues review panel of the American Association of Neuromuscular & Electrodiagnostic Medicine. Neurology 83:1453–1463, 2014. (review)

Newsway V, Fish M, Rohrer JD, Majounie E, Williams N, Hack M, et al. Perry syndrome due to the DCTN1 G71R mutation: a distinctive levodopa responsive disorder with behavioral syndrome, vertical gaze palsy, and respiratory failure. Mov Disord 25:767–770, 2010.

Nisijima K, Shioda K, Iwamura T. Neuroleptic malignant syndrome and serotonin syndrome. Progr Brain Res 162:81–104, 2007. (review)

Olanow CW, Kieburtz K, Rascol O, Poewe W, Schapira AH, Emre M, et al. Factors predictive of the development of levodopa-induced dyskinesia and wearing-off in Parkinson's disease. Mov Disord 28:1064–1071, 2013.

Osame M. Pathological mechanisms of human T-cell lymphotropic virus type I-associated myelopathy (HAM/TSP). J Neurovirol 8:359–364, 2002. (review)

Ozawa T, Koide R, Nakata Y, Saitsu H, Matsumoto N, Takahashi K, et al. A novel WDR45 mutation in a patient with static encephalopathy of childhood with neurodegeneration in adulthood (SENDA). Am J Med Genet Part A 164A:2388–2390, 2014.

Paudel R, Li A, Wiethoff S, Bandopadhyay R, Bhatia K, de Silva R, et al. Neuropathology of Beta-propeller protein associated neurodegeneration (BPAN): a new tauopathy. Acta Neuropath Comm 3 (39): 1–8, 2015.

Pierrot-Deseilligny E, Burke D. The Circuitry of the Human Spinal Cord: Its Role in Motor Control and Movement Disorders. Cambridge University Press, New York, 2005.

Pilliod J, Moutton S, Lavie J, Maurat E, Hubert C, Bellance N, et al. New practical definitions for the diagnosis of autosomal recessive spastic ataxia of Charlevoix-Saguenay. Ann Neurol 78:871–886, 2015.

Pilo-de-la-Fuente B, Jimenez-Escrig A, Lorenzo JR, Pardo J, Arias M, Ares-Luque A, et al. Cerebrotendinous xanthomatosis in Spain: clinical, prognostic, and genetic survey. Eup J Neurol 18:1203–1211, 2011.

Planté-Bordeneuve V, Guiochon-Mantel A, Lacroix C, Lapresle J, Said G. The Roussy-Lévy family: from the original description to the gene. Ann Neurol 46:770–773, 1999.

Raju R, Rakocevic G, Chen Z, Hoehn G, Semino-Mora C, Shi W, et al. Autoimmunity to GABAA-receptor-associated protein in stiff-person syndrome. Brain 129:3270–3276, 2006.

Ramirez-Zamora A, Zeigler W. Desai N, Biller J. Treatable causes of cerebellar ataxia. Mov Disord 30:614–623, 2015. (review)

Renton AE, Majounie E, Waite A, Simon-Sanchez J, Rollinson S, Gibbs JR, et al. A hexanucleotide repeat expansion in C9ORF72 is the cause of chromosome 9p21–linked ALS-FTD. Neuron 72:257–268, 2011.

Respondek G, Stamelou M, Kurz C, Ferguson LW, Rajput A, Chiu WZ, et al. The phenotypic spectrum of progressive supranuclear palsy: A retrospective multicenter study of 100 definite cases. Mov Disord 29:1758–1766, 2014.

Rohrer JD, Isaacs AM, Mizielinska S, Mead S, Lashley T, Wray S, et al. C9orf72 expansions in frontotemporal dementia and amyotrophic lateral sclerosis. Lancet Neurol 14:291–301, 2015. (review)

Ruts L, Drenthen J, Jacobs BC, van Doorn PA, Dutch GBS Study Group. Distinguishing acute-onset CIDP from fluctuating Guillain-Barré syndrome: A prospective study. Neurology 74:1680–1686, 2010.

Samaranch L, Riverol M, Masdeu JC, Lorenzo E, Vidal-Taboada JM, Irigoyen J, et al. SPG 11 compound mutations in spastic paraparesis with thin corpus callosum. Neurology 71:332–336, 2008.

Sato DK, Callegaro D, Lana-Peixoto MS, Waters PJ, de Haidar Jorge FM, Takahashi T, et al. Distinction between MOG antibody-positive and AQP4 antibody-positive NMO spectrum disorders. Neurology 82:474–481, 2014.

Schipper HM, Neurodegeneration with brain iron accumulation—clinical syndromes and neuroimaging. Biochimica Biophysica Acta 1822:350–360, 2012. (review)

Schneider SA, Hardy J, Bhatia KP. Syndromes of neurodegeneration with brain iron accumulation (NBIA): an update on clinical presentations, histological and genetic underpinnings, and treatment considerations. Mov Disord 27:42–53, 2012. (review)

Seto-Salvia N, Pagonabarraga J, Houlden H, Pascual-Sedano B, Dols-Icardo O, Tucci A, et al. Glucocerebrosidase mutations confer a greater risk of dementia during Parkinson's disease course. Mov Disord 27:393–399, 2012.

Shibasaki H. Cortical activities associated with voluntary movements and involuntary movements. Clin Neurophysiol 123:229–243, 2012. (review)

Shibasaki H, Endo C, Kuroda Y, Kakigi R, Oda K-I, Komine S-I. Clinical picture of HTLV-I associated myelopathy. J Neurol Sci 87:15–24, 1988.

Shibasaki H, Kakigi R, Ohnishi A, Kuroiwa Y. Peripheral and central nerve conduction in subacute myelo-optico-neuropathy. Neurology 32:1186–1189, 1982.

Shibasaki H, Kuroiwa Y. Painful tonic seizure in multiple sclerosis. Arch Neurol 30:47–51, 1974.

Shibasaki H, Nagae K. Mirror movement: application of movement-related cortical potentials. Ann Neurol 15:299–302, 1984.

Shibasaki H, Sadato N, Lyshkow H, Yonekura Y, Honda M, Nagamine T, et al. Both primary motor cortex and supplementary motor area play an important role in complex finger movement. Brain 116:1387–1398, 1993.

Shimizu J, Hatanaka Y, Hasegawa M, Iwata A, Sugimoto I, Date H, et al. IFNβ–1b may severely exacerbate Japanese optic-spinal MS in neuromyelitis optica spectrum. Neurology 75:1423–1427, 2010.

Siebert M, Sidransky E, Westbroek W. Glucocerebrosidase is shaking up the synucleinopathies. Brain 137:1304–1322, 2014. (review)

Smets K, Deconinck T, Baets J, Sieben A, Martin J-J, Smouts I, et al. Partial deletion of AFG3L2 causing spinocerebellar ataxia type 28. Neurology 82:2092–2100, 2014.

Spencer AH, Rickards H, Fasano A, Cavanna AE. The prevalence and clinical characteristics of punding in Parkinson's disease. Mov Disord 26:578–586, 2011.

Stamelou M, Mencacci NE, Cordivari C, Batia A, Wood NW, Houlden H, et al. Myoclonus-dystonia syndrome due to tyrosine hydroxylase deficiency. Neurology 79:435–441, 2012.

Sugihara K, Maruyama H, Morino H, Miyamoto R, Ueno H, Matsumoto M, et al. The clinical characteristics of spinocerebellar ataxia 36: a study of 2121 Japanese ataxia patients. Mov Disord 27:1158–1163, 2012.

Tawil R, Kissel JT, Heatwole C, Pandya S, Gronseth G, Benatar M. Evidence-based guideline summary: evaluation, diagnosis, and management of facioscapulohumeral muscular dystrophy. Neurology 85:357–364, 2015.

Thevathasan W, Cole MH, Graepel CL, Hyam JA, Jenkinson N, Brittain JS, et al. A spatiotemporal analysis of gait freezing and the impact of pedunculopontine nucleus stimulation. Brain 135:1446–1454, 2012.

Todd PK, Paulson HL. RNA-mediated neurodegeneration in repeat expansion disorders. Ann Neurol 67:291–300, 2010. (review)

Ueki Y, Mima T, Oga T, Ikeda A, Hitomi T, Fukuyama H, et al. Dominance of ipsilateral corticospinal pathway in congenital mirror movements. J Neurol Neurosurg Psychiatry 76:276–279, 2005.

Valentino P, Annesi G, Ciro Candiano IC, Annesi F, Civitelli D, Tarantino P, et al. Genetic heterogeneity in patients with pantothenate kinase-associated neurodegeneration and classic magnetic resonance imaging eye-of-the-tiger pattern. Mov Disord 21:252–254, 2006.

Voon V, Sohr M, Lang AE, Potenza MN, Siderowf AD, Whetteckey J, et al. Impulse control disorders in Parkinson disease: a multicenter case-control study. Ann Neurol 69:986–996, 2011.

Weintraub D, David AS, Evans AH, Grant JE, Stacy M. Clinical spectrum of impulse control disorders in Parkinson's disease. Mov Disord 30:121–127, 2015. (review)

Wheaton LA, Shibasaki H, Hallett M. Temporal activation pattern of parietal and premotor areas related to praxis movements. Clin Neurophysiol 116:1201–1212, 2005.

Wingerchuk DM, Banwell B, Bennett JL, Cabre P, Carroll W, Chitnis T, et al. International consensus diagnostic criteria for neuromyelitis optica spectrum disorders. Neurology 85:177–189, 2015.

Wise RA. Roles for nigrostriatal—not just mesocorticolimbic—dopamine in reward and addiction. Trends Neurosi 32:517–524, 2009. (review)

Yamashita S, Ando Y. Genotype-phenotype relationship in hereditary amyotrophic lateral sclerosis. Translat Neurodegen 4:13. doi: 10.1186/s40035–015-0036-y. eCollection 2015. (review)

Yayama T, Uchida K, Kobayashi S, Nakajima H, Kubota C, Sato R, et al. Cruciate paralysis and hemiplegia cruciata: report of three cases. Spinal Cord 44:393–398, 2006.

Yis U, Cirak S, Hiz S, Cakmakçi H, Dirik E. Heterogeneity of Marinesco-Sjögren syndrome: report of two cases. Pediatr Neurol 45:409–411, 2011.

Yokoseki A, Ishihara T, Koyama A, Shiga A, Yamada M, Suzuki C, et al. Genotype-phenotype correlations in early onset ataxia with ocular motor apraxia and hypoalbuminemia. Brain 134:1387–1399, 2011.

Young NP, Weinshenker BG, Parisi JE, Scheithauer B, Giannini C, Roemer SF, et al. Perivenous demyelination: association with clinically defined acute disseminated encephalomyelitis and comparison with pathologically confirmed multiple sclerosis. Brain 133:333–348, 2010.

Zamel R, Khan R, Pollex RL, Hegele RA. Abetalipoproteinemia: two case reports and literature review. Orphanet J Rare Dis 3:19, 2008.

17.

TENDON REFLEXES AND PATHOLOGICAL REFLEXES

1. PHYSIOLOGICAL MECHANISM OF THE TENDON REFLEX

The tendon reflex (**deep tendon reflex**, **muscle stretch reflex**, myotatic reflex) is a monosynaptic proprioceptive reflex. The afferent arc of the reflex starts from the **stretch receptor** in the muscle called the **muscle spindle**. The receptor is activated by sudden stretch, and an electric impulse generated there is conducted through **Ia fibers** to the anterior horn cells of the same segment, where the α motor neurons are monosynaptically activated. The efferent impulse is conducted through the α motor fibers to contract the muscle fibers from which the afferent impulse originated (see Figure 16-31). An electric impulse generated in the tension receptor in the muscle tendon called the **tendon organ** as a result of the reflex muscle contraction is conducted through the **Ib fibers** to the anterior horn of the same segment and via the interneurons inhibits the α motor neurons disynaptically (postsynaptically). Furthermore, the anterior horn cell is also inhibited by its own recurrent branch via an interneuron called the **Renshaw cell** (Figure 17-1).

As the conduction velocity of both the afferent and efferent fibers of the tendon reflex is as fast as 50 m/s, the latency of the tendon reflex of the hand is about 25 ms. When recorded with EMG, the tendon reflex is called the **T reflex** ("T" from tendon). A similar reflex can be produced by electrical stimulation of the afferent nerve trunk, and is called the **H reflex** ("H" from Hoffmann).

The tendon reflex is decreased or lost by a lesion of either the afferent arc or the efferent arc of the reflex. In addition, as the tone of the muscle spindle is modulated by the γ motor fibers, the tendon reflex can be decreased also by impairment of the γ motor fibers. Therefore, patients who are considered to have impairment of the peripheral nervous system with loss of tendon reflexes and yet no abnormality in the muscle strength or somatosensory function may have involvement of the γ motor fibers.

There is some evidence for this situation with acute cerebellar lesions.

As the lower motor neuron is inhibited by a component of the supraspinal drive presynaptically via spinal interneurons, impairment of the supraspinal drive is expected to cause an increase in the excitability of the anterior horn cells and consequently an enhancement of the tendon reflex (see Chapter 16-3D).

In a localized lesion of the cervical cord, either within the cord substance (intramedullary) or compressing the spinal cord or its blood supply (extramedullary), the tendon reflex of the affected segment is decreased or lost while the tendon reflexes of the immediately caudal segments may be increased. For example, if the biceps brachii reflex is lost and the triceps brachii reflex is overactive due to a lesion at the C6 segment, a tendon tap to the biceps muscle might elicit elbow extension instead of flexion because of the hyperactive triceps reflex. This phenomenon is called the **inverted biceps reflex**. In contrast, if a segmental lesion at the C7 segment is associated with disseminated lesions as seen in the neuromyelitis optica spectrum disorders (see Box 35), a tendon tap to the triceps muscle might elicit the elbow flexion instead of elbow extension because of the hyperactive biceps reflex due to the presence of a more rostral lesion (**inverted triceps reflex**).

2. EXAMINATION OF TENDON REFLEXES

There is no general rule in the order of examining tendon reflexes, but it is practical to start with the jaw jerk, and then to examine the biceps brachii, triceps brachii, radial and finger flexor muscles for the upper limbs, and the quadriceps femoris, gastrocnemius-soleus and toe flexor muscles for the lower limbs, in this order, each comparing the left and right. The hamstring reflex and abdominal muscle reflex may also be examined as necessary.

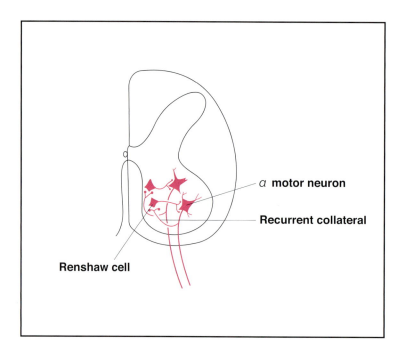

Figure 17-1 Schematic diagram to show the recurrent inhibitory pathway of the spinal cord. Although it is not shown in this figure, the Renshaw cell also inhibits other motor neurons that supply muscles with similar action. (Modified from Brodal, 2010, with permission)

For examining a tendon reflex, the muscle to be tested should be placed in a relaxed state with an intermediate length (Figure 17-2). For testing the **biceps brachii reflex**, for example, the elbow should be placed in a mildly flexed position (Figure 17-2b). When testing the **quadriceps femoris reflex (patellar tendon reflex, knee jerk)** in a supine position, the knees should be mildly flexed and gently supported from below by the examiner's hand (Figure 17-2d). Then the tendon should be gently tapped by a tendon hammer toward the direction so that the muscle can be stretched. For eliciting the **masseter reflex (jaw jerk)**, for example, the jaw should be tapped downward (Figure 17-2a). Practically speaking, however, for most muscles of the extremities, straight tapping of the tendon at a right angle has a sufficient effect for stretching the muscle spindle. Generally speaking, for the flexor muscles like the biceps brachii, it is easier to put an examiner's thumb on the tendon and to tap the thumb instead of directly tapping the tendon (Figure 17-2b). By contrast, for the extensor muscles like the triceps brachii and the quadriceps femoris, it is easier to tap the skin over the tendon directly (Figure 17-2c, d).

Regarding tendon hammers, a slightly flexible hammer is ideal, but the use of a metal hammer is perfectly all right. What is most important for the hammer is to use a relatively soft material for the head. A hard material is painful to the patient and is not effective for eliciting the tendon reflex efficiently. As for the way of tapping, leaving the hammer on the tendon for a moment after tapping is more effective than tapping in a bouncing way. For examining the tendon reflexes in newborns and infants, it is more practical to tap the skin with the examiner's finger instead of a hammer.

Tendon Reflex of the Distal Extremity Muscles

For examining the **finger flexor reflex** (Box 42), while the examiner's fingers are placed on the palmer aspect of the gently flexed fingers, tapping should be applied on the examiner's fingers. As this reflex may not be clearly visible even in healthy subjects, it is difficult to prove a loss of this reflex clinically. By contrast, if this reflex is abnormally enhanced and accompanied by flexion of the thumb, it is called the **Wartenberg reflex** and provides an important clue for the presence of pyramidal signs. A similar reflex can be elicited by grabbing a middle finger of the patient with the examiner's thumb and middle fingers and then flip a quick extension of the distal phalanx. An enhanced state of this reflex is called the **Hoffmann reflex**.

The **ankle jerk (Achilles tendon reflex)** is often decreased in healthy aged subjects, and may not be detectable by visual inspection. For eliciting the **toe flexor reflex**, the metatarsal bones can be tapped on their dorsal aspect or plantar aspect. If this reflex is abnormally enhanced, it is called the **Mendel-Bechterew reflex** for the dorsal tap and the **Rossolimo reflex** for the plantar tap. Like the finger

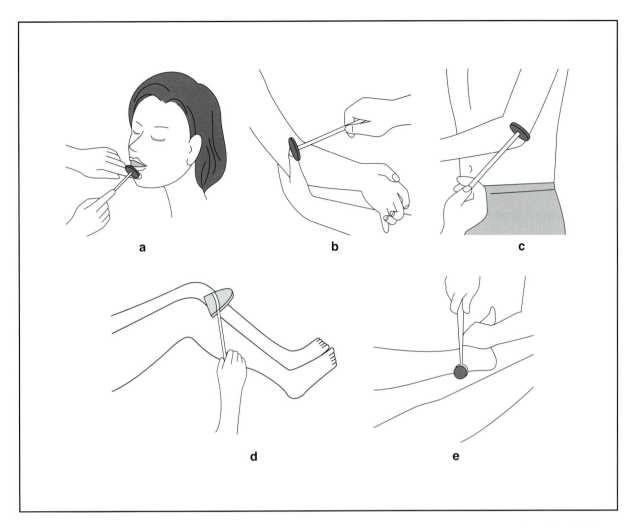

Figure 17-2 Methods for testing the representative tendon reflexes. (a) masseter reflex (jaw jerk), (b) biceps brachii reflex, (c) triceps brachii reflex, (d) knee jerk (quadriceps femoris reflex), (e) ankle jerk (Achilles tendon reflex). The ankle jerk can be also tested with the patient in a sitting position with the ankle free. In this figure, different kinds of tendon hammer are illustrated.

flexor reflex, it is often difficult to prove a loss of the toe flexor reflex clinically.

How to Confirm Loss of Ankle Jerk

In order to confirm loss of ankle jerk in patients with possible diagnosis of peripheral neuropathy, it is important to apply a **reinforcement** technique. For example, while a patient is asked to clasp hands together in front of the chest either in a sitting or supine position, the examiner gives a verbal order to pull them apart hard, and the Achilles tendon is tapped immediately after the verbal order is given. In fact, even in healthy older subjects, the ankle jerk may be elicited only by this maneuver (**Jendrassik maneuver**). If the ankle jerk is not elicited even by this reinforcement in a sitting or supine position, the tendon tap can be tried while the patient is kneeling down on a chair with the feet

protruding backward from the edge of the chair. If the ankle jerk is not elicited even after the above change of position, then the reinforcement technique can be applied in this new position. If the ankle jerk is not elicited after all those trials, then it is judged to be lost. In this regard, if the ankle jerk is unilaterally absent, as in a case of lumbar disc herniation, then its diagnostic significance is much higher (Box 43).

Significance of Hyperactive Tendon Reflexes

If symmetric increase of tendon reflexes is the only pyramidal sign, its diagnostic significance may not be specific. If it is accompanied by spasticity with clasp-knife phenomenon, clonus and/or pathological reflexes like the Babinski sign, then hyperreflexia is certainly regarded as a sign suggestive of a lesion of upper motor neuron or pyramidal tracts. Of course, if hyperreflexia is seen asymmetrically, its diagnostic significance is high.

As was described in relation to reinforcement, excitability of motor neurons is increased throughout the body by intended movement of any part of the body. Therefore, if a patient is nervous or emotionally excited, excitability of motor neurons might be increased even in the resting condition, thus lowering the threshold of motor neurons. In that case, therefore, it is worth examining the tendon reflexes after the patient is relaxed. However, no matter how nervous the patient is, hyperreflexia is never asymmetric in healthy conditions.

3. PATHOLOGICAL REFLEXES AND THEIR GENERATING MECHANISMS

Some reflexes seen in healthy newborns are pathological when seen in adults. There are two groups of pathological reflexes. One is the **pathological reflex** in a narrow sense, and its presence indicates an impairment of the upper motor neurons or the pyramidal tract. The other group is the primitive reflex (see Chapter 10-2E). Representative forms of the pathological reflex are the Babinski sign, Chaddock sign, and Strumpell sign of the lower extremities. Overactive tendon reflexes called by the investigator's name, such as Wartenberg, Hoffmann, Trömner, Mendel-Bechterew, and Rossolimo, do not belong to the pathological reflexes. The pathological reflex is a polysynaptic reflex formed of complex somatosensory afferents and multisegmental motor efferents.

The **plantar reflex** is elicited by stroking the sole of a foot with the blunt end of the handle of a tendon hammer or a key, and is manifested as toe flexion in healthy adults. The **extensor plantar reflex** consists of extension of the big toe associated with fanning and/or extension of other toes (Figure 17-3). It is elicited by stroking the lateral aspect of a sole from the heel toward the toes (**Babinski sign**) or by stroking the lateral dorsal aspect of a foot also from the heel toward the toes (**Chaddock sign**). For eliciting the Babinski sign, it is useful to grab the dorsum of foot with the examiner's hand while stroking the sole. When the Babinski sign is exaggerated, gentle pressure of the sole by the handle of the hammer is just enough to elicit the sign. Furthermore, when the pyramidal sign is exaggerated, a **flexor withdrawal reflex** may be seen in the proximal leg on the side of the stimulated sole (Box 44). In patients whose upper and lower motor neurons are both involved, if the extensor hallucis longus muscle is completely paralyzed as a result of a lower motor neuron lesion, the big toe is not expected to extend in response to the plantar stimulus. In that case, the proximal leg muscles might contract, eliciting the flexor withdrawal reflex, which can be interpreted to suggest the presence of upper motor neuron involvement.

THE NEUROLOGIC EXAMINATION

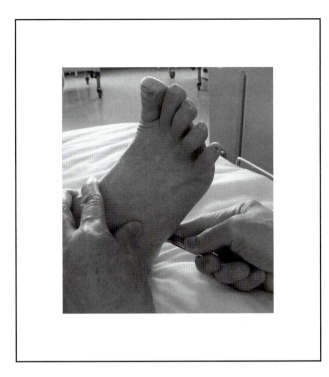

Figure 17-3 Typical Babinski sign elicited in a patient with multiple sclerosis. Mainly the big toe is dorsiflexed while the other toes show fanning. When it is difficult to elicit the sign, it is useful to grab the dorsum of foot with the examiner's other hand while stroking the sole as shown in this photo.

Significance of Babinski Sign

The Babinski sign is the most specific sign among all neurologic signs. Its presence always indicates a lesion of the pyramidal tract or the upper motor neurons. However, there are many false negatives (Isaza Jaramillo et al, 2014). Another problem with the Babinski sign is considerable interobserver variability. In spite of the fact that this is the most important sign in neurology, the mechanism underlying its generation has not been clearly elucidated. The Babinski sign is seen in healthy infants under the age of 6 months, and it disappears as myelination of the pyramidal tract is completed. Although other reflexes such as snout, sucking, and grasping are also seen in healthy infants, the occurrence of these reflexes in adults has nothing to do with a pyramidal lesion, and they belong to the primitive reflexes (see Chapter 10-2E).

4. LOSS OF SUPERFICIAL REFLEX AS A PYRAMIDAL SIGN

Among superficial reflexes, the abdominal reflex and the cremasteric reflex can be lost by a lesion of the pyramidal tract.

BOX 44 COMPLETE MOTOR PARALYSIS OF TOES AND BABINSKI SIGN

In patients with complete motor paralysis of toes, special caution is necessary for judging the presence or absence of the Babinski sign. If the toe extensor muscles are completely paralyzed due to impairment of the anterior horn cells or the α motor fibers innervating those muscles, the Babinski sign is not expected to occur even with the presence of the upper motor neuron impairment, because the reflex circuit is interrupted. In that case, however, if the muscle strength of the pelvic girdle and proximal legs is preserved to a certain extent, those muscles will contract in response to the plantar stimulus and produce the flexed posture of the legs. This is called **flexor withdrawal reflex** and may be interpreted as a pyramidal sign. By contrast, if the toe extensor muscles are paralyzed by a lesion of the corticospinal tracts or the upper motor neurons, the Babinski sign is expected to be positive even if the degree of motor paralysis is complete. An exception to this is the so-called **spinal shock**, which is seen in the acute stage of severe vascular or inflammatory insult to the central nervous system. In spinal shock, the tendon reflexes and superficial reflexes are all lost.

BOX 45 ABDOMINAL REFLEX AND ABDOMINAL MUSCLE REFLEX

The **abdominal reflex (abdominal wall reflex)** is a superficial reflex elicited by stroking the abdominal wall from lateral to medial and judged by observing a lateral shift of the umbilicus. By contrast, the **abdominal muscle reflex** is elicited by tapping the rectus abdominis muscle on either side and judged by observing the contraction of that muscle. In a lesion of the pyramidal tract above the lower thoracic segment, the abdominal reflex is lost whereas the abdominal muscle reflex is exaggerated. Therefore, it is conceivable that the abdominal muscle reflex is a muscle stretch reflex whereas the abdominal reflex is a polysynaptic superficial reflex involving the central nervous system at least above the lower thoracic cord. If the thoracic cord or thoracic nerves of the segments Th8-Th12 are involved by a lesion, both of the above two reflexes are lost, because the final common pathway is interrupted. Both reflexes may be difficult to elicit in aged subjects, obese subjects, multipara, and those having past history of abdominal surgery. Loss of the abdominal reflex or enhancement of the abdominal muscle reflex is especially meaningful when it is asymmetric.

Abdominal Reflex (Abdominal Wall Reflex)

The **abdominal reflex** is a reflex shift of the umbilicus elicited by a superficial stimulus of the abdominal wall. To elicit this reflex, the abdominal wall is stroked or lightly scratched by the handle of a hammer from lateral toward the umbilicus. As a normal response, the umbilicus shifts toward the side of stimulus presentation. However, if the abdominal wall is stroked away from the umbilicus, it may confuse the judgment because the umbilicus might be mechanically pulled laterally. It is useful to test the upper, middle, and lower segments of the abdomen, each comparing the left and right.

Tapping of the rectus abdominis muscle causes a reflex contraction of that muscle (**abdominal muscle reflex**), and this reflex is enhanced in a lesion of the pyramidal tract (Box 45). However, this reflex might not be easily elicited even in healthy subjects depending on the condition of the abdominal wall, and its diagnostic significance is not as high as the tendon reflexes of extremities, unless there is a clear asymmetry.

Cremasteric Reflex

This is a superficial reflex that can be tested only in males. The stimulus is given by stroking the skin of the proximal medial aspect of the thigh with the handle of a hammer downward and the reflex is observed as an ascent of the testis. Like the abdominal reflex, its loss indicates a lesion of either the spinal cord or spinal nerves of the corresponding segments or a lesion of the pyramidal tract. The stimulus can be applied upward as well, but it is easier to judge the reflex if it is applied toward the opposite direction from the response. The diagnostic significance is higher if this reflex is lost just on one side.

BIBLIOGRAPHY

Brodal P. The Central Nervous System: Structure and Function. 4th ed. Oxford University Press, New York, 2010.

Isaza Jaramillo SP, Uribe Uribe CS, Garcia Jimenez FA, Comejo-Ochoa W, Alvarez Restrepo JF, Romàn GC. Accuracy of the Babinski sign in the identification of pyramidal tract dysfunction. J Neurol Sci 343:66–68, 2014.

18.

INVOLUNTARY MOVEMENTS

nvoluntary movements are defined as abnormal unintended movements. It should be defined as "abnormal" because not all unintended movements are abnormal. For example, movements like blinks, spontaneous eye movements, chewing, swallowing, yawning, breathing, walking, and habits can be executed voluntarily, but they may occur spontaneously without involving "will to move." Involuntary movements are grouped into several categories depending on the characteristic clinical features of each involuntary movement. Those include tremor, chorea, ballism, athetosis, dystonia, myoclonus, dyskinesia, tics, and asterixis, and many of them were described more than 100 years ago based on clinical observation. Usually it is possible to classify involuntary movements by visual inspection, but electrophysiological tests are useful in confirming the diagnosis of some of them (Shibasaki, 2012, for review). It should be kept in mind that many of the involuntary movements can occur as side effects of pharmaceutical drugs.

1. EXAMINATION OF INVOLUNTARY MOVEMENTS

Involuntary movements can be examined systematically as shown in a flow chart (Figure 18-1). Physical examination of involuntary movements may be started by paying attention to the rhythmicity as to whether the movements in question repeat themselves at a steady rhythm (**rhythmic**) or with a steady interval between the movements (**periodic**), or whether they are **irregular**. The distinction between rhythmic and periodic movements may not be clear in some cases, especially when the movements are repeated at relatively high frequency. A typical example of rhythmic involuntary movement is **tremor**, and a typical example of periodic involuntary movements is periodic myoclonus as seen in Creutzfeldt-Jakob disease. **Myoclonus** is usually irregular, but it may appear

rhythmic when it repeats itself with short intervals. In this case, however, each individual movement may look shock-like and it can be confirmed by palpating the contracting muscle, whereas each movement of tremor is associated with relatively slow muscle contraction. Recording of the surface EMG is helpful for distinguishing the two conditions.

Most other involuntary movements occur irregularly. **Ballism (ballismus)** is a violent movement and is usually seen unilaterally (hemiballism [hemiballismus]). Among the involuntary movements associated with relatively slow muscle contraction, **athetosis** and **dystonia** are characterized by a twisting or writhing nature. **Dyskinesia** is composed of complex movements, and **chorea** is made of relatively simple movements.

When one encounters an involuntary movement, it is not always necessary to try to classify it into a known category. This is because some patients may have a mixed feature of more than one involuntary movement; for example, coexistence or mixture of tremor, myoclonus, and dystonia, and some patients may have a hitherto undescribed involuntary movement. What is most important is to precisely describe what is observed. If the examiner can describe the clinical manifestation appropriately, that will often lead to a correct diagnosis.

2. TREMOR

Tremor is characterized by repetition of the same movements at a certain pace (**rhythmicity**). Tremor was formerly described first in the 17th century, but its concept was established when Parkinson described **paralysis agitans** in 1817. In most cases of tremor, the surface EMG correlate of muscle contraction is usually a brief burst of action potentials. It commonly shows alternating contraction of agonist and antagonist muscles, but in some cases the agonist and antagonist contract almost at the same

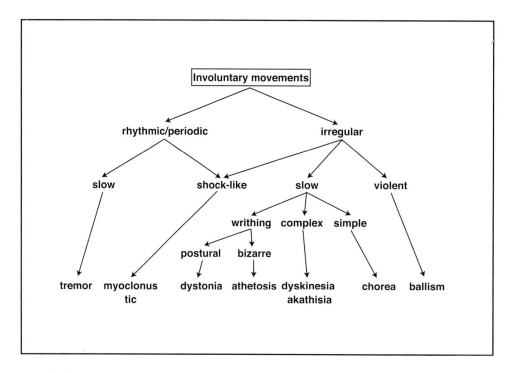

Figure 18-1 Classification of involuntary movements based on the clinical features, and an example flow of steps for visual inspection.

time, although not exactly synchronously. Furthermore, these EMG findings may vary depending on the clinical stage and the position of extremities. Even in a single case, reciprocal contraction may be seen in one hand and simultaneous contraction in the other hand at the same time (Figure 18-2). Tremor is largely classified into **physiological tremor** and pathological tremor, and **pathological**

tremor is classified into resting tremor, postural tremor, and action tremor (Deuschl et al, 2001, for review).

A. RESTING TREMOR

Tremor seen in the resting condition is called resting tremor. Resting tremor is commonly seen at about 5 Hz, and the

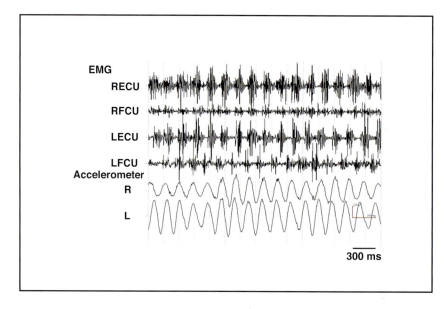

Figure 18-2 Records of the surface EMG and accelerometer in a patient with essential tremor. ECU: extensor carpi ulnaris muscle, FCU: flexor carpi ulnaris muscle. In the right hand (R), the wrist flexor and extensor muscles are contracting nearly at the same time while, in the left hand (L), they are contracting alternately. (Courtesy of Dr. Zoltan Mari)

typical resting tremor is seen in **Parkinson disease**. Similar resting tremor may be seen in parkinsonism other than idiopathic Parkinson disease, and its presence indicates a lesion or dysfunction of basal ganglia. "Resting" of the resting tremor does not imply psychological or emotional resting at all, because the resting tremor is rather enhanced by mental activity, emotional excitation, and physical exercises involving other parts of the body. For example, a patient with Parkinson disease may have no tremor when at complete rest, but once he/she starts talking or walking, the tremor often appears in hands. For another example, in a Parkinson patient having resting tremor in the right hand, the tremor may stop once he/she starts moving the right hand while the resting tremor may appear in the left hand. Physiologically, therefore, resting tremor is defined as a tremor seen in the muscles that are not actively contracting (Box 46). The resting tremor may be seen in the lips, which may be called **rabbit syndrome** because of its resemblance to the lips of a rabbit.

Generating Mechanism of Tremor in Parkinson Disease

Although the generating mechanism of tremor in Parkinson disease has not been completely clarified, it is considered to be mediated by the sensorimotor cortex. There is a significant correlation of frequency between the cortical rhythmic activities of the hand area of the motor cortex recorded by electroencephalogram (EEG) or magnetoencephalogram (MEG) and the EMG discharges of tremor of the contralateral hand (Figure 18-3). This phenomenon is called **corticomuscular coherence**. Here a question arises as to whether this correlation might be due to proprioceptive feedback from the peripheral muscle to the sensorimotor cortex as a result of the tremor. However, as a result of mathematical analysis, this cortical rhythm is believed to be a cause of tremor rather than its result. Namely, it is postulated that the tremor is driven by the cortical rhythm.

Although there is corticomuscular coherence in Parkinson tremor, the pacemaker of the tremor is thought to be subcortical with involvement of the basal ganglia but not in the sensorimotor cortex. In patients with Parkinson disease who have resting tremor, positive correlation has been found at the tremor frequency between the tremor of a hand and the neuronal discharge recorded from the contralateral subthalamic nucleus during deep brain stimulation (DBS) (Figure 18-4) (Wang et al, 2006). In a functional MRI study, functional correlation between the subthalamic nucleus and the ipsilateral sensorimotor cortex has been

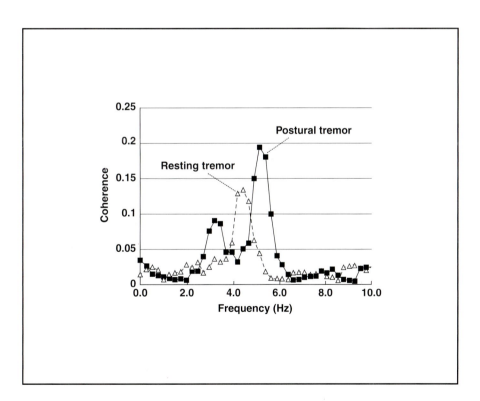

Figure 18-3 Coherence between EEG and EMG in a 78-year-old patient with essential tremor who developed Parkinson disease 50 years after the clinical onset of essential tremor. EMG discharges associated with resting tremor of a hand show a peak of coherence with EEG recorded from the contralateral central region at 4.3 Hz, and those associated with postural tremor show a peak of correlation at 5.2 Hz. (Modified from Inoue et al, 2007, with permission)

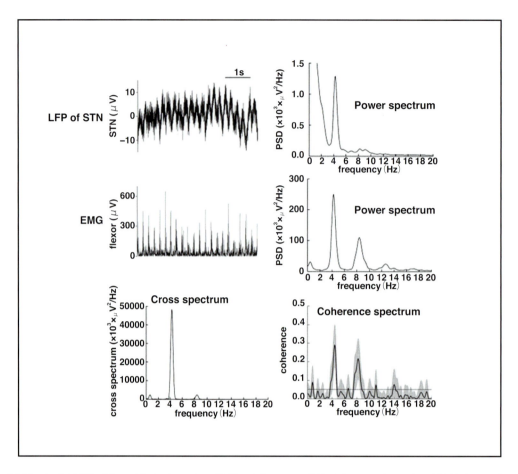

Figure 18-4 Local field potential (LFP) of the subthalamic nucleus (STN) and the tremor EMG of the contralateral hand (EMG) in a patient with Parkinson disease. Both LFP and EMG have maximum power at the peak frequency of 4.5 Hz, and there is a correlation between the two at that peak frequency. (Reproduced from Wang et al, 2006, with permission)

found greater in the Parkinson patients with tremor than those without tremor (Baudrexel et al, 2011).

Recently, a role of the cerebellum in the generation of tremor has drawn increasing attention. Clinically, deep brain stimulation of the Vim nucleus of the thalamus (cerebellar relay nucleus) is more effective for Parkinson tremor than that of the Vop nucleus (striatal relay nucleus). A functional MRI study of Parkinson patients with tremor by Helmich et al. (2011) showed that activity in the contralateral sensorimotor cortex, Vim, and ipsilateral cerebellum is increased in proportion to the magnitude of the resting tremor. In a study with transcranial magnetic stimulation (TMS), it was shown that the inhibitory effect of the cerebellum on the contralateral motor cortex is decreased in Parkinson patients (Ni et al, 2010). Recently, Helmich et al. (2012, for review) explained parkinsonian tremor as resulting from the combined actions of two circuits: the basal ganglia that trigger tremor episodes and the cerebello-thalamo-cortical circuit that produces the tremor.

B. POSTURAL TREMOR

Postural tremor is defined as a tremor seen while the corresponding extremity is assuming a certain posture, in other words during the isometric contraction of the corresponding muscles. Typical examples are seen in the hands while the upper extremities are kept extended forward or in the arms while they are kept in front of the chest with the elbows flexed, and in legs while the knees are kept flexed in the supine position. It usually starts a few seconds after taking a certain posture and increases in amplitude. In contrast, in patients with Parkinson disease, the resting tremor disappears after taking a certain posture and some seconds later it might reappear. This phenomenon is called **re-emergent tremor** (Jankovic et al, 1999).

Tremor seen in the hands while sitting in a chair with the hands placed on the knees is usually resting tremor, but essential tremor (see below) involving contraction of the proximal upper extremities may mechanically cause shaking of hands, which may resemble resting tremor of hands. In this case, it is useful to determine which muscles are actually contracting.

Essential Tremor

Essential tremor is the most common cause of postural tremor (Elble, 2006). It is commonly seen in hands at the frequency of 5 Hz on average. In the typical case of essential tremor, although the tremor may continue throughout motor execution like the nose-finger-nose test, it is especially pronounced when the movement stops at the nose or at the examiner's finger (Box 47).

Essential tremor often appears to be an autosomal dominant hereditary disease with high penetrance, but finding genes is proving very difficult. The age of onset varies from young adults to aged people. There are no significant movement abnormalities other than the tremor, although there might be a little ataxia or dystonia in some cases. Its progression is very slow, but it can cause a significant disability for daily life. Characteristically, essential tremor is ameliorated by ethanol intake (Box 48). Furthermore, about 20% of the patients with essential tremor also have migraine.

Pathophysiology of essential tremor has not been completely elucidated, but it is postulated, like the resting tremor in Parkinson disease, that it is also mediated by the sensorimotor cortex based on the demonstration of corticomuscular coherence (Figure 18-3).

The pacemaker of essential tremor is postulated to exist in the cerebellum. In patients with essential tremor, the neuronal discharge of the Vim nucleus of the thalamus (cerebellar relay nucleus) is increased with the same peak frequency as the tremor EMG of the contralateral hand, and both activities show a significant correlation at the same frequency (Figure 18-5). Furthermore, the tremor is suppressed by DBS of that thalamic region. A patient with essential tremor was reported in whom tremor disappeared and was replaced by ataxia and slow action tremor after hemorrhage in the ipsilateral cerebellar hemisphere (Rajput et al, 2008). Kinesiologic analysis of patients with essential tremor disclosed intention tremor and hypermetria suggesting cerebellar dysfunction. Furthermore, a functional neuroimaging study with positron emission tomography (PET) in patients with essential tremor revealed increased blood flow in the cerebellum and red nucleus at rest, and increased glucose metabolism in the cerebellum. Further, MR spectroscopy revealed a decrease in the ratio of N-acetyl aspartate/creatine in the cerebellar cortex. These findings are interpreted to suggest impairment of cerebellar cortex and disinhibition of the cerebellar efferent pathway. Furthermore, tremor induced in animals by harmaline is known to be suppressed by ethanol and β blockers, and in this condition increased neuronal activity was shown in the olivo-cerebellar system.

Recently an increasing number of autopsy cases of essential tremor have been reported. Axelrad et al. (2008) reported a decrease in the number of Purkinje cells in the cerebellum, but other reports have not shown consistent abnormalities in the cerebellum (Shill et al, 2008; Elble & Deuschl, 2011, for review; Symanski et al, 2014). A pathological study in 23 cases showed decreased parvalbumin, which is a marker of GABAergic neurons, in the locus coeruleus but no abnormality in the cerebellum (Shill et al, 2012). More recent pathological studies of essential tremor demonstrated significant reduction in dendritic complexity of Purkinje cells compared with normal age-matched control subjects (Louis et al, 2014).

There is increasing evidence suggesting an overlap between essential tremor and Parkinson disease (Jiménez-Jiménez et al, 2012, for review). However, this issue still remains controversial (Adler et al, 2011, for review).

Other Conditions Presenting with Postural Tremor

Tremor seen in **Wilson disease** is most commonly a typical postural tremor (Wilson, 1912). In this condition, the tremor mainly involves the distal upper extremities in the early clinical stage, but in the advanced stage it shows gross tremor in the arms, which is called **wing beating tremor**. The wing beating tremor may not be detected unless the arms are held in flexion in front of the chest or unless the legs are kept in flexion in the supine position or the legs are held apart in the sitting position.

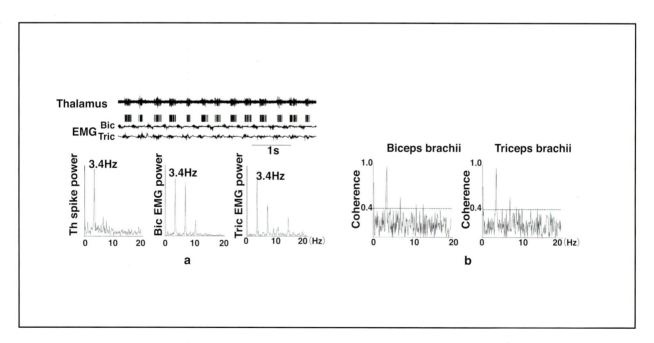

Figure 18-5 Simultaneous recording of neuronal discharge of the cerebellar relay nucleus of thalamus (Th) and the surface EMG associated with tremor of the contralateral hand and their frequency analysis (a) and correlation between the thalamic activity and the tremor EMG (b) in a patient with essential tremor. In (a), the thalamic data are shown both as a raw recording and then with another record below showing the firing of the identified neuron within the burst. Both the thalamic activity and the tremor EMG show peak frequency at 3.4 Hz, and the two activities show a significant correlation at the same frequency. (Courtesy of Professor Y. Katayama and Dr. K. Kobayashi of Department of Neurosurgery, Nihon University School of Medicine)

In contrast, tremor seen with hepatic encephalopathy is formed of repetitive drops of extended hands or extended fingers, and the term **asterixis** was coined by Adams and Foley in 1953 (Young & Shahani, 1986). This is caused by repetitive interruptions of EMG discharges of extensor muscles and is also called negative myoclonus. It is especially common in the state associated with hyperammonemia. The asterixis is different from the wing beating tremor of Wilson disease. The term "flapping" may be used to mean both wing beating tremor and asterixis, but this term may not be very appropriate.

Hyperthyroidism is also known to cause postural tremor. Thus, when a patient has tremor of undetermined cause, it is worthwhile checking the liver and thyroid functions. Whenever the wing beating tremor is encountered in young subjects, it is particularly important to test the blood level of ceruloplasmin and urinary copper. In Wilson disease, ceruloplasmin and total copper are decreased in the serum, and urinary excretion of copper is elevated (see also the section of dystonia).

Titubation

Oscillation of head in the anteroposterior or vertical direction in the standing position is called titubation. This phenomenon is seen in association with a cerebellar lesion and is considered to be a kind of postural tremor because it involves the neck and axial muscles during isometric contraction.

Physiological Tremor

In healthy subjects, fine tremor of fingers might be seen at a frequency of about 10 Hz when they hold the upper limbs straight forward, especially when the subjects are excited or nervous. Physiologically, both the mechanical factor and the central factor are considered to be involved in this tremor. Pure **mechanical tremor** is due to a resonance of the peripheral structures without involving muscle contraction, and thus it can be recorded with an accelerometer but not with EMG. By contrast, Parkinson tremor and essential tremor are **central tremors**. In **enhanced physiological tremor**, not only the mechanical but also the reflex mechanism is considered to be involved.

C. ACTION TREMOR

Tremor involving a muscle that is changing its length by isotonic contraction is called **action tremor**. Action tremors occur during kinetic or intentional movement (**kinetic tremor** or **intention tremor**). The intention tremor may be related to the fact that the excitability of motor cortex starts increasing before the actual movement starts. A typical example of action tremor is cerebellar tremor due to a lesion of the cerebellar efferent pathway or the dentatothalamic tract. It is usually seen in upper extremities as tremor of large amplitude. Its frequency varies but is most commonly about 3 Hz. The frequency tends to be low for action tremor involving the proximal muscles and relatively high for that of distal muscles. In most cases, cerebellar ataxia is also seen, but dysmetria is difficult to confirm because of the presence of tremor. Common causes of a lesion of the superior cerebellar peduncle are multiple sclerosis and vascular lesions (Boxes 49 and 50). A combination of scanning speech, intention tremor, and nystagmus was called the Charcot triad of multiple sclerosis.

Task-Specific Tremor

Tremor seen during execution of a specific task includes voice tremor, primary writing tremor, and orthostatic tremor. **Voice tremor** occurs in a subject who has to speak all the time, and the voice oscillates in its amplitude while speaking. **Primary writing tremor** is seen in the hand only when writing. These conditions may be variants of focal dystonia. Shaking of legs while standing is called **orthostatic tremor** and is seen in patients with Parkinson disease, parkinsonism, essential tremor, and cerebellar ataxia, but the underlying condition of undetermined etiology is called **primary orthostatic tremor** (Mestre et al, 2012; Hassan

---

BOX 49 TREMOR CAUSED BY MIDBRAIN LESION

Infarction involving the medial part of the midbrain causes complex tremor composed of resting, postural, and kinetic tremor at a frequency of less than 4.5 Hz in the contralateral upper extremity. Resting tremor is caused by a lesion of the nigrostriatal pathway in the midbrain tegmentum, and postural and kinetic tremor is due to a lesion of the dentatothalamic tract or red nucleus. This tremor complex corresponds to Holmes' tremor (Gajos et al, 2010; Raina et al, 2016). It may also be called "peduncular rubral tremor" (Remy et al, 1995), but this terminology might be a little confusing. The resting tremor in this condition responds to L-dopa in some cases. If unilateral oculomotor nerve palsy is associated with involuntary movement in the contralateral extremity, it is called Benedikt syndrome (see Chapter 9-1A and Table 8-1).

et al, 2016). The condition is primarily seen while standing still, and little if any during walking or during other activities. Recording with the surface EMG discloses symmetric oscillation at 13 ~ 18 Hz not only in the legs but also in the upper limbs. Treatment with gabapentin or clonazepam has been reported to be effective. Occurrence among siblings has been reported (Virmani et al, 2012).

3. CHOREA

Chorea is formed of irregular, relatively quick movements involving the hands, mouth, and tongue, and is characterized in the beginning by a quasi-purposive appearance. In other words, the movement may appear purposeful and can be easily imitated. Sydenham in 1686 described small movements of fingers, toes, and lips in children with rheumatic fever (**Sydenham chorea**). This form of chorea is different from the gross dancing movements described by Huntington in 1872.

Hereditary diseases presenting with chorea include Huntington disease, neuroacanthocytosis, and dentato-rubro-pallido-luysian atrophy. **Huntington disease** is a representative form of autosomal dominant hereditary disease and is characterized by chorea and progressive cognitive decline which often starts in the 30s (Box 51). It is due to a triplet repeat of the huntingtin gene, and its main pathological abnormality includes neuronal degeneration of the caudate nucleus and atrophy of the frontal lobe. In patients with young onset, rigidity may predominate over other symptoms.

Neuroacanthocytosis (chorea-acanthocytosis, Levine-Critchley syndrome) can be clinically similar to Huntington disease, but its mode of inheritance is variable. Its X-linked form is called McLeod syndrome. It is characterized by acanthocytosis in the peripheral blood, and the orolingual chorea is so severe that it often causes tongue bite (see Figure 3-14). **Dentato-rubro-pallido-luysian**

atrophy (**DRPLA**) is an autosomal dominant hereditary disease and shows myoclonus, generalized convulsions, cognitive decline, chorea, and cerebellar ataxia. It is caused by abnormal expansion of a CAG repeat and its gene product is atrophin-1. The main clinical picture is different depending on the age of onset. Patients with onset in childhood show myoclonus, generalized convulsion, and mental deterioration, whereas those with adult onset tend to show chorea and cerebellar ataxia in addition to myoclonus.

Symptomatic Chorea

Chorea may be seen in a variety of systemic conditions such as vascular disease of basal ganglia, rheumatic fever, pregnancy (chorea gravidarum), thyrotoxic chorea, and senile chorea. It is also important to note that chorea can occur as a side effect of neuroleptics. Chorea seen in association with rheumatic fever (**Syndenham chorea**) is considered to be caused by an autoimmune mechanism against striatal antigen in relation to streptococcal infection. A series of conditions seen in children in association with streptococcal infection is coined **pediatric autoimmune neuropsychiatric disorders associated with streptococcal infection (PANDAS)** (Brilot et al, 2011), but many experts do not believe that this is really a definable separate syndrome.

A question as to whether chorea is, like essential tremor and Parkinson tremor, mediated by the sensorimotor cortex or not has not been solved. As D2-blocker is effective on chorea in most cases, it is considered that a relative hyperexcitable state of the dopaminergic system is postulated for the underlying mechanism. The central monoamine inhibitor tetrabenazine has been reported to be effective for chorea.

4. BALLISM

Gross violent movements of extremities that look like throwing out or kicking away were first described as ballism(us) by Greiff in 1883. It is commonly caused by a vascular lesion of the subthalamic nucleus or striatum and thus involves contralateral upper and lower limbs (**hemiballism**). Vigorous muscle contractions irregularly involve the shoulder and pelvic girdles and the proximal limbs. It may be so severe that the patient may fall down from bed, and if hemiballism continues, it may even be life threatening. However, it usually responds to medication with diazepam or a D2-blocker like haloperidol. In the chronic stage, each movement becomes less violent and resembles chorea, although it still involves primarily the proximal muscles.

Ballism-like involuntary movements can be seen as a manifestation of a transient ischemic attack (TIA), and it is called **limb-shaking TIA**. It is commonly seen in patients with marked narrowing or occlusion of the internal carotid artery, and gross violent movements involve the contralateral upper or lower extremity, lasting less than 5 minutes. It is often induced by physical activities like standing up and may be accompanied by mild hemiparesis. Its underlying mechanism is undetermined, but it is postulated to be related to a hemodynamic disturbance (Persoon et al, 2010).

Hemichorea-hemiballism is seen in patients with uncontrolled diabetes mellitus, especially the **nonketotic hyperglycemic state** (Li & Chen, 2015). They may show high signal intensity lesions in the striatum on T1-weighted MRI.

5. ATHETOSIS

Athetosis was described by Hammond in 1871 as irregular, slow, writhing movements seen in hands and feet. The movement is often bizarre and cannot be imitated. It is caused by an organic lesion of the striatum, including cerebral palsy, a residual state of encephalitis or anoxic encephalopathy. In these conditions, athetosis is commonly seen in combination with dystonia. Indeed, there may not really be any important physiological difference between athetosis and dystonia.

6. DYSTONIA

In many cases of dystonia, the affected part of the body shows abnormal posture of a writhing nature in the resting condition, and slow, writhing involuntary movements are superimposed on the abnormal posture upon voluntary movement. In many other cases, there is no dystonia at rest, but only action dystonia. For childhood-onset patients, dystonia is generalized and mainly involves the trunk and proximal extremities (**generalized dystonia**), but there is also **focal dystonia**, which is usually of adult onset. Focal dystonia includes **blepharospasm**, **oromandibular dystonia**, **cervical dystonia (spasmodic torticollis)**, **spasmodic dysphonia**, **writer's cramp**, **musician's cramp**, and so forth. Writer's cramp and musician's cramp of the hand are put together as **focal hand dystonia**.

At the early clinical stage of blepharospasm and cervical dystonia, repetitive phasic movements like blinks and neck rotation, respectively, may predominate, resembling tremor. In the advanced stage, the eyelids can not be opened and the neck might remain rotated. In writer's cramp, tremor and myoclonus may superimpose onto the dystonia.

Writer's cramp and musician's cramp occur only when writing or only when playing a specific musical instrument, respectively, at least in the early clinical stage. This **task specificity** is characteristic of focal dystonia. For example, a patient with **embouchure dystonia** (lips) suffers from oral dystonia only when playing a certain kind of pipes but not when playing other kinds of pipes (Haslinger et al, 2010). Hand tremor occurring only when writing is called primary writing tremor, and this phenomenon might be caused by the same mechanism as focal dystonia.

The condition in which blepharospasm and oropharyngeal dystonia are combined is called **cranial dystonia** (formerly called Meige syndrome). In this condition, the bulbar muscles may show abnormal contraction while speaking or swallowing, causing **spasmodic dysphonia** and **spasmodic dysphagia**, respectively (see Chapter 14-7). Abrupt interruption of hitting movement of golf club (**yips**) may be another example of task specific dystonia.

Functional Abnormality of the Sensorimotor Cortex in Focal Dystonia

Functional abnormality of the somatosensory cortex and the motor cortex, or abnormality of functional coupling between the two cortical areas has been proposed as the pathophysiology of focal dystonia. For example, in patients with musician's cramp, fusion of finger areas in the primary somatosensory cortex has been demonstrated by an MEG study (Figure 18-6). A TMS study showed a decrease in the GABA-A mediated inhibitory functions in the primary motor cortex. A question as to whether these abnormalities of the sensorimotor cortex are a cause of focal dystonia or

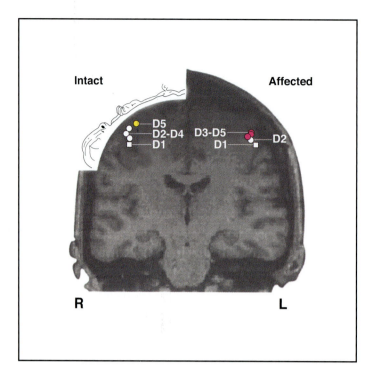

Figure 18-6 Abnormal somatotopic organization in the primary somatosensory cortex in a patient with musician's cramp, demonstrated by recording of the somatosensory evoked magnetic field following stimulation of each individual finger. Areas corresponding to the digit 1-5 (D1-D5) are separate in the intact cortex but fused in the affected cortex. (Reproduced from Elbert et al, 1998, with permission)

a plastic change secondary to dystonia has not been completely solved (Box 52).

Fixed Dystonia

The condition in which an extremity is fixed in a dystonic posture is called **fixed posture dystonia** or **fixed dystonia** (Figure 18-7). Sometimes it is fixed so hard that it is impossible to passively return it to the normal position. It is common in young females, and it often follows trauma or complex regional pain syndrome (Schrag et al, 2004). It is usually localized, but it may spread widely. Its most common cause is considered to be psychogenic (Hawley & Weiner, 2011, for review), but it may be an organic disorder modified by a psychogenic factor. In some cases of typical fixed dystonia, an excitability study of the motor cortex by TMS disclosed abnormal inhibitory function, which may suggest that those patients may have a predisposition to dystonia (Avanzino et al, 2008).

Sensory Trick

A phenomenon called **sensory trick** is another characteristic feature of focal dystonia (Ramos et al, 2014, for review). It is commonly seen in cervical dystonia. For example, as soon as the back of the patient's head is touched by the examiner's hand or by the patient's own hand, or as soon as the patient stands against a wall to which the head is attached, the head returns to normal position. Sometimes, the head might return to normal position even before the actual touching if the patient can predict the touching. In patients with blepharospasm, rubbing the forehead may help opening the eyelids. The mechanism underlying the sensory trick has not been fully elucidated. In some cases, intended movement of adjacent muscles might be effective (**motor trick**). For example, a patient with blepharospasm might learn to move his/her own mouth to help opening the eyelids.

Furthermore, some paradoxical phenomena might be seen in patients with generalized dystonia. Patients having great difficulty in walking forward because of generalized dystonia might be able to run forward or to walk backward or sideways more easily. This might be another manifestation of task specificity.

Causes of Generalized Dystonia

Generalized dystonia is seen in organic lesions of striatum such as cerebral palsy, Wilson disease, residual state of encephalitis, Creutzfeldt-Jakob disease, and hereditary or

GENERATING MECHANISM OF DYSTONIA

Generalized dystonia is considered to be caused by abnormal function of the sensorimotor cortex secondary to an organic lesion of basal ganglia. Deep brain stimulation of the internal segment of globus pallidus (GPi) is known to improve dystonia (Sako et al, 2008). In focal dystonia, by contrast, functional abnormality of the sensorimotor cortex as a result of plastic change is considered to play a major role (Abbruzzese & Berardelli, 2011, Hallett, 2011, and Quartarone & Hallett, 2013, for review). For example, writer's cramp is common among people who are engaged in writing, and musician's cramp commonly affects musicians who play a special kind of musical instrument over a long period of time. Furthermore, in patients with musician's cramp, fusion of finger areas in the primary somatosensory cortex has been demonstrated by an MEG study (Figure 18-6), and a TMS study showed a decrease in the GABA-A-mediated inhibitory functions in the primary motor cortex (Hallett, 2011 for review). In relation to these clinical observations, Merzenich and his group trained monkeys to continue strain hand movements, and they observed motor deterioration in the hand and physiological abnormality in the sensorimotor cortex. These findings suggest development of plastic change in the sensorimotor cortex as a result of continuous strain exercise. Although a possibility of these changes being secondary to the long-standing dystonia remains, it is more plausible to consider these plastic changes as a cause of dystonia.

Intramuscular injection of botulinum toxin is effective in many cases of focal dystonia (Hallett et al, 2013, for review). This effect is likely produced both by weakening the muscles directly related to dystonia and by changing the excitability of the sensorimotor cortex (Dresel et al, 2011).

sporadic neurodegenerative diseases primarily affecting the basal ganglia. It is especially common in patients who are taking antipsychotic drugs for a long period of time (**tardive dystonia**). It should be kept in mind that patients with focal dystonia might develop generalized dystonia during the clinical course, and it is especially so in subjects having a DYT1 gene mutation.

As **Wilson disease** is a treatable condition if the diagnosis is made early enough, its possibility should be considered whenever young subjects present with dystonia of undetermined etiology or postural tremor (Figure 18-8). Diagnosis can be made by finding a Kayser-Fleischer ring in the cornea due to copper deposit and a decrease of the blood ceruloplasmin. Although extremely rare, patients with Wilson

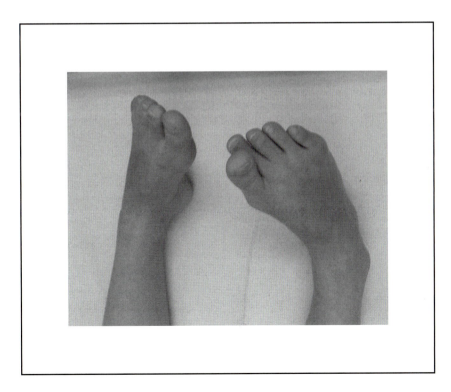

Figure 18-7 Fixed dystonia of the right leg following the posttraumatic complex regional pain syndrome. (Courtesy of Dr. Takahiro Mezaki)

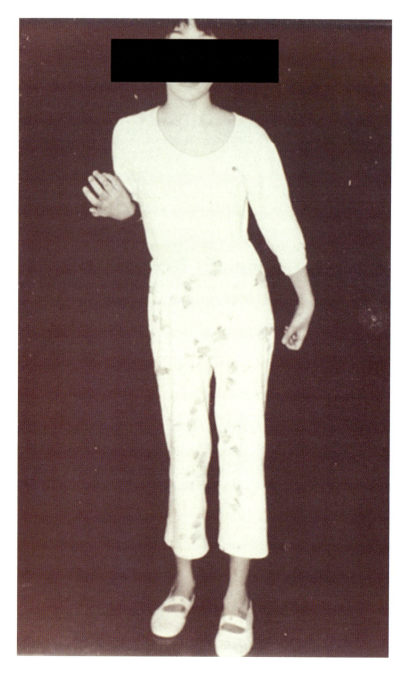

Figure 18-8 Abnormal posture of a patient with generalized dystonia due to Wilson disease. (Courtesy of the Department of Neurology, Kyushu University)

disease may have neither a Kayser-Fleischer ring nor a decreased ceruloplasmin level, in which case measurement of urinary copper or liver biopsy may be warranted.

Hereditary Dystonia

A number of hereditary disorders presenting with dystonia have been reported, and genetic abnormalities have been disclosed in many of them (Charlesworth et al, 2013, for review). **Torsion dystonia** was first reported by Oppenheim in 1911 as dystonia musculorum deformans. This is inherited in an autosomal dominant trait and is called **DYT1** with torsin gene mutation, but sporadic cases are not rare. The age of onset varies from childhood to young adults, and clinical forms are also variable. In some cases, the clinical symptoms may begin with focal dystonia and later spread to develop generalized dystonia. Muscles of the cranial nerve territory are rarely involved at first. Like the cases of hereditary myoclonus-dystonia syndrome (Box 53), DYT1 is often associated with depression. DYT6 due to mutation of THAP1 is also common.

There are three types of hereditary dopamine-responsive dystonia: **hereditary progressive dystonia with marked diurnal fluctuation (Segawa's disease), autosomal recessive dopamine-responsive dystonia with Segawa syndrome,** and **sepiapterin reductase deficiency.** Segawa's disease is autosomal dominant due to mutation of GTP cyclohydrolase I gene, and it occurs in childhood (Figure 18-9). It is characterized by marked improvement of the symptoms immediately after awakening from sleep. Sepiapterin reductase deficiency occurs in infancy or childhood with motor and language delays, axial hypotonia, dystonia, weakness, oculogyric crises, and diurnal fluctuation of symptoms with sleep benefit (Friedman et al, 2012).

X-kinked recessive dystonia-parkinsonism (DYT3) seen in the Philippines is called lubag (meaning "twisted"). Clinically, the patients present with dystonia, but later during the clinical course parkinsonism predominates. Pathologically, Goto et al. (2013) found a decrease in the number of neuropeptide Y-positive cells in the striatum. **Pantothenate kinase-associated neurodegeneration (PKAN)** is known as a neurodegeneration with brain iron accumulation (NBIA) and includes a condition previously named Hallervorden-Spatz syndrome (see Box 28). **Beta-propeller protein associated neurodegeneration (BPAN)** is another form of NBIA, which is characterized by learning disability and progressive gait abnormalities from childhood followed by progressive dystonia in adulthood (Paudel et al, 2015). **Machado-Joseph disease** is a type of spinocerebellar degeneration (SCA3) with ataxin as the gene product, but in some cases dystonia may be a predominant clinical sign (see Chapter 16-2C) (Box 53).

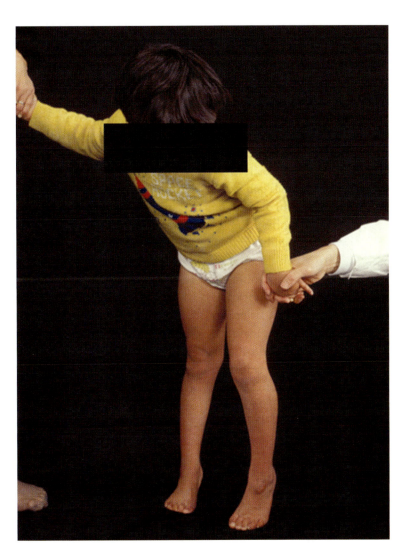

Figure 18-9 Dystonic posture of the left leg in a patient with Segawa's disease. (Courtesy of the Department of Neurology, Kyushu University)

HEREDITARY MYOCLONUS-DYSTONIA SYNDROME

This is an autosomal dominant hereditary disease characterized by myoclonus and dystonia occurring in childhood or puberty. It is not always progressive, and some cases might have a relatively benign clinical course.

Dystonia is generalized while myoclonus mainly involves the trunk and proximal extremities. In most cases, myoclonus and dystonia occur independently, but in some cases myoclonus and dystonia may appear in combination (myoclonic dystonia or dystonic myoclonus). **Mutation of the epsilon-sarcoglycan gene** has been found in many families with this condition (Nardocci et al, 2008). The symptoms may improve after ethanol intake. Patients with this disease may also have depression. Electrophysiological studies of many cases of this syndrome disclosed no evidence of cortical origin for myoclonus (Roze et al, 2008). This condition might have been included among the cases previously diagnosed as familial essential myoclonus. **Tyrosine hydroxylase deficiency** is another cause of familial myoclonus-dystonia syndrome, but this is transmitted in an autosomal recessive fashion (Stamelou et al, 2012a).

7. DYSKINESIA

Dyskinesia is often used to encompass complex involuntary movements that do not fit into another category. Dyskinesia is characterized by relatively quick, irregular involuntary movements involving lips, tongue, extremities, and trunk, and is often caused by pharmaceutical drugs. Focal dyskinesia is commonly seen in the lips and tongue (**orolingual dyskinesia** or **oral dyskinesia**). Orolingual dyskinesia is also commonly induced by drugs (**tardive dyskinesia**), but it may also be due to multiple small infarctions in the striatum. This type of dyskinesia is also common among aged subjects, and its etiology is often undetermined.

The condition in which a patient cannot keep sitting still is called **akathisia**. Akathisia is commonly induced by long-term administration of antipsychotic drugs or L-dopa. It is important to prevent this condition, because, once it develops, it may be resistant to drug control.

A common side effect seen in patients with Parkinson disease during L-dopa treatment is dyskinesia (see Box 41). Since this phenomenon is more common in relatively young patients with Parkinson disease, a dopamine agonist may be preferred for young patients instead of L-dopa. It is believed that L-dopa acts on both the D2 and D1 receptors, whereas the commonly used dopamine agonists act predominantly on the D2 receptor (Box 54).

HEREDITARY PAROXYSMAL DYSKINESIA

This is an autosomal dominant hereditary disorder characterized by paroxysmal attacks of dystonic, choreic, and ballistic movements, which was previously called paroxysmal kinesigenic choreoathetosis. The age at onset is commonly in puberty, and it is more common in males than in females. It is often the case that the patient's father might not have been aware of his own trouble until he sees the same problem in his son. Three forms are recognized in this category. One is a brief episode induced by sudden movement or intention to move (**paroxysmal kinesigenic dyskinesia, PKD**). The second form is **paroxysmal nonkinesigenic dyskinesia (PNKD)**, in which the attacks are triggered by coffee, alcohol, mental stress, and fatigue. The third form is **paroxysmal exercise-induced dyskinesia (PED)**, which is induced by prolonged exercise. At least four genes have been identified including proline-rich transmembrane protein 2 (PRRT2) which typically causes PKD, but there is no complete phenotype-genotype correlation (Wang et al, 2011; Méneret et al, 2012; Erro et al, 2014; Huang et al, 2015). A functional MRI study disclosed increased activity in putamen during the intervals, suggesting a possibility of epileptic dysfunction (Zhou et al, 2010). A small dose of carbamazepine is effective except for the paroxysmal exercise-induced dyskinesia. These conditions may belong to the category of ion channel disorder, but this is not clear (see Chapter 25-4A).

8. MYOCLONUS

Myoclonus is defined as shock-like involuntary movements of face and extremities. It was first described in 1881 by Friedreich, who reported a case with the term "Paramyoklonus multiplex" (Friedreich, 1881). Myoclonus is usually caused by abrupt, instantaneous contraction of muscles (**positive myoclonus**), but it can also be caused by transient interruption of ongoing muscle contraction (**negative myoclonus**). In fact, the two kinds of myoclonus often occur in combination, namely an abrupt muscle contraction immediately followed by a silent period of muscle discharge, or vice versa. Negative myoclonus is also called asterixis. Asterixis was originally described for hand tremor seen in patients with hepatic encephalopathy, but nowadays this term is also used for nonrhythmic negative myoclonus.

Involuntary movements fulfilling the criteria of myoclonus can also occur in physiological situations such as **hiccup** and **nocturnal myoclonus**. Nocturnal myoclonus is a shock-like movement seen unilaterally during the early stage of sleep. It is distinguished from periodic limb movement in sleep (PLMS) (see Chapter 24-3E) in that nocturnal myoclonus is more shock-like and not periodic.

Myoclonus can be classified into three types depending on its estimated sites of origin: cortical, brainstem, and spinal, but some myoclonia remain unclassified (Shibasaki & Hallett, 2005, and Shibasaki, 2007a, 2007b, for review). There might be myoclonus originating from the thalamus, basal ganglia, and cerebellum, but if any, those are estimated to be mediated by the sensorimotor cortex, and thus those might be classified into a category of cortical myoclonus.

A. MYOCLONUS OF CORTICAL ORIGIN

Cortical myoclonus in most cases is considered to be based on the abnormal increased excitability of the primary motor cortex (MI). Physiologically, myoclonus of the hand is preceded by a cortical spike generated in the hand area of the contralateral MI and is caused by abrupt contraction of the hand muscle via the fast conducting corticospinal tract (Figure 18-10) (Shibasaki & Hallett, 2005, and Shibasaki, 2012, for review). Thus, cortical myoclonus is commonly seen in the fingers, feet, and face, which are innervated by a large area of MI. If multiple sites of MI are activated, myoclonus involves the

corresponding multiple sites, and as the cortical discharge spreads within MI, myoclonus may also spread to adjacent muscles rapidly.

Excitability of MI can be studied by TMS. By using a paired stimulus with the interstimulus interval of several milliseconds (ms), impairment of GABA-Aergic intracortical inhibition has been demonstrated in cortical myoclonus. A similar phenomenon is seen also in focal dystonia, but Hanajima et al. (2008) found a qualitatively different abnormality in the inhibitory system between the two conditions.

Cortical Reflex Myoclonus

In most cases of cortical myoclonus, the excitability of the primary somatosensory cortex (SI) is also abnormally enhanced, and the incoming stimulus from the periphery produces a **giant evoked potential** and a reflex myoclonus through a **transcortical reflex** mechanism (Shibasaki & Hallett, 2005, for review). This is called **cortical reflex myoclonus** as against **spontaneous cortical myoclonus**, and both conditions are considered to be caused by involvement of MI either spontaneously or by the reflex mechanism (Figure 18-10). Most myoclonus epilepsies are considered to be caused by involvement of the whole strip of MI by this epileptogenic discharge. Thus, cortical myoclonus may be

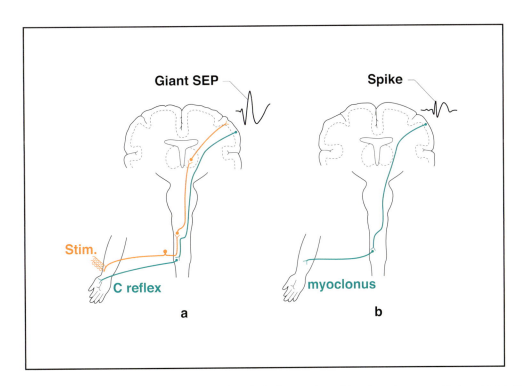

Figure 18-10 Schematic illustration showing generating mechanism of cortical reflex myoclonus (a) and spontaneous cortical myoclonus (b). Giant SEP: giant somatosensory evoked potential, Stim.: stimulus, C reflex: cortical reflex mediated by the transcortical reflex loop.

TABLE 18-1 CAUSES OF CORTICAL MYOCLONUS

1. Progressive myoclonus epilepsy
2. Juvenile myoclonic epilepsy
3. Postanoxic myoclonus
4. Alzheimer disease
5. Creutzfeldt-Jakob disease (in advanced stage)
6. Metabolic encephalopathy (especially uremia)
7. Corticobasal degeneration
8. Olivo-ponto-cerebellar atrophy
9. Rett syndrome

TABLE 18-3 GENE ABNORMALITIES OF PROGRESSIVE MYOCLONUS EPILEPSY

Disease	Inheritance	Chromosome	Gene	Protein
U-L	AR	21q22.3	CSTB	Cystatin B
Lafora	AR	6q24	EPM2A	Laforin
		6q22	NHLRC1	
MERRF	Mat.	mtDNA	MTTK	tRNALys
Sialidosis				
Type 1	AR	6p21.3	NEU1	Sialidase 1
Type 2	AR	20	NEU1	Sialidase 1
DRPLA	AD	12p13.31	DRPLA	Atrophin 1
NCL (5 types)	AR			

U-L: Unverricht-Lundborg disease, MERFF: myoclonus epilepsy associated with ragged-red fibers, DRPLA: dentato-rubro-pallido-luysian atrophy, NCL: neuronal ceroid lipofuscinosis (Williams & Mole, 2012 for classification of NCL), AR: autosomal recessive, Mat.: maternal inheritance, AD: autosomal dominant. (Modified from Shahwan et al, 2005)

called **epileptic myoclonus**. Reflex myoclonus may be also elicited by photic stimulus (**photic cortical reflex myoclonus**) (Shibasaki & Neshige, 1987).

Causes of Cortical Myoclonus

Cortical myoclonus is seen in a variety of conditions (Table 18-1), and there is no disease specificity. Its representative condition is a group of diseases categorized into **progressive myoclonus epilepsy**, which includes a variety of hereditary neurodegenerative diseases and metabolic abnormalities (Table 18-2). Recently, gene abnormalities have been identified in many of these diseases (Table 18- 3) (Franceschetti et al, 2014, for review) (Boxes 55, 56 and 57).

Negative Myoclonus

Cortical myoclonus and cortical reflex myoclonus are usually positive, but negative myoclonus is also seen in some cases, either alone or in combination with positive myoclonus. Negative myoclonus of cortical origin is often generated by a transcortical reflex mechanism (**cortical reflex negative myoclonus**) (Shibasaki et al, 1994). It has to be kept in mind that negative myoclonus is often caused as a side effect of pharmaceutical drugs, especially anticonvulsants. Unilateral negative myoclonus is seen in patients with infarction in the contralateral thalamus (**thalamic asterixis**) (Tatu et al, 2000) (Boxes 58 and 59).

Postanoxic myoclonus (Lance-Adams syndrome) may also present with a mixture of positive and negative myoclonus, and is mostly considered to be of cortical origin (Lance & Adams, 1963; Shibasaki, 2010, for review). This condition is commonly encountered and is difficult to treat, but anticonvulsants, including levetiracetam, can be effective.

TABLE 18-2 CAUSES OF PROGRESSIVE MYOCLONUS EPILEPSY

1. Unverricht-Lundborg disease
2. Lafora disease
3. Neuronal ceroid lipofuscinosis
4. Mitochondrial encephalomyopathy*
5. Sialidosis
6. Dentato-rubro-pallido-luysian atrophy (DRPLA)
7. Benign adult familial myoclonus epilepsy (BAFME)
8. Angelman syndrome

* Myoclonus epilepsy associated with ragged-red fibers (MERRF, Fukuhara disease)

BOX 55 UNVERRICHT-LUNDBORG DISEASE

This is an autosomal recessive hereditary disease previously called ataxia cerebellaris myoclonica or Ramsay Hunt syndrome. It is characterized by progressive postural and action myoclonus, cerebellar ataxia, generalized convulsions, and mental deterioration starting between 6 and 14 years of age. Mutation of the CSTB gene (previously called EPM1) on chromosome 21q22 was found (Hyppönen et al, 2015). Some cases also show ocular motor apraxia, dystonia, and marked dementia (Chew et al, 2008).

It is important to note that cortical myoclonus is not nec-essarily due to an organic brain lesion. In uremic encephalop-athy, for example, typical positive myoclonus and negative myoclonus of cortical origin are seen, and they may improve completely after the treatment with dialysis. There might be cases of uremia whose myoclonus is of brainstem origin.

B. MYOCLONUS OF BRAINSTEM ORIGIN

Palatal tremor (previously called palatal myoclonus) (Box 60), reticular reflex myoclonus, startle disease, opso-clonus, and intractable hiccup belong to this category.

Reticular reflex myoclonus was first described by Hallett et al. (1977) in posthypoxic patients. In response to auditory or somatosensory stimulus, muscle contraction starts in the sternocleidomastoid and trapezius muscles and spreads rostrally to involve the facial muscles and caudally to involve extremity muscles (Figure 18-11).

Startle disease is an excessive startle reaction elicited by unexpected, sudden stimulus, and is considered to be an abnormal enhancement of an ordinary startle reflex. In this case, the response begins in the orbicularis oculi muscles and spreads generally. Familial occurrence of this condition by autosomal dominant transmission is called **hyperekplexia**. In many of these families, mutation of

UNILATERAL ASTERIXIS DUE TO THALAMIC LESION

Patients with a vascular lesion in the lateral thalamus may show asterixis in the contralateral hand. Many of those cases also show ataxia and loss of superficial as well as proprioceptive sense in the contralateral extremities, suggesting the presence of a lesion in the motor thalamus (Vim nucleus) and the sensory relay nucleus (see Chapter 27-1,2). Two cases of thalamic asterixis were reported in whom the β EEG rhythm was increased over the contralateral central region in association with each asterixis, which might suggest an increased inhibitory mechanism of the corresponding motor cortex (Inoue et al, 2012b). These findings suggest that thalamic asterixis is mediated by the sensorimotor cortex, probably as a result of impairment of the input from the cerebellar dentate nucleus to the motor cortex.

the gene coding the α1 or β subunit of inhibitory glycine receptor has been demonstrated (see Chapter 25-1A and Table 25-1) (Box 61).

Myoclonus of brainstem origin tends to be resistant to medical treatment. **Opsoclonus** (see Chapter 9-5D) has been treated symptomatically with clonazepam and gabapentin with some effect. Opsoclonus caused by an autoimmune pathogenesis including a paraneoplastic syndrome may be treated with plasmapheresis or intravenous administration of immunoglobulin (IVIg). For **essential palatal tremor**, the ear click can be symptomatic; no drug therapy

TRANSIENT MYOCLONIC STATE WITH ASTERIXIS IN ELDERLY PATIENTS

Hashimoto et al. (1992) reported seven aged patients who showed transient episodes of asterixis with the name of "transient myoclonic state with asterixis in elderly patients." In this condition, both positive and negative myoclonus are seen mainly in the upper extremities and spontaneously disappear in a week or two, but it may recur. It responds well to clonazepam. No metabolic abnormality or history of drug use was identified. A short burst of spike-and-wave complexes is seen on EEG over the central region in association with the asterixis, suggesting cortical origin. This condition is common in Japan, and so far there has been no report of similar conditions from other countries. Although there is no familial occurrence, it may be a kind of ion channel disorder just like benign adult familial myoclonus epilepsy (Box 56).

PALATAL TREMOR AND GUILLAIN-MOLLARET TRIANGLE

Palatal tremor is rhythmic vertical oscillation of the soft palate at frequency of about 3 Hz. It used to be called palatal myoclonus, but in a symposium of the first international congress of Movement Disorder Society organized by one of the authors (MH) in Washington, DC, in 1990, another author (HS) presented a case of palatal myoclonus due to brainstem lesion on video and suggested that the movement might fit the characteristics of tremor rather than myoclonus. At that time, Professor C. D. Marsden, as the chairman of the symposium, motioned for voting, and as a result the new term was approved by a majority of the audience. Palatal tremor is divided into symptomatic and essential groups. **Symptomatic palatal tremor** is caused by a lesion involving any part of the Guillain-Mollaret triangle, but most commonly by a lesion of the central tegmental tract in the pons, and then by a cerebellar lesion (Deuschl et al, 1994; Jang & Borruat, 2014). In this case, enlargement of the inferior olive is commonly observed on MRI, which is considered to be due to trans-synaptic degeneration. This condition is sometimes associated with synchronous vertical oscillation of eyes (ocular myoclonus) (see Chapter 9-5D), and in some cases it is also associated with rhythmic involuntary movements at the same frequency in the neck and/or upper extremities. Repetitive, rhythmic, slow (1-4 Hz) movement mainly affecting cranial and limb muscles is sometimes called **myorhythmia**, and this condition is due to various etiologies including Whipple disease (Baizabal-Carvallo et al, 2015, for review).

The **Guillain-Mollaret triangle** is a circuit connecting the cerebellar dentate nucleus with the contralateral inferior olive via the superior cerebellar peduncle and the central tegmental tract and back to the dentate nucleus via the inferior cerebellar peduncle. It is known that parvocellular neurons of the red nucleus receive main afferents from the contralateral dentate nucleus and send main efferents to the ipsilateral inferior olive through the central tegmental tract (see Brodal, 2010). However, it is also believed that there is a direct pathway from the dentate nucleus to the contralateral inferior olive, which passes by the red nucleus without forming synapses (Lapresle & Ben Hamida, 1970). In view of the occurrence of pseudohypertrophy of the inferior olive following not only a lesion of the central tegmental tract but also a lesion of the cerebellum, involvement of the direct dentato-olivary tract is more likely to play a primary role in generation of symptomatic palatal tremor.

Patients with **essential palatal tremor** often complain of hearing ear clicking due to periodic contraction of the tensor veli palatini muscle (Deuschl et al, 1994). Recently, it has been reported that many cases of essential palatal tremor are likely psychogenic (Richardson et al, 2006; Stamelou et al, 2012b). Local injection of botulinum toxin can be used for its treatment.

has been consistently effective, but injection of botulinum toxin may be useful (Box 60). **Hiccup** is a physiological myoclonus involving the diaphragm, but long-lasting, medically intractable hiccup is certainly abnormal, and may be caused by a lesion of the medulla oblongata. Various drugs including gabapentin, baclofen, olanzapine, and midazolam have been tried for intractable hiccup with some effect.

C. MYOCLONUS OF SPINAL CORD ORIGIN

There are two kinds of spinal myoclonus; spinal segmental myoclonus and propriospinal myoclonus. **Spinal segmental myoclonus** is irregular or periodic positive myoclonus localized to the muscles innervated by one or two spinal segments, and it is stimulus-sensitive in some cases. Although its etiology is not always identifiable, some cases are thought to have myelitis. Prognosis is favorable with good response to clonazepam.

Propriospinal myoclonus manifests irregular shock-like movements of the trunk, mainly causing abrupt flexion of the trunk. Physiologically, it is characterized by slow spread from a certain thoracic segment to rostral as well as caudal segments. It may be stimulus-sensitive and often requires differentiation from a psychogenic disorder, which now seems the most frequent etiology (Kang & Sohn, 2006; Williams et al, 2008; Esposito et al, 2014; van der Salm et al, 2014).

D. MYOCLONUS OF UNDETERMINED ORIGIN

The source of myoclonus in some conditions has not been fully determined. This includes periodic myoclonus seen in Creutzfeldt-Jakob disease and subacute sclerosing panencephalitis (SSPE), hereditary myoclonus-dystonia syndrome (Box 53), and drug-induced myoclonus.

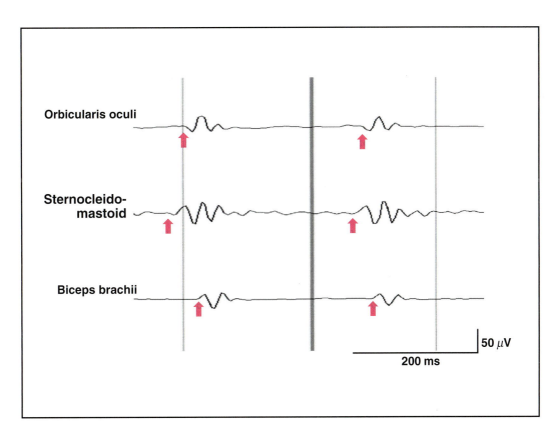

Figure 18-11 Surface EMG of reticular reflex myoclonus recorded from three muscles in a 60-year-old woman who showed spontaneous as well as reflex myoclonus in the face, neck, and upper extremities following an episode of anoxic encephalopathy. Arrows indicate the onset of each EMG discharge. (Reproduced from Inoue et al, 2012a, with permission)

Creutzfeldt-Jakob Disease

Periodic myoclonus is seen in the initial stage of this disease. It repeats with an interval of about 1 second, although its interval varies to a considerable degree within the same patient. The EMG discharge associated with the myoclonus also varies in length, and the sites of involvement may also vary. It is commonly accompanied by periodic synchronous discharge (PSD) on EEG, but either periodic myoclonus or PSD may appear independently. The relationship between the myoclonus and PSD also varies (Figure 18-12). In this disease, therefore, there is no causative relationship between the cortical activity and the peripheral motor phenomenon (Box 62).

Subacute Sclerosing Panencephalitis

Subacute sclerosing panencephalitis (SSPE) is chronic encephalitis that occurs years after infection with the measles virus. Periodic involuntary movements seen in this condition repeat at an interval of 4 to 13 seconds, and the frequency is quite constant at each stage of disease. Each movement is much longer in duration than ordinary myoclonus, and thus it might be called **periodic dystonic myoclonus**. It is commonly seen in extremities, but it may also be seen in eyes. On EEG, characteristic PSDs are seen in this condition. Unlike Creutzfeldt-Jakob disease, PSDs in this condition are quite constant in waveform and duration, and are constantly associated with the involuntary movements, suggesting cortical participation in their generation (Figure 18-13) (Oga et al, 2000).

9. MOTOR STEREOTYPIES

Repetitive occurrence of the same movements may be called motor stereotypies. Movements commonly encountered in this condition range from simple movements like shaking arms, nodding, and swinging body to complex movements, and they may look purposive, but actually they have no purpose or function (Edwards et al, 2012, for review). They tend to occur in clusters, each cluster lasting several seconds

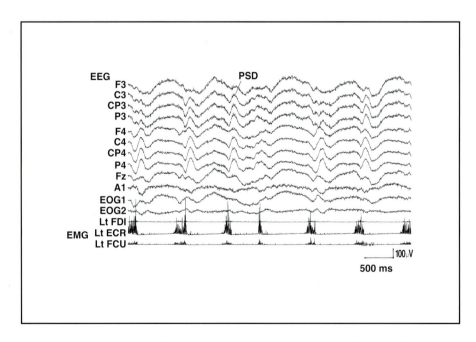

Figure 18-12 Polygraphic record of electroencephalogram (EEG) and electromyogram (EMG) in a patient with Creutzfeldt-Jakob disease.
EOG: electrooculogram, Lt: left, FDI: first dorsal interosseous muscle, ECR: extensor carpi radialis muscle, FCU: flexor carpi ulnaris muscle;
PSD: periodic synchronous discharge.

Prion disease is a group of diseases causing fatal neurodegeneration due to a deposit of prion protein. It was previously called subacute spongiform encephalopathy based on its pathological feature. Its representative form is **Creutzfeldt-Jakob disease (CJD)**. Most cases of CJD are sporadic, but 10–15% of cases are transmitted by autosomal dominant inheritance with mutation of the coding region of human prion protein gene (Roeber et al, 2008). Sporadic cases of CJD manifest cognitive decline, periodic myoclonus, and periodic synchronous discharges on EEG, and its clinical course is rapidly progressive. Another form of familial prion disease is **Gerstmann-Sträussler-Scheinker syndrome**, which initially presents with mild gait disturbance, abnormal sensation, loss of tendon reflexes in the lower extremities, and truncal ataxia. **Fatal familial insomnia** is also a familial prion disease, characterized by insomnia and MRI abnormality in the pulvinar (see Chapter 24-3G). A variant form of spongiform encephalopathy (variant Creutzfeldt-Jakob disease) is known as mad cow disease. Clinically it starts with psychiatric symptoms, and myoclonus is rare, if any, in this condition.

Cases of rapidly progressive dementia tend to be diagnosed as CJD, but other conditions including Alzheimer disease, vascular dementia, autoimmune encephalitis, brain tumor like lymphoma, infectious disease, and metabolic encephalopathy could present with similar symptoms. Therefore, diagnosis of CJD has to be made with caution (Chitravas et al, 2011).

to several minutes. The patient's consciousness is usually preserved, but the movements do not appear to be intentional, and distraction of the patient's attention to other objects may decrease the movements. They are called **motor stereotypies** in order to distinguish from stereotypic behavior encountered in psychiatric diseases.

Motor stereotypies are commonly observed in children with Asperger syndrome and other automatisms, and mental retardation. In adults, this abnormal behavior is seen in severe infectious encephalitis, autoimmune encephalitis like limbic encephalitis, cerebrovascular diseases, and neurodegeneration, among others frontotemporal lobar degeneration (see Chapter 22-2B) (Mateen & Josephs, 2009). It is postulated that motor stereotypies are seen when the circuit connecting the dorsolateral prefrontal cortex and the anterior striatum is interrupted.

Repetitive movements may be also seen in complex tics, obsessive-compulsive neurosis, and habits, but distinction of motor stereotypies from these conditions is not difficult

from the history and other accompanying symptoms and signs. In motor stereotypies, reciprocal innervation of agonist and antagonist muscles may be preserved because the movement appears quasi-purposive.

Rett Syndrome

This is a developmental disorder due to mutation of methyl-CpG binding protein 2 (MECP2) gene (Percy et al, 2010). It primarily affects female infants. Girls of this syndrome develop normally until 12 months of age and then manifest various neurologic symptoms including stereotypic movements of both hands such as washing, squeezing, and clapping. These stereotypic movements subside in several years, but the patients may show other involuntary movements such as tremor, chorea, myoclonus, and dystonia and also rigidity and ataxia. Dystonia may progress to cause scoliosis during the course of illness (Temudo et al, 2008).

10. INVOLUNTARY MOVEMENTS THAT CAN BE SUPPRESSED MOMENTARILY

Some involuntary movements can be suppressed for a short period of time if the patient wishes to do so. Those are tics, psychogenic involuntary movements, and restless legs syndrome.

A. TICS

Tics are irregular brisk movements ranging from shock-like simple movements resembling myoclonus (**simple tic**) to complex movements (**complex tic**). Patients with tics tend to repeat certain movements like blinking, grimacing, shrugging of shoulder, and twisting of fingers, but in patients with **Gilles de la Tourette syndrome**, tics appear as various kinds of movements. They often pout, smack, and vocalize (**vocal tic**), and utter obscene words (**coprolalia**). They can stop the movements for several seconds if they try, but it is often followed by rebound. The patients often feel the **urge** to move before a bout of tics, and feel release after the bout. Many families suggest a possibility of autosomal dominant transmission, but the genes have been elusive (State, 2011, for review). Tic disorders are usually associated with comorbid symptoms such as attention-deficit hyperactivity and obsessive-compulsive disorder/behavior, and multiple cerebral structures have been shown to be involved (Yael et al, 2015, for review).

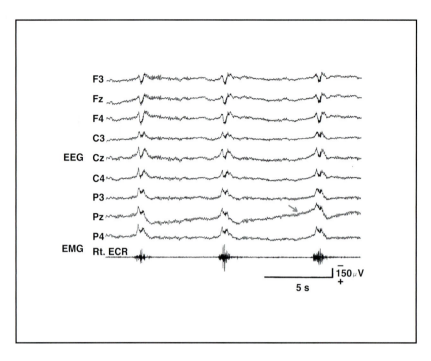

Figure 18-13 Polygraphic record of electroencephalogram (EEG) and electromyogram (EMG) in a patient with subacute sclerosing panencephalitis (SSPE). Rt. ECR: right extensor carpi radialis muscle. There is a fixed relationship between dystonic myoclonus and periodic synchronous discharge on EEG. (Reproduced from Oga et al, 2000, with permission)

B. PSYCHOGENIC INVOLUNTARY MOVEMENTS

Psychogenic involuntary movements are not infrequently encountered. They may look like tremor, myoclonus, or focal dystonia. Characteristics of psychogenic involuntary movements include the facts that it is difficult to explain as an ordinary involuntary movement (**incongruous**); it fluctuates in the pattern, degree, and distribution during the clinical course (**inconsistent**); it decreases or disappears when the patient's attention is drawn to others (**distraction**); and there is a **psychogenic background** in the patient's character or environment (Fahn, 2007, Lang & Voon, 2011, Czarnecki & Hallett, 2012, and Hallett et al, 2012, for review). In case of unilaterally predominant tremor, if the patient is requested to repeat voluntary movements with the intact or less affected hand at a certain pace, the tremor frequency might be replaced by the frequency of the voluntary movement (**entrainment**). In those cases in which it is difficult to confirm the psychogenic nature, it is useful and important to follow up the clinical course with repeated observations.

In cases showing repetitive shock-like movements with some time intervals in between, it may be worthwhile to record EEG and EMG simultaneously and to back average the EEG with respect to the EMG correlates of the involuntary movements. If a Bereitschaftspotential (readiness potential) is demonstrated before those movements, it suggests involvement of the mechanisms responsible for normal voluntary movement (Shibasaki & Hallett, 2006, and Shibasaki, 2012, for review). However, it should be noted that, in conversion, the movement is involuntary; hence, there is no intention.

C. RESTLESS LEGS SYNDROME

In this condition, the patients complain of unpleasant sensation in the lower extremities and trunk, and they feel a strong urge to move the legs. It tends to occur while taking a rest at night, and the symptoms are transiently relieved by moving the legs. It is said to be seen in 3 to 10% of population. About 60% of cases are said to be familial, and an increasing attention has been paid to this condition from a genetic point of view (Winkelmann et al, 2008; Ylikoski et al, 2015).

Many patients suffering from this phenomenon may also have periodic limb movement in sleep (Chapter 24-3E). Based on the fact that this phenomenon is suppressed by L-dopa or dopamine agonists, its possible relationship with Parkinson disease has been discussed, but the current consensus is that these two conditions are not related in pathogenesis (Fulda & Wetter, 2008).

Restless legs syndrome was considered in relation with peripheral nerve lesions. According to the study by Hattan et al. (2009) on a large number of patients with various neuropathies, it was shown that this phenomenon is seen more commonly in the group of hereditary neuropathies than in the control group, but not in the group of acquired neuropathies. Restless legs syndrome also occurs in association with various conditions including iron deficiency, pregnancy, uremia, and celiac disease.

11. INVOLUNTARY MOVEMENTS OF PERIPHERAL NERVE ORIGIN

Fasciculation and **myokymia** are abnormal muscle contractions due to an increase in the spontaneous excitability of anterior horn cells (see Chapter 16-3B). Repetitive muscle contraction seen in **hemifacial spasm** is myoclonus of peripheral nerve origin (see Chapter 11-1A). In **painful legs and moving toes syndrome**, irregular and slow involuntary movements are seen in toes associated with pain in the legs. This condition is often associated with peripheral nerve lesions like sciatica. A similar condition seen in upper extremities is called **painful hand and moving fingers syndrome**.

Some patients with inflammatory or hereditary polyneuropathies may show finger tremor, although its pathogenesis is not well known. Involuntary movements resembling athetosis might be seen in patients with proprioceptive loss if they keep the eyes closed, regardless of a lesion in the central or peripheral nervous system. This is called **pseudoathetosis** (see Chapter 19-2B). However, the above tremor associated with polyneuropathy is also seen while the eyes are kept open. A retrospective large case-control study by Ahlskog et al. (2012) showed that tremor was more frequently seen in patients with neuropathy associated with IgM-monocloncal gammopathy than those with neuropathy of other causes. Disabling tremor has been also reported in patients with CIDP positive for neurofascin IgG4 antibodies and poor response to IVIg (Querol et al, 2014).

BIBLIOGRAPHY

Abbruzzese G, Berardelli A. Further progress in understanding the pathophysiology of primary dystonia. Mov Disord 26:1185–1186, 2011. (review)

Adler CH, Shill HA, Beach TG. Essential tremor and Parkinson's disease: lack of a link. Mov Disord 26:372–377, 2011. (review)

Ahlskog MC, Kumar N, Mauermann ML, Klein CJ. IgM-monoclonal gammopathy neuropathy and tremor: a first epidemiological case control study. Parkinsonism Relat Disord 18:748–752, 2012.

Avanzino L, Martino D, van de Warrenburg BPC, Schneider SA, Abbruzzese G, Defazio G, et al. Cortical excitability is abnormal in patients with the "fixed dystonia" syndrome. Mov Disord 23:646–652, 2008.

Axelrad JE, Louis ED, Honig LS, Flores I, Ross GW, Pahwa R, et al. Reduced Purkinje cell number in essential tremor: a postmortem study. Arch Neurol 65:101–107, 2008.

Baizabal-Carvallo J, Cardoso F, Jankovic J. Myorhythmia: phenomenology, etiology, and treatment. Mov Disord 30:171–179, 2015. (review)

Bartolo M, Serrao M, Perrotta A, Tassorelli C, Sandrini G, Pierelli F. Lack of trigemino-cervical reflexes in progressive supranuclear palsy. Mov Disord 23:1475–1479, 2008.

Baudrexel S, Witte T, Seifried C, von Wegner F, Beissner F, Klein JC, et al. Resting state fMRI reveals increased subthalamic nucleus-motor cortex connectivity in Parkinson's disease. Neuroimage 55:1728–1738, 2011.

Berry-Kravis E, Abrams L, Coffey SM, Hall DA, Greco C, Gane LW, et al. Fragile X-associated tremor/ataxia syndrome: clinical features, genetics, and testing guidelines. Mov Disord 22:2018–2030, 2007.

Brilot F, Merheb V, Ding A, Murphy T, Dale RC. Antibody binding to neuronal surface in Sydenham chorea, but not in PANDAS or Tourette syndrome. Neurology 76:1508–1513, 2011.

Brodal P. The Central Nervous System: Structure and Function. 4th ed. Oxford University Press, New York, 2010.

Charlesworth G, Bhatia KP, Wood NW. The genetics of dystonia: new twists in an old tale. Brain 136:2017–2037, 2013. (review)

Chew NK, Mir P, Edwards MJ, Cordivari C, Martino D, Schneider SA, et al. The natural history of Unverricht-Lundborg disease: a report of eight genetically proven cases. Mov Disord 23:107–113, 2008.

Chitravas N, Jung RS, Kofskey DM, Blevins JE, Gambetti P, Leigh RJ, et al. Treatable neurological disorders misdiagnosed as Creutzfeldt-Jakob disease. Ann Neurol 70:437–444, 2011.

Czarnecki K, Hallett M. Functional (psychogenic) movement disorders. Curr Opin Neurol 25:507–512, 2012. (review)

Depienne C, Magnin E, Bouteiller D, Stevanin G, Saint-Martin C, Vidailhet M, et al. Familial cortical myoclonic tremor with epilepsy: the third locus (FCMTE3) maps to 5p. Neurology 74:2000–2003, 2010.

Deuschl G, Toro C, Valls-Solé J, Zeffiro T, Zee DS, Hallett M. Symptomatic and essential palatal tremor. 1. Clinical, physiological and MRI analysis. Brain 117:775–788, 1994.

Deuschl G, Raethjen J, Lindemann M, Krack P. The pathophysiology of tremor. Muscle Nerve 24:716–735, 2001. (review)

DiMauro S. Mitochondrial encephalomyopathies—fifty years on. The Robert Wartenberg Lecture. Neurology 81:281–291, 2013. (review)

Dresel C, Bayer F, Castrop F, Rimpau C, Zimmer C, Haslinger B. Botulinum toxin modulates basal ganglia but not deficient somatosensory activation in orofacial dystonia. Mov Disord 26:1496–1502, 2011.

Edwards MJ, Lang AE, Bhatia KP. Stereotypies: a critical appraisal and suggestion of a clinically useful definition. Mov Disord 27:179–185, 2012. (review)

Elbert T, Candia V, Altenmüller E, Rau H, Sterr A, Rockstroh B, et al. Alteration of digital representations in somatosensory cortex in focal hand dystonia. Neuroreport 9:3571–3575, 1998.

Elble RJ. Report from a U.S. Conference on essential tremor. Mov Disord 21:2052–2061, 2006.

Elble R, Deuschl G. Milestones in tremor research. Mov Disord 26:1096–1105, 2011. (review)

Erro R, Sheerin U-M, Bhatia KP. Paroxysmal dyskinesias revisited: a review of 500 genetically proven cases and a new classification. Mov Disord 29:1108–1116, 2014. (review)

Esposito M, Erro R, Edwards MJ, Cawley N, Choi D, Bhatia KP, et al. The pathophysiology of symptomatic propriospinal myoclonus. Mov Disord 29:1097–1099, 2014.

Fahn S. Psychogenic movement disorders. In Jankovic J, Tolosa E. (eds). Parkinson's Disease & Movement Disorders. 5th ed. Lippincott Williams & Wilkins, Philadelphia, 2007, pp. 562–566. (review)

Farkas Z, Csillik A, Szirmai I, Kamondi A. Asymmetry of tremor intensity and frequency in Parkinson's disease and essential tremor. Parkinsonism Relat Disord 12:49–55, 2006.

Franceschetti S, Michelucci R, Canafoglia L, Striano P, Gambardella A, Magaudda A, et al. Progressive myoclonic epilepsies: definitive and still undetermined causes. Neurology 82:405–411, 2014.

Friedman J, Roze E, Abdenur JE, Chang R, Gasperini S, Saletti V, et al. Sepiapterin reductase deficiency: a treatable mimic of cerebral palsy. Ann Neurol 71:520–530, 2012.

Friedreich N. Neuropathologische Beobachtungen. I. Paramyoklonus multiplex. Arch Path Anat (Virchow Arch) 86:421–430, 1881.

Frucht SJ, Houghton WC, Bordelon Y, Greene PE, Louis ED. A single-blind, open-label trial of sodium oxybate for myoclonus and essential tremor. Neurology 65:1967–1969, 2005.

Fulda S, Wetter TC. Where dopamine meets opioids: a meta-analysis of the placebo effect in restless legs syndrome treatment studies. Brain 131:902–917, 2008.

Gajos A, Bogucki A, Schinwelski M, Soltan W, Rudzinska M, Budrewicz S, et al. The clinical and neuroimaging studies in Holmes tremor. Acta Neurol Scand 122:360–366, 2010.

Garone C, Tadesse S, Hirano M. Clinical and genetic spectrum of mitochondrial neurogastrointestinal encephalomyopathy. Brain 134:3326–3332, 2011. (review)

Goto S, Kawarai T, Morigaki R, Okita S, Koizumi H, Nagahiro S, et al. Defects in the striatal neuropeptide Y system in X-linked dystonia-parkinsonism. Brain 136:1555–1567, 2013.

Hallett M, Chadwick D, Adam J, Marsden CD. Reticular reflex myoclonus: a physiological type of human post-hypoxic myoclonus. J Neurol Neurosurg Psychiatry 40:253–264, 1977.

Hallett M. Neurophysiology of dystonia: the role of inhibition. Neurobiol Dis 42:177–184, 2011. (review)

Hallett M, Weiner WJ, Kompoliti K. Psychogenic movement disorders. Parkinsonism Relat Disord 18S1:S155–S157, 2012. (review)

Hallett M, Albanese A, Dressler D, Segal KR, Simpson DM, Truong D, et al. Evidence-based review and assessment of botulinum neurotoxin for the treatment of movement disorders. Toxicon 67:94–114, 2013. (review)

Hanajima R, Okabe S, Terao Y, Furubayashi T, Arai N, Inomata-Terada S, et al. Difference in intracortical inhibition of the motor cortex between cortical myoclonus and focal hand dystonia. Clin Neurophysiol 119:1400–1407, 2008.

Hashimoto S, Kawamura J, Yamamoto T, Kinoshita A, Segawa Y, Harada Y, et al. Transient myoclonic state with asterixis in elderly patients: a new syndrome? J Neurol Sci 109:132–139, 1992.

Haslinger B, Altenmüller E, Castrop F, Zimmer C, Dresel C. Sensorimotor overactivity as a pathophysiologic trait of embouchure dystonia. Neurology 74:1790–1797, 2010.

Hassan A, Ahlskog JE, Matsumoto JY, Milber JM, Bower JH, Wilkinson JR. Orthostatic tremor. Clinical, electrophysiologic, and treatment findings in 184 patients. Neurology 86:458–464, 2016.

Hattan E, Chalk C, Postuma RB. Is there a higher risk of restless legs syndrome in peripheral neuropathy? Neurology 72:955–960, 2009.

Hawley JS, Weiner WJ. Psychogenic dystonia and peripheral trauma. Neurology 77:496–502, 2011. (review)

Helmich RC, Janssen MJR, Oyen WJG, Bloem BR, Toni I. Pallidal dysfunction drives a cerebellothalamic circuit into Parkinson tremor. Ann Neurol 69:269–281, 2011.

Helmich RC, Hallett M, Deuschl G, Toni I, Bloem BR. Cerebral causes and consequences of parkinsonian resting tremor: a tale of two circuits? Brain 135:3206–3226, 2012. (Review)

Huang X-J, Wang T, Wang J-L, Liu X-L, Che X-Q, Li, J, et al. Paroxysmal kinesigenic dyskinesia. Clinical and genetic analyses of 110 patients. Neurology 85:1546–1553, 2015.

Hyppönen J, Äikiä M, Joensuu T, Julkunen P, Danner N, Koskenkorva P, et al. Refining the phenotype of Unverricht-Lundborg disease (EPM1): a population-wide Finnish study. Neurology 84:1529–1536, 2015.

Inoue M, Mima T, Kojima Y, Satoi H, Makino F, Kanda M, et al. A case presenting with both features of essential tremor and Parkinson tremor. Clin Neurol 47:413–418, 2007. (Abstract in English)

Inoue M, Kojima Y, Kinboshi M, Kanda M, Shibasaki H. A case of post-anoxic reticular reflex myoclonus. Clin Neurol 52:557–560, 2012a.

Inoue M, Kojima Y, Mima T, Sawamoto N, Matsuhashi M, Fumuro T, et al. Pathophysiology of unilateral asterixis due to thalamic lesion. Clin Neurophysiol 123:1858–1864, 2012b.

Jang L, Borruat FX. Oculopalatal tremor: variations on a theme by Guillain and Mollaret. Eur Neurol 72:144–149, 2014.

Jankovic J, Schwartz KS, Ondo W. Re-emergent tremor of Parkinson's disease. J Neurol Neurosurg Psychiatry 67:646–650, 1999.

Jiménez-Jiménez FJ, Alonso-Navarro H, Garcia-Martin E, Aqundez JA. The relationship between Parkinson's disease and essential tremor: review of clinical, epidemiologic, genetic, neuroimaging and neuropathological data, and data on the presence of cardinal signs of parkinsonism in essential tremor. Tremor Other Hyperkinet Mov (NY) 2012;2. pii: tre-02-75-409-3 (Epub 2012 Sep 12). (review)

Kang SY, Sohn YH. Electromyography patterns of propriospinal myoclonus can be mimicked voluntarily. Mov Disord 21:1241–1244, 2006.

Kim DS, Fung VS. An update on Huntington's disease: from the gene to the clinic.Curr Opin Neurol 27:477–483, 2014. (review)

Lake NJ, Compton AG, Rahman S, Thorburn DR. Leigh syndrome: one disorder, more than 75 monogenic causes. Ann Neurol 79:190–203, 2016.

Lance JW, Adams RD. The syndrome of intention or action myoclonus as a sequel to hypoxic encephalopathy. Brain 86:111–136, 1963.

Lang AE, Voon V. Psychogenic movement disorders: past developments, current status, and future directions. Mov Disord 26:1175–1182, 2011. (review)

Lapresle J, Ben Hamida M. The dentato-olivary pathway: somatotopic relationship between the dentate nucleus and the contralateral inferior olive. Arch Neurol 22:135–143, 1970.

Li J-Y, Chen R. Increased intracortical inhibition in hyperglycemic hemichorea-hemiballism. Mov Disord 30:198–205, 2015.

Louis ED, Lee M, Babij R, Ma K, Cortés E, Vonsattel JG, et al. Reduced Purkinje cell dendritic arborization and loss of dendritic spines in essential tremor. Brain 137:3142–3148, 2014.

Mateen FJ, Josephs KA. The clinical spectrum of stereotypies in frontotemporal lobar degeneration. Mov Disord 24:1237–1240, 2009.

Méneret A, Grabli D, Depienne C, Gaudebout C, Picard F, Dürr A, et al. PRRT2 mutations: a major cause of paroxysmal kinesigenic dyskinesia in the European population. Neurology 79:170–174, 2012.

Mestre TA, Lang AE, Ferreira JJ, Almeida V, de Varvalho M, Miyasaki J, et al. Associated movement disorders in orthostatic tremor. J Neurol Neurosurg Psychiatry 83:725–729, 2012.

Muraga K, Suda S, Nagayama H, Okubo S, Abe A, Aoki J, et al. Limb-shaking TIA: cortical myoclonus associated with ICA stenosis. Neurology 86:307–309, 2016.

Nahab FB, Wittevrongel L, Ippolito D, Toro C, Grimes GJ, Starling J, et al. An open-label, single-dose, crossover study of the pharmacokinetics and metabolism or two oral formulations of 1–octanol in patients with essential tremor. Neurotherapeutics 8:753–762, 2011.

Nardocci N, Zorzi G, Barzaghi C, Zibordi F, Ciano C, Ghezzi D, et al. Myoclonus-dystonia syndrome: clinical presentation, disease course, and genetic features in 11 families. Mov Disord 23:28–34, 2008.

Ni Z, Pinto AD, Lang AE, Chen R. Involvement of the cerebellothalamocortical pathway in Parkinson disease. Ann Neurol 68:816–824, 2010.

Oga T, Ikeda A, Nagamine T, Sumi E, Matsumoto R, Akigushi I, et al. Implication of sensorimotor integration in the generation of periodic dystonic myoclonus in subacute sclerosing panencephalitis (SSPE). Mov Disord 15:1173–1183, 2000.

Paudel R, Li A, Wiethoff S, Bandopadhyay R, Bhatia K, de Silva R, et al. Neuropathology of Beta-propeller protein associated neurodegeneration (BPAN): a new tauopathy. Acta Neuropath Comm 3 (39): 1–8, 2015.

Percy AK, Neul JL, Glaze DG, Motil KJ, Skinner SA, Khwaja O, et al. Rett syndrome diagnostic criteria: lessons from the Natural History Study. Ann Neurol 68:951–955, 2010.

Persoon S, Kappelle LJ, Klijn CJM. Limb-shaking transient ischaemic attacks in patients with internal carotid artery occlusion: a case-control study. Brain 133:915–922, 2010.

Quartarone A, Hallett M. Emerging concepts in the physiological basis of dystonia. Mov Disord 28:958–967, 2013. (review)

Querol L, Nogales-Gadea G, Rojas-Garcia R, Diaz-Manera J, Pardo J, Ortega-Moreno A, et al. Neurofascin IgG4 antibodies in CIDP associated with disabling tremor and poor response to IVIg. Neurology 82:879–886, 2014.

Raina GB, Cersosimo MG, Folgar SS, Giugni JC, Calandra C, Paviolo JP, et al. Holmes tremor. Clinical description, lesion localization, and treatment in a series of 29 cases. Neurology 86:931–938, 2016.

Rajput AH, Maxood K, Rajput A. Classic essential tremor changes following cerebellar hemorrhage. Neurology 71:1739–1740, 2008.

Ramos VF, Karp BI, Hallett M. Tricks in dystonia: ordering the complexity. J Neurol Neurosurg Psychiatry 85:987–993, 2014. (review)

Remy P, de Recondo A, Defer G, Loc'h C, Amarenco P, Planté-Bordeneuve V, et al. Peduncular "rubral" tremor and dopaminergic denervation: a PET study. Neurology 45:472–477, 1995.

Richardson SP, Mari Z, Matsuhashi M, Hallett M. Psychogenic palatal tremor. Mov Disord 21:274–278, 2006.

Roeber S, Grasbon-Frodl E-M, Windl O, Krebs B, Xiang W, Vollmert C, et al. Evidence for a pathogenic role of different mutations at codon 188 of PRNP. PloS ONE 3 (e2147):1–8, 2008.

Roze E, Apartis E, Clot F, Dorison N, Thobois S, Guyant-Marechal L, et al. Myoclonus-dystonia: clinical and electrophysiologic pattern related to SGCE mutations. Neurology 70:1010–1016, 2008.

Russell JF, Steckley JL, Coppola G, Hahn AF, Howard MA, Kornberg Z, et al. Familial cortical myoclonus with a mutation in NOL3. Ann Neurol 72:175–183, 2012.

Sako W, Goto S, Shimazu H, Murase N, Matsuzaki K, Tamura T, et al. Bilateral deep brain stimulation of the globus pallidus internus in tardive dystonia. Mov Disord 23:1929–1931, 2008.

Schrag A, Trimble M, Quinn N, Bhatia K. The syndrome of fixed dystonia: an evaluation of 103 patients. Brain 127:2360–2372, 2004.

Shahwan A, Farrell M, Delanty N. Progressive myoclonic epilepsies: a review of genetic and therapeutic aspect. Lancet Neurol 4:239–248, 2005. (review)

Shibasaki H, Neshige R. Photic cortical reflex myoclonus. Ann Neurol 22:252–257, 1987.

Shibasaki H, Ikeda A, Nagamine T, Mima T, Terada K, Nishitani N, et al. Cortical reflex negative myoclonus. Brain 117:477–486, 1994.

Shibasaki H, Hallett M. Electrophysiological studies of myoclonus. Muscle Nerve 31:157–174, 2005. (review)

Shibasaki H, Hallett M. What is the Bereitschaftspotential? Clin Neurophysiol 117:2341–2356, 2006. (review)

Shibasaki H. Myoclonus and startle syndrome. In Jankovic J, Tolosa E (eds.). Parkinson's Disease and Movement Disorders. 5th ed. Lippincott Williams & Wilkins, Philadelphia, 2007a, pp. 377–386.

Shibasaki H. Myoclonus. In Schapira AHV (ed.). Neurology and Clinical Neuroscience. Mosby, Philadelphia, 2007b, pp. 435–442.

Shibasaki H. Lance-Adams syndrome. In Kompoliti K, Verhagen M (eds.). Encyclopedia of Movement Disorders. Vol. 2. Academic Press, Oxford, pp. 116–119, 2010. (review)

Shibasaki H, Thompson PD. Milestones in myoclonus. Mov Disord 26:1142–1148, 2011. (review)

Shibasaki H. Cortical activities associated with voluntary movements and involuntary movements. Clin Neurophysiol 123:229–243, 2012. (review)

Shill HA, Adler CH, Sabbagh MN, Connor DJ, Caviness JN, Hentz JG, et al. Pathologic findings in prospectively ascertained essential tremor subjects. Neurology 70:1452–1455, 2008.

Shill HA, Adler CH, Beach TG, Lue LF, Caviness JN, Sabbagh MN, et al. Brain biochemistry in autopsied patients with essential tremor. Mov Disord 27:113–117, 2012.

Stamelou M, Mencacci NE, Cordivari C, Batia A, Wood NW, Houlden H, et al. Myoclonus-dystonia syndrome due to tyrosine hydroxylase deficiency. Neurology 79:435–441, 2012a.

Stamelou M, Saifee TA, Edwards MJ, Bhatia KP. Psychogenic palatal tremor may be underrecognized: reappraisal of a large series of cases. Mov Disord 27:1164–1168, 2012b.

State MW. The genetics of Tourette disorder. Curr Opin Genetics Develop 21:302–309, 2011. (review)

Stogmann E, Reinthaler E, El Tawil S, El Etribi MA, Hemeda M, El Nahhas N, et al. Autosomal recessive cortical myoclonic tremor and epilepsy: association with a mutation in the potassium channel associated gene CNTN2. Brain 136:1155–1160, 2013.

Symanski C, Shill HA, Dugger B, Hentz JG, Adler CH, Jacobson SA, et al. Essential tremor is not associated with cerebellar Purkinje cell loss. Mov Disord 29:496–500, 2014.

Tatu L, Moulin T, Martin V, Monnier G, Rumbach L. Unilateral pure thalamic asterixis: clinical, electromyographic, and topographic patterns. Neurology 54:2339–2342, 2000.

Temudo T, Ramos E, Dias K, Barbot C, Vieira JP, Moreira A, et al. Movement disorders in Rett syndrome; an analysis of 60 patients with detected MECP2 mutation and correlation with mutation type. Mov Disord 23:1384–1390, 2008.

van der Salm SMA, Erro R, Cordivari C, Edwards MJ, Koelman JHTM, van den Ende T, et al. Propriospinal myoclonus. Clinical reappraisal and review of literature. Neurology 83:1862–1870, 2014.

van Rootselaar AF, van der Salm SM, Bour LJ, Edwards MJ, Brown P, Aronica E, et al. Decreased cortical inhibition and yet cerebellar pathology in "familial cortical myoclonic tremor with epilepsy." Mov Disord 22:2378–2385, 2007.

Virmani T, Louis ED, Waters C, Pullman SL. Familial orthostatic tremor: an additional report in siblings. Neurology 79:288–289, 2012.

Wang J-L, Cao L, Li X-H, Hu Z-M, Li J-D, Zhang J-G, et al. Identification of PRRT2 as the causative gene of paroxysmal kinesigenic dyskinesias. Brain 134:3490–3498, 2011.

Wang S, Aziz TZ, Stein JF, Bain PG, Liu X. Physiological and harmonic components in neural and muscular coherence in Parkinsonian tremor. Clin Neurophysiol 117:1487–1498, 2006.

Wild EJ, Mudanohwo EE. Sweeney MG, Schneider SA, Beck J, Bhatia KP, et al. Huntington's disease phenocopies are clinically and genetically heterogeneous. Mov Disord 23:716–720, 2008.

Williams DR, Cowey M, Day B. Psychogenic propriospinal myoclonus. Mov Disord 23:1312–1313, 2008.

Williams RE, Mole SE. New nomenclature and classification scheme for the neuronal ceroid lipofuscinoses. Neurology 79:183–191, 2012.

Wilson SAK. Progressive lenticular degeneration: a familial nervous disease associated with cirrhosis of the liver. Brain 34:295–509, 1912.

Winkelmann J, Lichtner P, Schormair B, Uhr M, Hauk S, Stiasny-Kolster K, et al. Variants in the neuronal nitric oxide synthase (nNOS, NOS1) gene are associated with restless legs syndrome. Mov Disord 23:350–358, 2008.

Yael D, Vinner E, Bar-Gad I. Pathophysiology of tic disorders. Mov Disord 30:1171–1178, 2015. (review)

Yeetong P, Ausavarat S, Bhidayasiri R, Piravej K, Pasutharnchat N, Desudchit T, et al. A newly identified locus for benign adult familial myoclonic epilepsy on chromosome 3q26.32–3q28. Eur J Hum Genet 21:225–228, 2013.

Ylikoski A, Martikainen K, Partinen M. Parkinson's disease and restless legs syndrome. Eur Neurol 73:212–219, 2015.

Young RR, Shahani BT. Asterixis: one type of negative myoclonus. Adv Neurol 43:137–156, 1986.

Zhou B, Chen Q, Zhang Q, Chen L, Gong Q, Shang H, et al. Hyperactive putamen in patients with paroxysmal kinesigenic choreoathetosis: a resting-state functional magnetic resonance imaging study. Mov Disord 25:1226–1231, 2010.

19.

SOMATOSENSORY FUNCTION

Sensation (sense) is defined as the primary reception of input from the external environment and that of change in the internal condition, whereas **perception** is defined as recognition of the above inputs. Sensation is divided into somatic sensation and visceral sensation. **Somatic sensation** is further divided into general somatic sensation, which receives sensory input from skin, skeletal muscles, and joints, and special somatic sensations such as visual, auditory, and equilibrium. **Visceral sensation** is divided into general visceral sensation, which receives sensory input from visceral organs and smooth muscles, and special visceral sensation like taste and olfactory sense. Among these sensations, general somatic sensation is described in this chapter as the somatosensory system. There are three kinds of sensation in the somatosensory system: **superficial**, **deep/proprioceptive**, and **cortical** sensation. Each sense is further classified into several modalities (Table 19-1).

1. STRUCTURE AND FUNCTIONS OF THE SOMATOSENSORY SYSTEM

A. SOMATOSENSORY RECEPTORS

Different kinds of receptors are known for the somatosensory system. Receptors for superficial sensation are free nerve endings for pain as well as temperature sense, hair follicle endings, Krause corpuscles, Ruffini corpuscles, and free nerve endings for light touch, and Meissner corpuscles, Merkel disks, and Pacinian corpuscles for touch. **Modality specificity** of these receptors is not mutually exclusive, and it is determined by the lowest threshold of each receptor. In other words, all receptors can be activated to a certain degree if stimulated with sufficiently high intensity. The kind of stimulus that activates a receptor with the lowest threshold is an adequate stimulus for that receptor. Receptors for deep/proprioceptive sensation are muscle spindles, Golgi tendon organs, and joint receptors (see Chapter 17-1).

Sensory receptors generate a local potential called **receptor potential** or **generator potential** in response to the stimulus. When the receptor potential exceeds a certain threshold, an action potential is generated in the nerve terminal attached to the receptors. The discharge rate of action potentials is proportional to the stimulus intensity. Physiologically, the sensory receptors are classified into two types depending on the mode of excitation; rapidly adapting and slowly adapting. **Rapidly adapting receptors** are phasic receptors, which rapidly diminish their receptor potentials in response to continuous stimulus presentation, thus rapidly diminishing the discharge rate of action potentials generated in the afferent nerve fibers. **Slowly adapting receptors** are tonic receptors, which slowly diminish the receptor potentials and the nerve discharge.

B. PERIPHERAL SOMATOSENSORY NERVES

Primary neurons of the somatosensory system for limbs and trunk are in the **dorsal root ganglion**. For the cranial nerve territory, the primary neurons are in the semilunar ganglion of the trigeminal nerve (see Figure 10-1), the geniculate ganglion of the facial nerve (see Figure 11-1), and the superior ganglion and petrous ganglion of the glossopharyngeal nerve (see Figure 14-4). All these neurons are bipolar cells, and impulses are conducted through the peripheral axon and the central axon to enter the spinal cord or brainstem. As described in each relevant chapter, the extramedullary axons are surrounded by a myelin sheath of Schwann cell origin whereas the intramedullary axons are made by a myelin sheath of oligodendroglia (Figure 19-1). Histologically, therefore, a peripheral somatosensory nerve belongs to the central nervous system once it enters the spinal cord or brainstem.

The peripheral nerves are classified into four groups based on their diameter, conduction velocity, and

TABLE 19-1 MODALITIES OF SOMATOSENSORY SYSTEM

1. Superficial sensation
Pain
Warm sense
Cold sense
Touch, tactile sense
2. Deep/proprioceptive sensation
Vibratory sense
Joint position sense
Movement sense, kinesthesia
Deep pressure pain
3. Cortical sensation
Stereognosis
Graphesthesia
Two-point discrimination
Baroesthesia
Touch localization

function (Table 19-2). The largest fibers are Aα fibers, to which Group I and Group II fibers belong. Proprioceptive fibers (Ia and Ib) and α motor fibers belong to Group I. Group II includes the sensory fibers for light touch and touch, fibers from the secondary sensory ending of muscle spindle, and γ motor fibers. Aδ (Group III) fibers and C (Group IV) fibers are related to the nociceptive sensation. Aδ fibers are myelinated, and C fibers are unmyelinated. The larger the fiber diameter, the higher is the conduction velocity.

C. SOMATOSENSORY PATHWAY IN THE SPINAL CORD

After entering the spinal cord through the dorsal root entry zone, the somatosensory fibers are separated into two groups (Figure 19-2). Nociceptive small fibers send their branches up and down for 1 ~ 3 segments through the Lissauer tract to enter the dorsal horn gray matter, where they make synapses with the secondary neurons. Deep/proprioceptive large fibers enter the **dorsal column** from the dorsal root entry zone, and ascend to the lower medullary tegmentum, where they make synapses with the secondary neurons. Fibers related to the sensation of the lower limbs and lower trunk ascend through the medial part of the dorsal column (**gracile fascicle**, fasciculus gracilis, **Goll column**) and reach the **gracile nucleus** (nucleus gracilis) at the medulla. Fibers related to the sensation of the upper limbs and upper trunk ascend through the lateral part of the dorsal column (**cuneate fascicle**, fasciculus cuneatus,

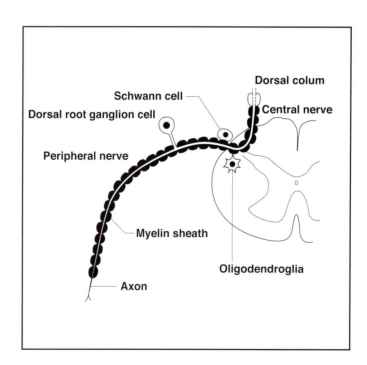

Figure 19-1 Schematic illustration of a peripheral somatosensory nerve fiber. The dorsal root ganglion cell is a bipolar cell, and its peripheral axon and the extramedullary part of the central axon have its myelin sheath made of Schwann cells, whereas the intramedullary part of the central axon has its myelin sheath made of oligodendroglia.

TABLE 19-2 CLASSIFICATION OF PERIPHERAL NERVE FIBERS BASED ON THE DIAMETER

Nerve fibers	Diameter (μm)	Conduction (m/s)	Functions
Aα fiber			
Group I	12 ~ 20	72 ~120	Proprioception (Ia, Ib), α motor fibers
Group II	6 ~ 11	30 ~ 72	Light touch, touch, secondary terminal of muscle spindle, γ motor fibers
Aδ fiber			
Group III	1 ~ 5	4 ~ 30	Fast pain
C fiber			
Group IV	0.3 ~ 1.5	0.4 ~ 2.0	Slow pain

Burdach column) and reach the **cuneate nucleus** (nucleus cuneatus) at the medulla (Figure 19-2, see also Figure 5-3). There is a laminar structure in the dorsal column with the fibers innervating the caudal part of the body located medially and those innervating the rostral part of the body located laterally (see Figure 16-3).

D. NOCICEPTIVE PATHWAY

The secondary neurons of the nociceptive pathway are in the substantia gelatinosa of the dorsal horn (layer II and III of Rexed), where they receive synaptic transmission from the central axon of the primary neurons. Substance P is considered to be the neurotransmitter for this synapse. Axons of the secondary neurons either make synaptic contact with other neurons in the dorsal horn or cross through the anterior white commissure to the anterior part of the lateral column of the other side, where they ascend as the **lateral spinothalamic tract**. This tract ascends through the lateral part of the brainstem to reach the **ventral posterolateral nucleus (VPL)** of the thalamus (Figure 19-2). In the transverse section of the lateral spinothalamic tract, fibers are arranged in laminar layers, with the caudally originating fibers located laterally and the rostrally originating fibers located medially (see Figure 16-3). Therefore, when the spinal cord is compressed from the lateral side, numbness and nociceptive loss appear first in the distal part of the contralateral lower limb, and spread proximally as the compression increases. In an intramedullary lesion, by contrast, those sensory symptoms are limited to a certain segment of the body depending on which layers are damaged. If the most lateral layer of the spinothalamic tract is spared

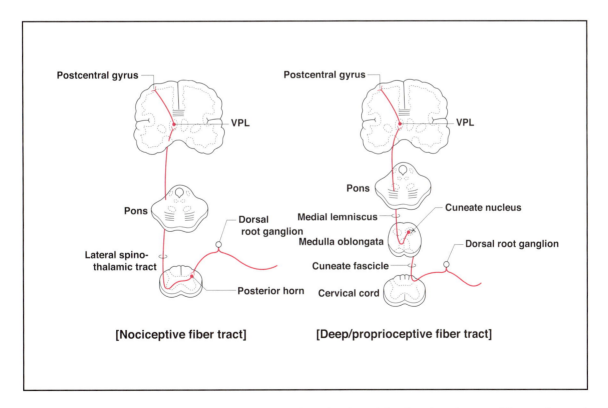

Figure 19-2 Schematic diagram of the somatosensory pathways comparing the nociceptive and deep/proprioceptive tracts. VPL: ventral posterolateral nucleus of thalamus.

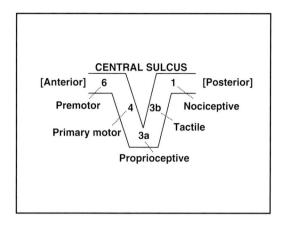

by an intramedullary lesion, the perianal skin innervated by the sacral segments may remain unaffected. This phenomenon is called **sacral sparing** and suggests the presence of an intramedullary cord lesion. Thus, even in a brainstem lesion, if only a certain layer of the spinothalamic tract is involved, it might cause nociceptive loss restricted to the corresponding parts of the trunk or limbs. Even in this case, distinction from the dissociated segmental sensory loss due to a lesion of the spinal cord gray matter is possible from other accompanying symptoms and signs.

E. PROPRIOCEPTIVE PATHWAY

The secondary neurons of the proprioceptive pathway are in the gracile nucleus and the cuneate nucleus located in the medullary tegmentum. Axons arising from those nuclei cross at the same level and ascend the ventral medial part of the brainstem tegmentum as the **medial lemniscus** to reach the VPL (Figure 19-2, also see Figures 5-2 and 5-3). As the medial lemniscus is located near the midline of brainstem, it is not damaged by external compression of the brainstem. Thus, selective impairment of tactile or proprioceptive sense in the contralateral limbs in patients with posterior fossa lesion suggests the presence of an intramedullary brainstem lesion.

F. THE THIRD SENSORY NEURON AND CORTICAL RECEPTIVE AREAS

The third sensory neurons are in the VPM and VPL of the thalamus (see Chapter 10-1), and their axons pass through the posterior limb of internal capsule and reach the **primary somatosensory cortex** (SI) in the postcentral gyrus as the thalamocortical fibers. In SI, like the primary motor cortex, there is **somatotopic organization** in the upside

down homunculus (see Figure 10-2). In the clinical setting, it is rare to encounter a localized lesion in the postcentral gyrus. Based on the experimental studies by using evoked potentials and evoked magnetic fields, it is postulated that S1 plays a role in the sensation itself and its localization and perception of intensity.

As for the functional localization in SI, the tactile input is mainly received in the posterior wall of the central sulcus (area 3b), the proprioceptive input in its trough (area 3a), and the nociceptive input in the crown of the postcentral gyrus (area 1) (Figure 19-3). For somatosensory function, however, functional specificity of these cortical areas may not be very high.

Nerve fibers originating from SI project bilaterally to the **secondary somatosensory cortex** (SII) located in the superior bank of the sylvian fissure, and also to the ipsilateral areas 5 and 7 located posterior to SI. SII is known to play a role in selective attention, and the areas 5 and 7 are thought to be involved in somatosensory perception and recognition.

Nociceptive cortical areas are unique because the nociception is closely related to the affect and emotional reaction. The SI is primarily related to perception of the intensity and localization of pain, and the SII is engaged in distinction of the nature of pain. In addition, the amygdala, insula, and cingulate gyrus are related to the emotion-related nociceptive perception and the emotional reaction to pain (Shibasaki, 2004, for review) (Figure 19-4). In a lesion of these limbic areas, the patient becomes indifferent to pain even if the pain can be perceived (**indifference to pain**), or the patient becomes unable to express the pain in language or behavior (**asymbolia for pain**). This condition, however, has to be distinguished from **congenital insensitivity to pain**, which is due to an ion channel disorder of the peripheral nerve (see Chapter 25-1B).

In relation to pain, itch is a complex sensory and emotional experience, and its functional neuroimaging studies disclosed that multiple cortical areas similar to those related to pain perception are involved in its perception and emotional response (Mochizuki & Kakigi, 2015, for review).

2. EXAMINATION OF SOMATOSENSORY FUNCTION AND ABNORMAL FINDINGS

As sensory examination of the face is described in the section on the trigeminal nerve (Chapter 10-2B), sensory examination of extremities is described here.

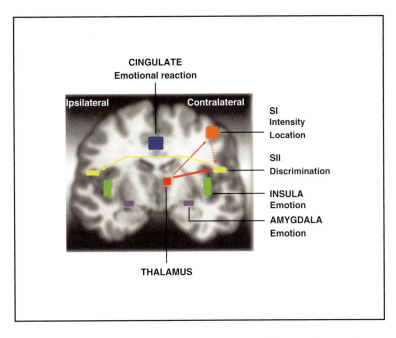

Figure 19-4 Nociceptive cortical areas and their functions. SI: primary somatosensory cortex, SII: secondary somatosensory cortex. (Based on Shibasaki, 2004)

A. EXAMINATION OF SOMATOSENSORY FUNCTION

For the sensory examination of extremities, the pain and temperature sense, light touch, vibration sense, and joint position sense are usually examined. How much in detail the sensory examination should be performed differs depending on the results of history taking. If there is no sensory symptom in the history of the present illness, it may be sufficient to screen some or all of the above modalities in the extremities.

Pain sense may be examined by sterile pins in order to avoid infection and injury. Breaking the thin wooden stick holding a cotton swab sometimes reveals a sharp wooden point that can also be used for testing pain. **Temperature sense** is tested by using flasks filled with hot or cold water. For testing cold sensation, often the side of a tuning fork is used; this is not actually cold, but feels cold due to rapid absorption of heat. **Tactile sense** can be tested in two ways, light touch and a little stronger touch. Light touch can be tested with tissue paper, and a little stronger touch may be tested by rubbing the skin with a soft material. **Vibration sense** is usually tested by placing a vibrating tuning fork over the bone. Vibration sense differs depending on which part of the body is tested and on the age of subjects. **Joint position sense** is tested by flexing or extending a finger or a toe while the subject keeps the eyes closed and is asked to tell the position of the finger or toe. It is important to grab a finger or toe from both sides instead of front and back in order to avoid the effect of pressure sense. In relation to joint position sense, joint movement sense (**kinesthesia**) can be tested by asking a patient to report any movement of the finger or toe regardless of the direction of movement. Occasionally there is dissociation between the results of joint position sense and kinesthesia. In sensory testing, it is always important to compare the left and right homologous areas.

Examination of Cortical Sensation

Examination of cortical sensation is important because its loss might be the only abnormality of the sensory functions in some cases of a localized lesion in the postcentral area or in patients with corticobasal degeneration (see Box 79). In order to mask the visual information, all cortical senses must be tested while the subject's eyes are kept closed. **Stereognosis** is tested by asking a patient to touch an object with a hand and to tell its name or shape. If a patient is weak or clumsy and cannot manipulate the object themselves, then the examiner should move it across the hand. **Graphesthesia** is tested by asking a patient to read a letter or number scripted on the skin. **Two-point discrimination** is tested by asking a patient to judge one or two by presenting a single stimulus or two stimuli simultaneously to the skin with various distances between the two. The distinguishable distance between the two stimuli is longer in the affected extremity than in the homologous part of the contralateral extremity. **Baroesthesia** is tested by asking a subject to judge the weight of an object placed in the supported hand. **Touch localization** is tested by asking a patient to report what part of the body was touched. Again it is important to compare each sense between the two homologous sites.

B. SOMATOSENSORY SYMPTOMS/SIGNS

If joint position sense or joint movement sense is lost, voluntary movement cannot be executed with appropriate sensory feedback, resulting in incoordination of movement. This condition is called **sensory ataxia**, and can be corrected by visual input. In this condition, if the patient holds the arms straight ahead and closes his eyes, the fingers may show an athetosis-like movement (**pseudoathetosis**). In the same principle, a patient with loss of joint senses in the lower limbs tends to fall if the eyes are closed in the standing position. This is called a **positive Romberg sign** (Figure 19-5). Likewise, the patient may have to hold on to a basin to keep balance when washing the face (**basin phenomenon**).

When a patient complains of sensory symptoms like pins and needles, it is better to describe what the patient is actually feeling instead of just saying "numbness." Spontaneous abnormal sensation is called **dysesthesia**, and unusual sensation caused by stimulus is called **paresthesia**. Hypersensitivity to a painful stimulus is called **hyperalgesia**. Uncomfortable painful sensation elicited by a light stimulus such as exposure to a breeze is called **hyperpathia**. In this condition, the pain induced by a pin prick might spread much wider and last much longer than usually expected. Hyperpathia is characteristically seen in association with **central pain** such as thalamic pain, although it may also be seen in a peripheral nerve lesion. Decrease in the somesthetic sense is called **hypesthesia**, and loss of sensation is called **anesthesia**, and likewise **hyp(o)algesia** and **analgesia** for decrease and loss of pain sense, respectively.

Pain and Neuralgia

Pain is one of the most common symptoms in clinical medicine. Pain is often caused by a lesion of the nervous system, but it is also induced by algesic (algogenic) substance without a direct lesion of the nervous system.

Instantaneous, radiating, shock-like pain along the pathway of a peripheral nerve is called **neuralgia** such as trigeminal neuralgia (see Chapter 10-2B), glossopharyngeal neuralgia (see Chapter 14-2), intercostal neuralgia, and postherpetic neuralgia (Box 63). Radiating pain seen in cervical spondylosis and lumbar disc herniation is also a typical neuralgia (**root pain**). In cervical spondylosis, radiating pain is induced or aggravated by flexing the neck posterolaterally, because the mechanical compression of the nerve root by the narrowed intervertebral foramen is worsened by this maneuver (**Spurling sign**). When the fifth lumbar or the first sacral root is

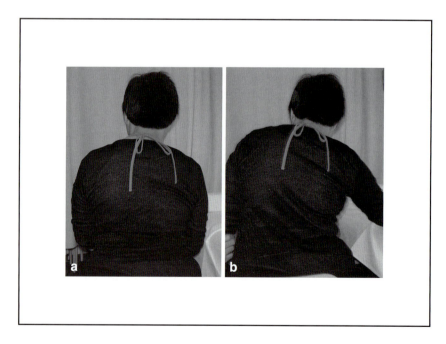

Figure 19-5 Romberg sign seen in a patient with congenital sensory neuropathy. (a) Eyes kept open, (b) eyes closed. As the proprioceptive sense is totally lost below the neck in this patient, Romberg sign is positive even in the sitting position. (See Shibasaki et al, 2004, with permission of the patient)

THE NEUROLOGIC EXAMINATION

involved by lumbar disc herniation, passive straight leg raising causes a radiating pain along the sciatic nerve (**Lasègue sign**).

In the mechanical entrapment of a peripheral nerve like carpal tunnel syndrome (Box 64) and tarsal tunnel syndrome, tapping of the entrapped site elicits radiating pain in the distal part of the nerve (**Tinel sign**). Pain, burning sensation, and numbness or sensory loss over the lateral aspect of thigh is called **meralgia paresthetica**. This is due to mechanical compression of the lateral femoral cutaneous nerve, and is commonly seen in obese, aged, or diabetic subjects (Parisi et al, 2011). This kind of neuropathy caused by mechanical compression is generally called **entrapment neuropathy**.

Radiating pain starting from the back and descending down along the posterior aspect of the legs induced by neck flexion is called the **Lhermitte sign** (see Chapter 15-1). This phenomenon is commonly seen in patients with demyelinating diseases such as multiple sclerosis, and is postulated to be due to nonsynaptic (ephaptic) transmission of impulses across the demyelinated nerve fibers within the dorsal column.

Painful dysesthesia symmetrically involving the distal limbs, especially the distal lower limbs, is a common symptom in polyneuropathy, often due to **diabetic polyneuropathy** or **alcohol vitamin deficiency polyneuropathy**. In these conditions, burning pain in the feet is commonly experienced at night. Sensory dominant polyneuropathy due to a deficiency of vitamins such as thiamine, cobalamin, and folate is not uncommon (Koike et al, 2015). Pain was thought to be relatively uncommon in Guillain-Barré syndrome (see Chapter 16-3C), but in fact it may not be so rare, and pain may be even the initial symptom of this

---

---

condition (Ruts et al, 2010). Pain in this condition includes root pain, painful dysesthesia, and myalgia.

Following a vascular lesion in the thalamus or brainstem, an extremely uncomfortable pain might occur in the contralateral limbs. This condition is called **thalamic pain** and is often associated with hyperpathia. This is a cardinal symptom of **Dejerine-Roussy syndrome** (Box 65).

When the distal part of a limb is lost due to trauma or surgical procedure, the patient might feel as if the lost part still exists (**phantom limb**). If pain is felt in the lost part of the limb, it is called **phantom limb pain**. Its mechanism has not been clarified. Injection of botulinum toxin was reported to be effective for phantom limb pain (Kollewe et al, 2009), but the reason for its efficacy is obscure (Box 66).

C. IMPAIRMENT OF THE SOMATOSENSORY NERVOUS SYSTEM AND DISTRIBUTION OF THE SENSORY SYMPTOMS

Distribution of the somatosensory symptoms gives an important clue to the anatomical diagnosis. Abnormality of facial sensation is described in Chapter 10-2B. Symmetric sensory impairment of distal lower limbs or distal four limbs (**glove and stocking distribution**) suggests the presence of a diffuse involvement of the peripheral nerves (**polyneuropathy**)

(Figure 19-6). Sensory symptoms usually start in the toes or in both the fingers and toes, and they tend to spread proximally. The sensory symptoms are usually more severe in the distal part of limbs. It may be associated with muscle weakness of the distal limbs, and tendon reflexes are usually lost (Box 67).

Polyneuropathy Primarily Presenting with Sensory Symptoms

Sensory predominant polyneuropathy is caused by a variety of etiologies. Among metabolic diseases, diabetes mellitus is the most common cause and the neuropathy is characterized by severe burning dysesthesia. Toxins primarily involving the dorsal root ganglion include arsenic, organic mercury, cisplatin, and n-hexane (see Chapter 16-3C). Malnutrition also causes sensory-dominant polyneuropathy. Examples are vitamin deficiency polyneuropathy due to gastrointestinal diseases, chronic alcoholism, and niacin deficiency. Vitamin B1 (thiamine) deficiency causes **beriberi**, which is characterized by axonal sensory-dominant polyneuropathy with severe burning dysesthesia of feet and marked tenderness of calf muscles, associated with congestive heart failure. Niacin deficiency causes **pellagra**, which is characterized by ruby erythema of tongue, diarrhea, dermatitis, and dementia in addition to sensory polyneuropathy. Vitamin B12 deficiency may also cause polyneuropathy in addition to the subacute combined degeneration of spinal cord (see Chapter 16-2C). Folate deficiency also causes sensory dominant axonal polyneuropathy (Koike et al, 2015).

If the sensory symptoms are localized to a certain part of limbs or trunk, it is important to determine whether the affected region corresponds to the territory innervated by a single peripheral nerve, a dermatome innervated by a certain spinal segment, or a region innervated by the brachial plexus for the upper limb or the lumbosacral plexus for the lower limb. For this purpose, diagrams of the sensory nerve innervation (Figure 19-7) and the plexus (see Figures 16-28 and 16-29) are useful.

Segmental Sensory Impairment

Sensory impairment localized to a dermatome innervated by one or more segments of the spinal cord is caused by a lesion of the spinal cord or the corresponding nerve roots. If the pain and temperature senses are selectively impaired in that

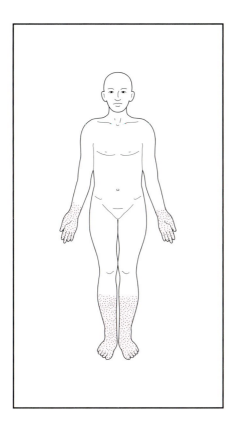

Figure 19-6 Glove and stocking distribution of the sensory symptoms due to polyneuropathy.

distribution, it is called **segmental dissociated sensory loss**. The responsible lesion for this condition is in the gray matter of the spinal cord, because a lesion of the dorsal root entry zone or roots is expected to impair the tactile and deep/proprioceptive senses as well. A typical example manifesting segmental dissociated sensory loss is **syringomyelia** (Figure 19-8).

When a cervical cord lesion is localized to the central region around the central canal as shown in Figure 19-8, dissociated sensory loss is seen in the dermatomes innervated by the corresponding segments bilaterally, but the tendon reflexes of biceps and triceps brachii muscles are preserved. This is because the reflex circuit passes through the lateral part of the spinal gray matter and thus is not damaged by the lesion. If the lesion extends a little more laterally, the corresponding tendon reflexes are lost. However, this principle does not apply to the thoracic cord, because there is no testable tendon reflex in the thoracic segments.

Sensory Impairment in a Transverse Spinal Cord Lesion

In a transverse lesion of the spinal cord, somatic senses of all modalities are diminished below the affected segment, because both the spinothalamic tracts and dorsal columns are transected at that level (Figure 19-9). In addition, as the gray matter is also damaged in the affected segment(s), pain and temperature senses are lost at the corresponding level in a sash-shaped distribution. In this condition, the patient may complain of a tight sensation around the trunk at the corresponding segments (**girdle sensation**). Based on the length of the analgesic area or of the girdle sensation, it is possible to estimate the length of the transverse lesion. As the corticospinal tracts are also damaged in this case, the trunk and limbs caudal to the affected segments are paralyzed. Furthermore, the autonomic pathways are also impaired, resulting in sphincter disturbance and loss of sweating below the affected level (see Chapter 20-3).

Brown-Séquard Syndrome

If either the left or right half of the spinal cord is damaged at a certain segment, motor paralysis is seen below the affected segment only on the affected side due to a lesion of the corticospinal tract, and vibratory sense and joint position sense are diminished below that level also on the affected side due to a lesion of the dorsal column. By contrast, pain and

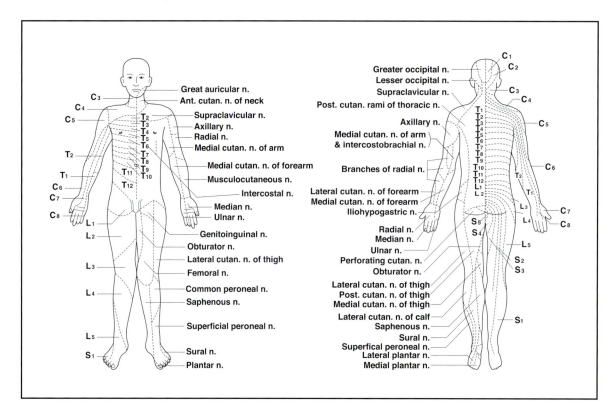

Figure 19-7 Somatosensory innervation by the peripheral nerves and spinal dermatomes. (a) Frontal view, (b) back view. n.: nerve, C: cervical, T: thoracic, L: lumbar, S: sacral. (Modified from Mayo Clinic and Mayo Foundation, 1998)

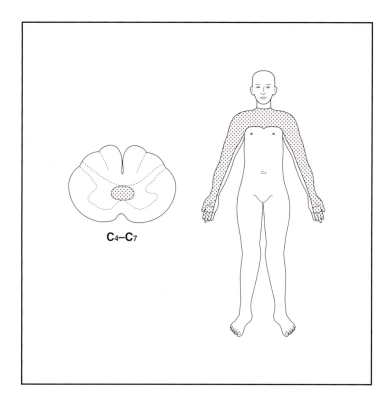

C4–C7

Figure 19-8 Segmental dissociated sensory loss due to a lesion of the central gray matter at the fourth to seventh cervical (C) segment of the spinal cord.

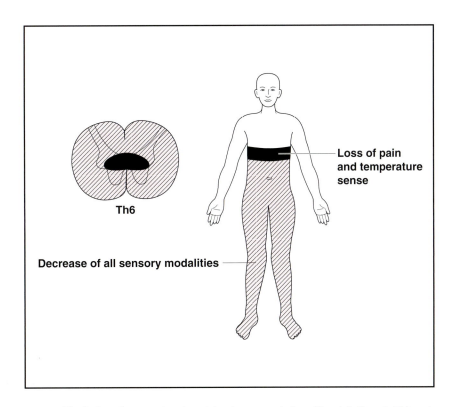

Figure 19-9 Distribution of sensory impairment in a transverse lesion of the sixth thoracic (Th) cord.

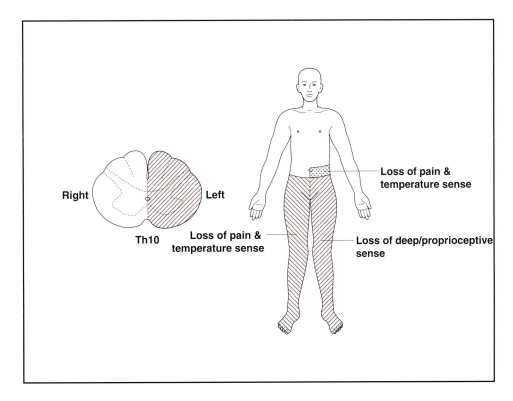

Figure 19-10 Brown-Séquard syndrome due to a lesion of the left half of the tenth thoracic (Th) cord.

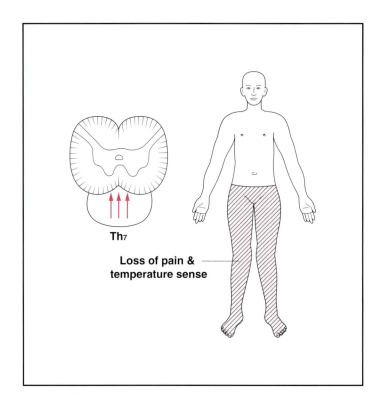

Figure 19-11 An example distribution of nociceptive loss due to anterior compression of the spinal cord. Although the cord is compressed at the seventh thoracic (Th) segment in this case, the pain and temperature sense is lost below the eleventh thoracic segment due to laminar structure of the spinothalamic tract (see Figure 16-3).

temperature senses are diminished below the affected segment on the contralateral side, because the fibers forming the spinothalamic tract already crossed from the other side below the affected segment. This clinical picture is called Brown-Séquard syndrome (Figure 19-10). In this case, since the gray matter is also damaged on the affected side, pain and temperature senses may be segmentally lost at the dermatomes on the affected side, again corresponding to the length of lesion (see "Segmental Dissociated Sensory Loss" described above).

In fact, it is quite rare to see a transection that is exactly limited to either half of the spinal cord. It is more common to see a bilateral lesion with considerable asymmetry. In the clinical setting, a modified form of Brown-Séquard syndrome is commonly encountered in an extramedullary compression of the spinal cord, because lateral compression of the spinal cord from one side has a contrecoup effect on the other side of the cord. Namely, motor paralysis is present bilaterally but more severe on the compressed side, and likewise for the proprioceptive sensory impairment, but the nociceptive impairment is more severe on the contralateral side. In an extramedullary compression, motor paralysis starts from the distal lower limb, because, in the corticospinal tract, the more

caudally projecting fibers are located more laterally (see Figure 16-3). Likewise, the nociceptive impairment on the contralateral side starts distally and ascends as the compression increases in its degree because of the laminar structure of the lateral spinothalamic tract (Figure 19-11, see also Figure 16-3).

In a Brown-Séquard syndrome due to an external cord compression, segmental sensory loss at the affected segment may not be just for the pain and temperature sense but also might include other modalities, because the dorsal root may be directly compressed.

When the spinal cord is compressed from anteriorly, the corticospinal tracts and the lateral spinothalamic tracts may be bilaterally affected (Figure 19-11). This is considered to be due to the fact that the spinal cord is bilaterally fixed to the spinal canal with the denticulate ligament, so that anterior compression causes mechanical distortion of the cord (see Chapter 16-1B).

The sympathetic tract of the autonomic nervous system descends through the medial part of the lateral column close to the gray matter (see Chapter 20-1). Therefore, if sphincter disturbance is present in a case of external cord compression, it suggests that the compression is strong enough to affect the intramedullary structure. In fact, the presence or absence of sphincter disturbance provides an important clue, in addition to the degree of motor weakness, for judging the necessity of surgical decompression.

Hemianalgesia is commonly seen in psychogenic disorders such as conversion reaction, which is described in the relevant chapter (see Chapter 26).

BIBLIOGRAPHY

Henry JL, Lalloo C, Yashpal K. Central poststroke pain: an abstruse outcome. Pain Res Manage 13:41–49, 2008.

Hongo Y, Onoue H, Takeshima S, Kamakura K, Kaida K. A case of Sjögren syndrome with subacute combined degeneration-like posterior column lesion on cervical MRI. Clin Neurol 52:491–494, 2012. (Abstract in English).

Igata A. Clinical studies on rising and re-rising neurological diseases in Japan. A personal contribution. Proc Jpn Acad Ser B 86:366–377, 2010. (review)

Koike H, Takahashi M, Ohyama K, Hashimoto R, Kawagashira Y, Iijima M, et al. Clinicopathologic features of folate-deficiency neuropathy. Neurology 84:1026–1033, 2015.

Kollewe K, Jin L, Krampfl K, Dengler R, Mohammadi B. Treatment of phantom limb pain with botulinum toxin type A. Pain Med 10:300–303, 2009.

Krarup-Hansen A, Helweg-Larsen S, Schmalbruch H, Rørth M, Krarup C. Neuronal involvement in cisplatin neuropathy: prospective clinical and neurophysiological studies. Brain 130:1076–1088, 2007.

Kusunoki S, Kaida K, Ueda M. Antibodies against gangliosides and ganglioside complexes in Guillain-Barré syndrome: new aspects of research. Biochim Biophys Acta 1780:441–444, 2008.

Lenders M, Karabul N, Duning T, Schmitz B, Schelleckes M, Mesters R, et al. Thromboembolic events in Fabry disease and the impact of factor V Leiden. Neurology 84:1009–1016, 2015.

Löhle M, Hughes D, Milligan A, Richfield L, Reichmann H, Mehta A, et al. Clinical prodromes of neurodegeneration in Anderson-Fabry disease. Neurology 84:1454–1464, 2015.

Mayo Clinic and Mayo Foundation. Mayo Clinic Examinations in Neurology, 7th ed. Mosby, St. Louis, 1998.

Mochizuki H, Kakigi R. Central mechanisms of itch. Clin Neurophysiol 126:1650–1660, 2015. (review)

Parisi TJ, Mandrekar J, Dyck PJB, Klein CJ. Meralgia paresthetica: relation to obesity, advanced age, and diabetes mellitus. Neurology 77:1538–1542, 2011.

Ruts L, Drenthen J, Jongen JLM, Hop WC, Visser GH, Jacobs BC, et al. Pain in Guillain-Barré syndrome: a long-term follow-up study. Neurology 75:1439–1447, 2010.

Shibasaki H, Kakigi R, Ohnishi A, Kuroiwa Y. Peripheral and central nerve conduction in subacute myelo-optico-neuropathy. Neurology 32:1186–1189, 1982.

Shibasaki H. Central mechanisms of pain perception. Clin Neurophysiol Suppl 57:39–49, 2004. (review)

Shibasaki H, Hitomi T, Mezaki T, Kihara T, Tomimoto H, Ikeda A, et al. A new form of congenital proprioceptive sensory neuropathy associated with arthrogryposis multiplex. J Neurol 251:1340–1344, 2004.

Toyooka K. Fabry disease. Curr Opin Neurology 24:463–468, 2011. (review)

20.

AUTONOMIC NERVOUS SYSTEM

Functions of the autonomic nervous system are control of vital signs, visceral control, and adjustment to the external environment. The autonomic nervous system consists of sympathetic and parasympathetic nervous systems, which are different from each other anatomically as well as pharmacologically. Both systems contain afferent and efferent systems.

1. STRUCTURE AND FUNCTION OF THE AUTONOMIC EFFERENT SYSTEM

The center of the autonomic nervous system is in the hypothalamus for both the sympathetic and parasympathetic systems (see Chapter 28-1).

A. SYMPATHETIC NERVOUS SYSTEM

The **sympathetic tract** arising from the hypothalamus descends through the brainstem tegmentum and the medial part of the lateral column of spinal cord, and enters the **intermediolateral nucleus**, which extends from the first thoracic (Th1) segment to the first lumbar (L1) segment (see Figures 8-4, 14-1 and 14-5). It is important to note that the whole body including the head and face is innervated by the sympathetic nervous system through the intermediolateral nucleus. For example, the intermediolateral nucleus at the Th1 segment projects its preganglionic fibers to the superior cervical ganglion, which innervates the pupils, and that nucleus is called the **ciliospinal center of Budge** (see Figure 8-4). For another example, the urinary bladder and genital organs are innervated by the intermediolateral nucleus at the Th12-L1 segment.

Thus, if the sympathetic tract is unilaterally damaged in the brainstem or cervical cord, sweating is lost and the skin temperature is elevated on the whole body (from head to feet) on the affected side. If the sympathetic tract is unilaterally damaged in the thoracic cord, the loss of sweating and the elevation of skin temperature are seen on the affected side below the affected segment. If the intermediolateral nucleus is damaged at a certain level between the Th1 and L1 segments, the loss of sweating and the elevation of skin temperature may be seen segmentally on the dermatomes corresponding to the affected segment.

Preganglionic fibers originating from the intermediolateral nucleus join the ventral root at each segment and exit the spinal canal through the intervertebral foramen, and they make synaptic contact with the postganglionic neurons in the **sympathetic ganglia** [Figure 20-1, see also Figure 16-6]. **Postganglionic fibers** are unmyelinated fibers and innervate pupils, blood vessels, sweat glands, endocrine glands, and visceral organs.

In the sympathetic nervous system, the preganglionic fibers are much shorter than the postganglionic fibers, because the sympathetic ganglion is situated near the spinal canal (Figure 20-2). An exception to this principle is the preganglionic fibers for the pupils, which make synaptic contact with the postganglionic neurons in the superior cervical ganglion (see Figure 8-4). By contrast, in the parasympathetic nervous system, the preganglionic fibers are much longer than the postganglionic fibers, because the parasympathetic ganglia are located near their target organs (Figure 20-2).

The neurotransmitter of the preganglionic fibers is acetylcholine with nicotinic transmission for both the sympathetic and parasympathetic nervous system. The neurotransmitter for the parasympathetic postganglionic fibers is acetylcholine with muscarinic transmission, and that for the sympathetic postganglionic fibers is noradrenaline. The only exception for the latter system is the postganglionic fibers for sweat glands, for which acetylcholine is the transmitter with muscarinic transmission (Figure 20-2).

B. PARASYMPATHETIC NERVOUS SYSTEM

The preganglionic neurons of the parasympathetic nervous system are located in the brainstem and in the second to fourth sacral segments of the spinal cord. In the

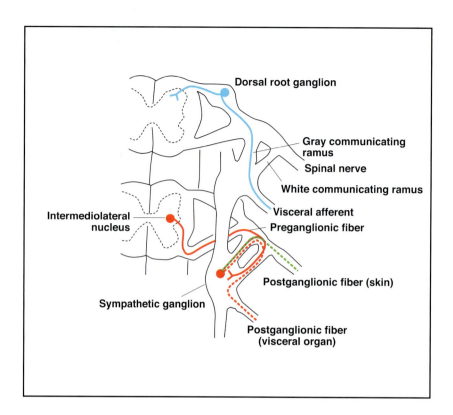

Figure 20-1 Schematic diagram showing the efferent pathway (in red) and afferent pathway (in blue) of the spinal sympathetic nervous system. The preganglionic fibers (solid red line) pass through the white communicating ramus to enter the sympathetic ganglion. The postganglionic fibers for skin (dotted green line) pass through the gray communicating ramus and join the spinal nerve, and those for visceral organs (dotted red lines) form the visceral nerve. The afferent sympathetic fibers are the peripheral axons of small bipolar cells in the dorsal root ganglion, which transmit the impulse from visceral organ through the gray communicating ramus to the dorsal root ganglion, and its central axons go to the dorsal horn of the spinal cord.

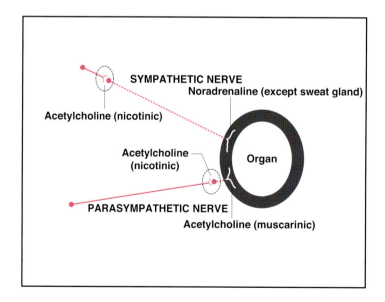

Figure 20-2 Schematic illustration of the sympathetic and parasympathetic ganglia with neurotransmitters. The preganglionic fiber shown in solid line is myelinated, and the postganglionic fiber shown in interrupted line is unmyelinated. The preganglionic fibers are much longer than the postganglionic fibers for the parasympathetic nervous system, and vice versa for the sympathetic nervous system.

brainstem, the parasympathetic nuclei of four cranial nerves (III, VII, IX, and X) project their preganglionic fibers to their respective ganglia. The Edinger-Westphal nucleus of the oculomotor nerve controls pupils and accommodation (see Chapter 8). The lacrimal nucleus and the superior salivatory nucleus of the facial nerve control lacrimation and salivation of the sublingual and submandibular glands, respectively (see Chapter 11-1D). The inferior salivatory nucleus of the glossopharyngeal nerve controls salivation of the parotid gland (see Chapter 14-4). The dorsal motor nucleus of the vagus controls visceral organs such as heart, lung, and gastrointestinal organs (see Chapter 14-5).

The parasympathetic nucleus of the sacral cord controls the urinary bladder and urinary tract, genital organs, and colon from the middle transverse colon to the rectum. As described in relation to the sympathetic nervous system (see above), the neurotransmitter for the parasympathetic preganglionic fibers is acetylcholine with nicotinic transmission and that for the postganglionic fibers is acetylcholine with muscarinic transmission (Figure 20-2).

When treating patients with myasthenia gravis with cholinesterase inhibitors, symptoms like miosis (small pupils), increased salivation, and upper respiratory secretion and abdominal pain may occur, because the drug enhances not only the cholinergic transmission at the neuromuscular junction but also the muscarinic transmission of the parasympathetic postganglionic fibers. In this case, sweating is also increased in spite of the fact the sweat gland is innervated by the sympathetic nervous system. This is because the sweat gland is exceptionally controlled by cholinergic transmission instead of noradrenergic transmission (see above). Furthermore, when giving atropine sulfate to myasthenic patients for preventing the autonomic side effects of cholinesterase inhibitors, there is no need to worry about its untoward effect on the neuromuscular junction, because atropine inhibits only the muscarinic transmission and does not inhibit the nicotinic transmission of acetylcholine at the neuromuscular junction.

C. DISORDERS OF THE PERIPHERAL AUTONOMIC NERVES

Some peripheral neuropathies affect primarily the autonomic nervous system. **Familial amyloid polyneuropathy** (Box 68) and **systemic amyloidosis** associated with multiple myeloma are well known to cause severe impairment of autonomic functions.

Autonomic ganglia might be affected by an autoimmune pathology, and this condition acutely causes severe autonomic disturbance, which is often intractable to medical treatment.

D. CORTICAL CENTER OF THE AUTONOMIC NERVOUS SYSTEM

Although no particular cortical areas have been identified as an autonomic center, the limbic areas including amygdala, insula, and cingulate gyrus are connected to the hypothalamic autonomic center. For urination, the **paracentral lobule** at the posterior mesial aspect of the frontal lobe is believed to play an important part in its voluntary control. In relation to this, bilateral compression of the mesial frontal lobes by a **falx meningioma** is known to cause bladder disturbance in addition to spastic paraparesis, thus resembling the spinal cord compression. Urinary incontinence seen in patients with **idiopathic normal-pressure hydrocephalus** might be due to dysfunction of the descending fibers from the mesial frontal cortex passing by the dilated lateral ventricles (see Box 71).

Patients with partial epilepsy may show cardiac arrhythmia or transient cardiac arrest during the ictal episode. The mesial temporal lobe or insula is believed to be responsible for this paroxysmal phenomenon, but the dominant hemisphere for this autonomic function has not been determined.

E. NEURAL CONTROL OF URINATION

Although urination (micturition) is a representative autonomic function, it can be controlled by intention as well. Thus a complex neuronal circuit from the frontal cortex through the brainstem to the sacral cord is involved in its control (Benarroch, 2010, for review). Among the cortical areas, the mesial prefrontal area, anterior cingulate gyrus, insular cortex, and motor cortices are considered to be involved in this function. In the spinal cord, the preganglionic neurons at the S2 to S4 segments, Onuf nucleus, and the intermediolateral nucleus at the Th12-L1 segments play major parts. Furthermore, the periaqueductal gray substance and the pontine micturition center are considered to play a role for connecting the cortex with the caudal spinal cord. Unilateral infarction in the lateral medulla or the dorsal lateral pontine tegmentum can cause urinary retention (Cho et al, 2015).

2. STRUCTURE AND FUNCTION OF THE AUTONOMIC AFFERENT SYSTEM

There are two kinds of autonomic afferent systems: visceral pain and visceral sensation. The primary neuron for **visceral pain** is a bipolar cell located in the dorsal root ganglion. Its peripheral axon transports impulses from a visceral organ to a ganglion along the sympathetic postganglionic fibers through the gray communicating ramus (Figure 20-1). The central axon enters the dorsal horn of the gray matter at the Th1 to L1 segments, from where the secondary neuron projects its axon centrally through the spinothalamic tract.

As the nociceptive impulse originating from the heart, for example, enters the dorsal horn at the Th2 segment, the pain is felt as if it came from the Th2 somatosensory dermatome as a **referred pain**, namely the left upper chest and the medial aspect of the left arm (Figure 20-3). For another example, the pain due to the urinary stones is felt in the inguinal region and the anterior aspect of the proximal thigh, because the sympathetic afferent fibers from the urinary tract enter the spinal cord at the L1 dermatome.

Visceral sensation like fullness of abdomen and bladder distention is centrally transmitted through the parasympathetic nerve fibers. For example, fullness of upper abdomen is transmitted through the vagus nerve to the solitary nucleus in the medulla, and the fibers from the solitary nucleus project to the thalamus and the brainstem reticular formation. Micturition desire is transmitted through the pelvic nerve to the S2 to S4 segments of the sacral cord, and then transmitted centrally through the lateral and

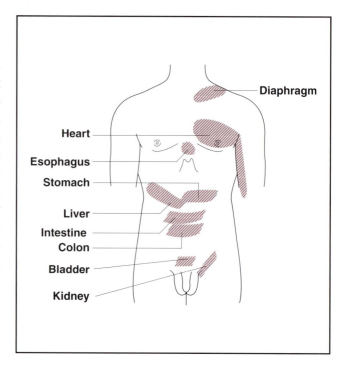

Figure 20-3 Dermatomes of referred pain originating from representative visceral organs.

posterior columns of the spinal cord. Micturition desire is considered to be partially transmitted also through the sympathetic nerve.

3. EXAMINATION OF THE AUTONOMIC NERVOUS FUNCTION

Examination of pupils can test an important autonomic function in the cranial nerve territory, but as it is described in Chapter 8-2, it is not repeated here.

A. AUTONOMIC SYMPTOMS OF SKIN

It is important to examine the color, temperature, and moisture of the skin. The skin temperature and moisture can be tested by palpating the skin by hand. In a unilateral lesion of the brainstem tegmentum like **Horner syndrome**, decreased sweating and elevated temperature of the skin are often seen ipsilaterally (see Chapter 8-1). Elevation of the skin temperature in this case is due to dilation of capillaries and arterioles due to a lesion of the sympathetic tract, causing an increased blood flow. In testing the skin moisture for Horner syndrome, move the hand from the possible dry side to the moist side. Movement in the other direction is less sensitive, since fluid could be moved along with the hand to the dry side. It is also possible to compare the homologous areas of the two sides with both hands of the examiner.

In **complex regional pain syndrome (CRPS)**, previously called reflex sympathetic dystrophy or causalgia, the affected part of skin is pale with increased sweating and decreased temperature. The CRPS is subdivided into two types: CRPS I is intended to encompass reflex sympathetic dystrophy and similar disorders without a nerve injury, and CRPS II occurs after damage to a peripheral nerve (Borchers & Gershwin, 2014, and Birklein et al, 2015, for review). In a transverse lesion of the spinal cord, sweating is decreased on the skin below the affected level. In a segmental lesion of the spinal cord, **dermographia** and abnormal **pilomotor reflex** might be seen at the corresponding dermatome. For all these tests, it is important to compare the homologous areas of the two sides, or in case of a spinal cord lesion, the skin regions above and below the affected segment should be compared.

B. MICTURITION AND SEXUAL FUNCTIONS

Micturition/defecation and sexual functions are some of the important autonomic functions. Careful history taking is most useful for checking these functions. Increased frequency of urination (**urinary frequency**) and **urge incontinence** are caused by a lesion of the central nervous system proximal to the sacral segment of the spinal cord. By contrast, a lesion of the sacral cord or cauda equina causes difficulty of micturition or **urinary retention**. In a lesion of the sacral cord, the anal sphincter reflex is decreased or lost, and in male patients, the bulbocavernous reflex is also lost. The **anal sphincter reflex** is tested by stimulating the perianal skin with a sterile pin and observing or digitally palpating a reflex contraction of the anal sphincter muscle. For testing the **bulbocavernous reflex**, glans penis is pinched and a reflex contraction of the anal sphincter muscle is confirmed by digital examination.

As the patient may not actively complain of sexual dysfunction, it is important in men to confirm the presence or absence of disturbance of penile erection (**impotence**) or disturbance of ejaculation by the history taking as necessary. In a lesion of the spinal cord rostral to the sacral segment, excessive erection may spontaneously occur and continue (**priapism**). In relation to this phenomenon, touching the legs might cause reflex urinary incontinence or profuse sweating in the legs.

C. GASTROINTESTINAL SYMPTOMS

Diarrhea associated with continuous abdominal pain or continuous constipation of unknown etiology might be due to disorders of the autonomic nervous system. However, pure disturbance of defecation due to neurological disorders without any disturbance of urination is extremely rare. **Alternating occurrence of diarrhea and constipation** is often seen in disorders of the autonomic nervous system. A triad of dysphagia, chest pain, and regurgitation is seen in **achalasia**. A combination of achalasia, alacrima (loss of tears), and adrenal failure is called triple A syndrome.

D. ORTHOSTATIC HYPOTENSION

This is one of the most common symptoms suggestive of the presence of autonomic failure, and the history taking might give an important clue. Generally, the symptom is feeling faint or a sense of impending loss of consciousness. For testing this function at the bedside, blood pressure can be measured first in the supine position and then in the upright position. After the patient takes the upright position, it is important to measure blood pressure, not just immediately after standing, but to keep measuring intermittently for at least about 3 minutes. If there is a drop of the systolic pressure by more than 20 mmHg, it can be judged to be orthostatic hypotension. It is important to measure the pulse rate simultaneously and to see whether or not the drop of blood pressure is compensated by an increase in the pulse rate. Since patients with movement disorders may require an excessive effort for standing up from the bed, it may have some effect on the blood pressure. Therefore, in order to determine the postural change of blood pressure precisely, it is ideal to use a tilt table.

For testing the physiological change of pulse rate with breathing, the patient may be asked to repeat taking deep breath slowly while the pulse rate is being measured. Quantitatively, the **R-R interval** may be calculated by electrocardiogram to quantitatively measure its variability. Complete loss of the variability in the R-R interval suggests the presence of autonomic failure.

Orthostatic hypotension is caused by various etiologies including neurodegenerative diseases such as **pure autonomic failure** and **multiple system atrophy (Shy-Drager syndrome)** (Box 69), and autonomic failure due to a lesion of the spinal cord or the peripheral nervous system. Orthostatic hypotension is also seen in Parkinson disease at various frequencies (up to 40% depending on the statistics). In fact, a deficiency of transmitter uptake at the sympathetic nerve terminals of myocardium has been demonstrated by single photon emission computed tomography (SPECT) using [123]metaiodobenzylguanidine (MIBG) as a tracer in patients with idiopathic Parkinson disease, although its

The Aschner eyeball pressure test and carotid sinus
pressure test are tests for evaluating autonomic function by
demonstrating reflex bradycardia in response to pressure of
the eyeballs and carotid artery, respectively. However, these
tests are not recommended especially for the patients with
autonomic failure, because these maneuvers may induce
cardiac arrest in them.

BIBLIOGRAPHY

Adams D, Coelho T, Obici L, Merlini G, Mincheva Z, Suanprasert N,
et al. Rapid progression of familial amyloidotic polyneuropathy: a
multinational natural history study. Neurology 85:675–682, 2015.
Ando Y, Nakamura M, Araki S. Transthyretin-related familial amyloidotic polyneuropathy. Arch Neurol 62:1057–1062, 2005. (review)
Benarroch EE. Neural control of the bladder: recent advances and neurologic implications. Neurology 75:1839–1846, 2010. (review)
Birklein F, O'Neill D, Schlereth T. Complex regional pain syndrome: an
optimistic perspective. Neurology 84:89–96, 2015. (review)
Borchers AT, Gershwin ME. Complex regional pain syndrome: a com-
prehensive and critical review. Autoimmun Rev 13:242–265, 2014.
(review)
Cho H-J, Kang T-H, Chang J-H, Choi Y-R, Park M-G, Choi K-D, et al.
Neuroanatomical correlation of urinary retention in lateral medullary infarction. Ann Neurol 77:726–733, 2015.
Gilman S, Wenning GK, Low PA, Brooks DJ, Mathias CJ, Trojanowski
JQ, et al. Second consensus statement on the diagnosis of multiple
system atrophy. Neurology 71:670–676, 2008.
Heckman MG, Schottlaender L, Soto-Ortolaza AI, Diehl NN, Ray-
aprolu S, Ogaki K, et al. LRRK2 exonic variants and risk of multiple
system atrophy. Neurology 83:2256–2261, 2014.
Jellinger KA. Neuropathology of multiple system atrophy: new thoughts
about pathogenesis. Mov Disord 29:1720–1741, 2014. (review)
King AE, Mintz J, Royall DR. Meta-analysis of ^{123}I-MIBG cardiac scin-
tigraphy for the diagnosis of Lewy body-related disorders. Mov Disord 26:1218–1224, 2011.
Koga S, Aoki N, Uitti RJ, van Gerpen JA, Cheshire WP, Josephs KA,
et al. When DLB, PD, and PSP masquerade as MSA: an autopsy
study of 134 patients. Neurology 85:404–412, 2015.
The Multiple-System Atrophy Research Collaboration. Mutations in
COQ2 in familial and sporadic multiple-system atrophy. N Engl J
Med 369:233–244, 2013.
Wenning GK, Stefanova N, Jellinger KA, Poewe W, Schlossmacher MG.
Multiple system atrophy: a primary oligodendrogliopathy. Ann Neu-
rol 64:239–246, 2008.
Yamashita T, Ando Y, Okamoto S, Misumi Y, Hirahara T, Ueda M, et al.
Long-term survival after liver transplantation in patients with famil-
ial amyloid polyneuropathy. Neurology 78:637–643, 2012.

relationship with orthostatic hypotension is not clear. It
is the current consensus that **decreased uptake of MIBG
in myocardium** is relatively characteristic of Lewy body-
associated disorders including Parkinson disease, Lewy
body dementia, and pure autonomic failure, and it is rare
in multiple system atrophy, progressive supranuclear palsy,
Alzheimer disease, and frontotemporal dementia (King
et al, 2011) (Box 69).

21.

POSTURE AND GAIT

1. CENTRAL CONTROL MECHANISM OF GAIT

In human walking, intention or attention takes part to various degrees, from fully attended walking to nearly automatic walking. Multiple structures of the central nervous system are known to be involved in the central control of walking (Figure 21-1) (Shibasaki et al, 2004, and Nutt et al, 2011, for review). In addition to the sensorimotor areas directly related to leg movement such as the pre-SMA, SMA proper, anterior cingulate gyrus, lateral premotor areas, and the foot areas of the primary sensorimotor cortices, the cortical areas related to the visual information processing such as the occipital cortex and the posterior parietal area are also important. Furthermore, the brainstem gait center, cerebellum, and basal ganglia also play an important part. In animals, the locomotion

center located in the dorsal part of the rostral brainstem plays an important role. The greater the intention and attention paid to the walking, the more widespread is the cortical activation.

2. EXAMINATION OF GAIT

Careful observation of walking provides important information in the clinical setting. Abnormal gait is classified into several typical patterns.

A. SPASTIC GAIT

Spastic gait is characterized by a stiff shuffling gait. The patient walks slowly, dragging both legs, without lifting

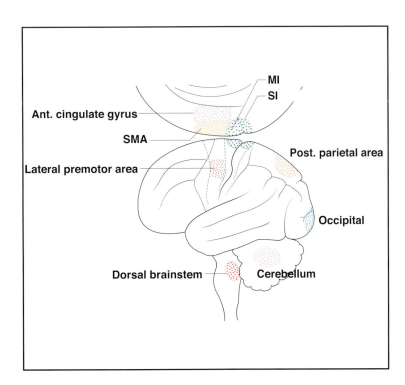

Figure 21-1 Schematic diagram showing the human brain areas activated during intended walking. (Based on Shibasaki et al, 2004)

the feet completely off the ground. When it is severe, the knees tend to cross with each step because of increased tightness of the hip adductors (**scissor gait**). The patient often complains of bouncing and trembling especially when going downstairs. This is considered to be due to patellar and ankle clonus, which is evoked by stretching the leg muscles when stepping downstairs (see Chapter 16-3D). Spastic gait is seen in patients with spasticity of leg muscles due to a lesion of the pyramidal tract or upper motor neurons.

B. PARKINSONIAN GAIT

Parkinsonian gait is characterized by delayed initiation, slow walking with small steps, loss of arm swing, and tendency to accelerate involuntarily (**festinating gait, propulsion**). It is not rare to festinate backward and fall

(**retropulsion**). In relation to the stooped posture, some patients might show markedly flexed posture while standing or walking, but the posture improves when lying down. This condition is called **camptocormia** or **bent spine syndrome** (see Chapter 15-2).

Freezing of Gait

Patients with Parkinson disease may suddenly become unable to move, particularly upon gait initiation or turning (**freezing phenomenon**) (Nutt et al, 2011, for review). The freezing phenomenon might improve by some types of visual input. For example, the patient can walk much better if transverse lines are drawn on the floor at short intervals so that the patient could walk across the lines. This phenomenon is called **kinésie paradoxale (paradoxical kinesia)** (Box 70).

Paradoxical kinesia is also seen in patients with **pure akinesia**, of which progressive supranuclear palsy (PSP) is believed to be the most likely cause (Park et al, 2009). As for the causes of frequent falls in patients with PSP, abnormalities of vestibulospinal function (which can be tested with vestibulo-ocular reflexes or vestibular-evoked myogenic potentials) have been reported (Liao et al, 2008) (Box 71).

It is noteworthy that Parkinson patients have greater difficulty in controlling the posture in the anteroposterior direction as seen in festinating gait, propulsion, and retropulsion, while patients with cerebellar ataxia have loss of equilibrium in all directions, especially in the lateral direction. Falls are not uncommon in patients with Parkinson disease, and this might be primarily related to impairment of the pedunculopontine nucleus (Bohnen et al, 2009) (see Box 27).

In order to examine postural stability, the **pull test** is performed while the patient stands with his feet side by side and the examiner stands behind the patient with one foot slightly behind the other. The patient should be given an explanation in advance that the examiner is going to pull the patient abruptly backward by his shoulders and that he is allowed to step backward in order to maintain balance. However, since there is a risk of falls during this test especially in patients with movement disorders, this test should be done with great caution.

C. ATAXIC GAIT

Unsteady, staggering gait due to loss of equilibrium is called ataxic gait. Patients with ataxia usually stand or walk with a wide base (**wide-based gait**). In patients with mild ataxia, ordinary walking might appear normal, but **tandem gait**

BOX 70 HOW DOES PARADOXICAL KINESIA OCCUR?

Patients who are unable to walk on the flat floor because of frozen gait may be able to climb upstairs. This phenomenon called **paradoxical kinesia (kinésie paradoxale)** may be also seen when the patient walks across the transverse lines drawn on the floor at short intervals, suggesting that the visual input of transverse lines in front of the body plays a primary role in improving the initiation of gait. A similar phenomenon is also seen in the upper limbs. A patient who has great difficulty in moving the arm in response to verbal instruction might be able to promptly catch a ball thrown toward him/her. There was a hypothesis that the cerebellum might take over the role of the basal ganglia immediately in response to visual input, but it has not been proved. Hanakawa et al. (1999a, 1999b) used a blood flow activation study with SPECT while patients with Parkinson disease walked on a treadmill, comparing transverse lines and parallel lines, and demonstrated a greater activation in the right lateral premotor area in association with transverse lines compared with parallel lines. This result was interpreted by postulating that, in Parkinson patients, self-initiated gait is impaired because of a deficient excitatory input to the SMA, but the lateral premotor area, which is relatively preserved in Parkinson disease and which is known to receive abundant visual input, might be activated by transverse lines (Shibasaki et al, 2004, for review). However, a question as to why only transverse lines, but not parallel lines, are effective remains to be solved. In general, paradoxical kinesia occurs because external triggering of movement is more effective than internal triggering in Parkinson patients.

BOX 71 IDIOPATHIC NORMAL-PRESSURE HYDROCEPHALUS

Progressive gait disturbance associated with urinary incontinence and cognitive impairment in the elderly patients may be due to idiopathic normal-pressure hydrocephalus (INPH), which is a treatable condition. This condition was first reported by Adams et al. in 1965. As a ventricular shunt is effective in some cases of this condition, how to determine its indication has been a practical problem (Torsnes et al, 2014, for review; Halperin et al, 2015). Having all three symptoms makes the diagnosis more likely. McGirt et al. (2008) investigated the effect of shunting in 132 cases who had at least two of the above three symptoms, dilated ventricles on imaging study, and β waves (slow rhythmic oscillation) of the cerebrospinal fluid. Other causes of secondary hydrocephalus such as subarachnoid hemorrhage, head trauma, and meningitis were excluded in those cases. After the mean follow-up period of a year and half, 75% of all patients showed improvement. It was found especially effective in patients in the relatively short period after clinical onset and in those predominantly presenting the gait disturbance. Among the triad, improvement was found to be most prominent in gait disturbance. It is important to keep this condition in mind whenever elderly subjects suffer from gait disturbance and falls of unknown etiology (Jaraj et al, 2014).

will disclose truncal ataxia. It is important to instruct the subject to put the heel of one foot just in front of the toes of the other foot. When testing the tandem gait, it may be anticipated that walking slowly might be easier than walking fast, but the fact is on the contrary. In ataxic gait due to an organic lesion, tandem gait can be executed easier with faster speed than with slower speed just as it is so for healthy subjects to walk on a balance beam. Some patients with psychogenic gait disturbance of ataxic nature tend to execute the tandem gait poorly with fast speed and much better with slower speed.

Ataxic gait is due to a lesion of the cerebellum, vestibular system, or proprioceptive system. When a patient complains of vertigo, the ataxic gait is often vestibular in nature. Presence of tinnitus, hearing loss, postural nystagmus, or rotatory nystagmus suggests vestibular ataxia (see Chapter 13-2). Patients with ataxic gait of cerebellar origin also tend to have abnormalities in ocular movements, dysarthria, and limb ataxia. Occasionally, a localized lesion confined to the cerebellum may cause vertigo due to involvement of the vestibular input to the cerebellum (see Chapter 13-1). **Sensory ataxia** is caused by interruption of proprioceptive input by a lesion of the dorsal column or

the peripheral nervous system (see Chapter 19-2B). As the effect of proprioceptive deficit may be compensated visually, interruption of visual input by closing eyes provokes or worsens the truncal ataxia (**Romberg sign** and **basin phenomenon**) (see Figure 19-5).

D. WADDLING GAIT AND STEPPAGE GAIT

Muscle weakness in the pelvic girdle causes excessive pelvic swing on walking (**waddling gait**). This phenomenon is typically seen in myopathy, especially in the limb-girdle muscular dystrophy, but it may be also seen in neurogenic muscle atrophy of proximal muscles like Kugelberg-Welander disease (see Chapter 16-3B).

Weakness of foot extensor muscles, especially that of the anterior tibial muscle, causes difficulty in lifting toes (**foot-drop**) and lifting legs high in order to avoid tripping during walking (**steppage gait**). A typical example of steppage gait is seen in Charcot-Marie-Tooth disease (see Chapter 16-3C).

Falls/falling is a big social problem in the aging society. When taking the medical history of patients with

BOX 72 INTERMITTENT CLAUDICATION

In this condition, the patient develops pain and numbness in the lower extremities after walking some distance, which disappears by taking rest.

Intermittent claudication is not uncommon in elderly subjects. There are two kinds of causes for this condition: obstructive disorders of the peripheral arteries like **Buerger disease** and neurological disorders related to the spinal cord or cauda equina. In the former condition, the skin of the affected limb appears pale with cold surface temperature, and pulsation of the dorsal artery of foot is deficient. **Neurogenic or spinal intermittent claudication** is commonly due to the spinal canal stenosis or arteriovenous malformation. As the symptoms may appear only when walking, it is important to examine the patient when the symptoms appear after walking. Segmental loss of superficial sensation, muscle weakness, or loss of tendon reflexes might be observed during the episode. Neurologic deficit during this episode might be due to direct mechanical compression of the lumbosacral cord or cauda equina on one hand, but on the other hand it may be due to the regional ischemia due to stealing of arterial perfusion from the narrowed artery to the skeletal muscles during walking (**steal phenomenon**). Whichever the cause, treatment of the underlying condition is important.

gait disturbance, it is important to confirm any episode of falling within the past year and the presence or absence of any disorders which might cause falling (Thurman et al, 2008) (Box 72).

BIBLIOGRAPHY

Bohnen NI, Müller MLTM, Koeppe RA, Studenski SA, Kilbourn MA, Frey KA, et al. History of falls in Parkinson disease is associated with reduced cholinergic activity. Neurology 73:1670–1676, 2009.

Halperin JJ, Kurlan R, Schwalb JM, Cusimano MD, Gronseth G, Gloss D. Practice guideline: Idiopathic normal pressure hydrocephalus: Response to shunting and predictors of response. Report of the Guideline Development, Dissemination, and Implementation Subcommittee of the American Academy of Neurology. Neurology 85:2063–2071, 2015.

Hanakawa T, Katsumi Y, Fukuyama H, Honda M, Hayashi T, Kimura J, et al. Mechanisms underlying gait disturbance in Parkinson's disease: a single photon emission computed tomography study. Brain 122:1271–1282, 1999a.

Hanakawa T, Fukuyama H, Katsumi Y, Honda M, Shibasaki H. Enhanced lateral premotor activity during paradoxical gait in Parkinson's disease. Ann Neurol 45:329–336, 1999b.

Jaraj D, Rabiei K, Marlow T, Jensen C, Skoog I, Wikkelso C. Prevalence of idiopathic normal-pressure hydrocephalus. Neurology 82:1449–1454, 2014.

Liao K, Wagner J, Joshi A, Estrovich I, Walker MF, Strupp M, et al. Why do patients with PSP fall? Evidence for abnormal otolith responses. Neurology 70:802–809, 2008.

McGirt MJ, Woodworth G, Coon AL, Thomas G, Williams MA, Rigamonti D. Diagnosis, treatment, and analysis of long-term outcomes in idiopathic normal-pressure hydrocephalus. Neurosurgery 62 (Suppl 2):670–677, 2008.

Nutt JG, Bloem BR, Giladi N, Hallett M, Horak FB, Nieuwboer A. Freezing of gait: moving forward on a mysterious clinical phenomenon. Lancet Neurol 10:734–744, 2011. (review)

Park HK, Kim JS, Im KC, Oh SJ, Kim MJ, Lee JH, et al. Functional brain imaging in pure akinesia with gait freezing: [^{18}F] FDG PET and [^{18}F] FP-CIT PET analyses. Mov Disord 24:237–245, 2009.

Shibasaki H, Fukuyama H, Hanakawa T. Neural control mechanisms for normal versus parkinsonian gait. Prog Brain Res 143:199–205, 2004. (review)

Thurman DJ, Stevens JA, Rao JK. Practice parameter: assessing patients in a neurology practice for risk of falls (an evidence-based review). Report of the Quality Standards Subcommittee of the American Academy of Neurology. Neurology 70:473–479, 2008. (review)

Torsnes L, Blafjelldal V, Poulsen FR. Treatment and clinical outcome in patients with idiopathic normal pressure hydrocephalus—a systematic review. Dan Med J 61:A4911, 2014. (review)

22.

MENTAL AND COGNITIVE FUNCTIONS

I f a patient has any mental disorders or cognitive disturbances, those symptoms are often noticed while taking the history. Therefore, when evaluating the mental and cognitive functions in detail, it may be efficient to do so after completing the physical examination, instead of spending a long time for the interview at the beginning of the examination. On the other hand, a number of clinicians do prefer to do the cognitive testing first. In fact, abnormalities of higher cortical functions, if any, are often detected while carrying out the physical examination, because verbal communication is necessary for physical examination.

There are various ways of quantitatively evaluating the mental state (Daffner et al, 2015). The **Mini-Mental State Examination (MMSE)** proposed by Folstein et al. (1975) is shown in Table 22-1 as an example. Another popular test is the **Montreal Cognitive Assessment (MoCA)** (Table 22-2) (Chiti & Pantoni, 2014, for review). The MoCA includes executive functions testing. What is most essential for the mental state examination is to obtain concrete information about daily life from the patient's family or to directly observe the patient's behavior in the clinic. The direct observation of actual behaviors often provides far more important information than examining the patient in the outpatient clinic.

Examination of the mental state and cognitive functions is only possible with conscious patients. Furthermore, it is important to confirm hearing ability, language comprehension, and spontaneous speech before starting the mental evaluation, because all the related tests are performed by using spoken or written language. When a patient has any difficulty in comprehending spoken language, he/she may still be able to communicate by using the written language. If the patient has difficulty in both spoken and written languages, then the test has to be done by gesture or with the aid of pictures.

1. EXAMINATION OF MENTAL/COGNITIVE FUNCTIONS

Cognitive testing is performed for the following items. The order of examination of these items can be freely chosen depending on the patient's condition and circumstances.

Orientation to time, place, and person

Memory; retention span, recent memory, old memory, and presence or absence of confabulation

Calculation

Common knowledge and judgment

Emotion and character

Presence or absence of illusion, hallucination, and delusion

State of daily living

A. ORIENTATION

This is to test how much a patient is aware of the situation in which he/she is placed in terms of time, place, and person. If the patient is suddenly asked what day it is, he/she may be unable to answer promptly because he/she is upset by the unexpected question. In that case, it is useful to make the patient relaxed before repeating the question. The presence of **disorientation** is often noticed while taking the history. In most patients with mental impairment, orientation is more impaired to time than to space.

Sometimes it may be difficult to distinguish whether the patient is disoriented to time or has disturbance of recent memory (see below). If the patient answers a wrong day, it is useful to give the correct day and ask to remember it. If the patient can recall the correct day a few minutes

TABLE 22-1 MINI-MENTAL STATE EXAMINATION (MMSE)

Category	Possible points	Description
Orientation to time	5	Year, season, day of the week, month, and day.
Orientation to place	5	State, county or prefecture, city, hospital, floor, and region.
Registration	3	Memory of three unrelated objects.
Attention and calculation	5	Serial sevens.
Recall	3	Registration recall of the three objects presented above.
Language	2	Naming a pencil and a watch.
Repetition	1	Repeating a phrase forward and backward.
Complex commands	6	Six complex commands, including drawing a presented figure.
Total score	30	

SOURCE: Modified from Folstein et al, 1975.

later, recent memory may not be a primary problem for that patient.

B. MEMORY

Memory is divided into **episodic memory** and **procedural memory**, and episodic memory is mainly composed of **semantic memory**. Acquisition (registration), retention, and retrieval of information are all necessary

TABLE 22-2 MONTREAL COGNITIVE ASSESSMENT (MoCA)

1. Alternating trail making

2. Visuoconstructional skills (cube)

3. Visuoconstructional skills (clock)

4. Naming

5. Memory

6. Attention: Forward digit span, Backward digit span, Vigilance, Administration

7. Sentence repetition

8. Verbal fluency

9. Abstraction

10. Delayed recall

11. Orientation

for each category of memory. According to the length of the information retention, memory can be divided either into short-term memory and long-term memory, or into immediate memory, recent memory, and remote memory. **Immediate memory** is a memory lasting seconds and almost equal to repetition. For example, it is tested by giving five digits and asking the patient to repeat them soon afterward. **Recent memory** is a memory lasting a few minutes. In transient global amnesia, recent memory is mainly impaired, so that the patient repeats the same questions (Box 73). **Remote memory** is a memory lasting years, and it is tested by asking past events related to the patient or from the news. In general, patients with memory disturbance can better recall events that occurred in childhood than more recent events.

Examination of Memory

The presence of memory disturbance is usually suspected when taking the history. In the clinical practice, three unrelated words can be given verbally or in a written form, and the patient is asked to recall them after a short while. For quantitative measurement, 10 pairs of unrelated words are presented for memorizing, and after a short period of time, the patient is asked to answer the paired word for each given word. If this test was poorly performed, then 10 pairs of related words may be used. As described above, if the patient is found to be disoriented to time, the correct information should be provided for memorizing.

In memory loss due to acute cerebral lesions such as strokes, acute encephalitis and head trauma, the patients often lose memory of events that occurred various lengths of time before the acute insult. In this case, the information preserved in the past cannot be retrieved (**retrograde amnesia**). How far back the memory is lost differs depending on the severity of the retrograde amnesia. In severe retrograde amnesia, all the previously acquired information is lost back to childhood, and during recovery, the memory gradually returns starting from the older events.

If consciousness is lost due to an acute brain insult due to trauma, for example, the patient is not expected to remember what happened during unconsciousness. Even in that case, however, if the memory center is not damaged by the insult, the patient is able to recall later what happened up to the exact moment of that injury. Therefore, if retrograde amnesia is present after the recovery from unconsciousness, it suggests that the memory center has also been damaged.

BOX 73 **TRANSIENT GLOBAL AMNESIA**

This episode suddenly occurs in healthy adults above middle age, and is characterized by confusion recognized for example by repetition of the same questions or comments during the episode. It is accompanied by retrograde amnesia of various lengths, but it recovers completely starting from the oldest memories. During such an episode, therefore, the patient is not only unable to acquire, retain, and retrieve the new information, but also unable to retrieve the old memory. In contrast with a psychomotor seizure, there is no behavioral abnormality during an attack of retrograde amnesia. Excessive emotional excitation may provoke the attack in some cases, but a precipitating factor may not be found in others. A release of glutamate from the amygdala to the hippocampus by emotional excitation was thought to cause spreading depression in the hippocampus. Hypotheses for its pathogenesis also include partial epilepsy and transient ischemic attack of hippocampus. A study of patients within 48 hours after the onset of the attack with diffusion MRI showed abnormality in the CA-1 region of hippocampus, which disappeared within 10 days (Bartsch et al, 2007). These data suggested ischemia as the most likely cause (Bartsch et al, 2010). Recurrence of this condition is relatively uncommon.

Memory function is usually tested by using verbal or written language. However, some patients may retain memory of the visual or auditory information, but not in language. In this case, it is useful to present a set of objects or a set of sounds, and after a short time, to present one of the objects to ask whether it was one of the presented objects or not. Theoretically, it is also possible to do a similar test for gustatory and olfactory information.

Korsakov (Korsakoff) Syndrome

When a patient has disorientation in time and loss of recent memory, it is important to check if there is any **confabulation** or not. If a patient has confabulation, the patient not only gives a clearly wrong answer to the examiner's question but also he/she believes that the given answer is correct. In an extreme situation, the patient might even agree with wrong information deliberately given by the examiner.

A combination of disorientation in time, loss of recent memory, and confabulation is called **Korsakov syndrome** (it may also be spelled Korsakoff), which is usually associated with a lesion of the mammillary bodies and hypothalamus. The most representative conditions manifesting this syndrome are **Wernicke encephalopathy** (Boxes 74 and 75)

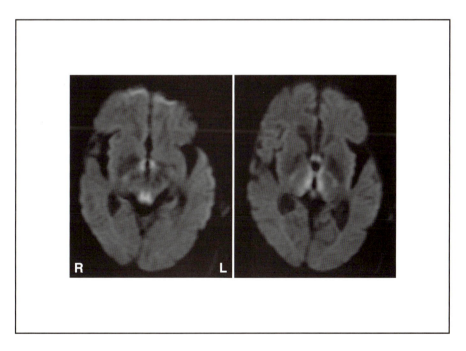

Figure 22-1 Diffusion MRI of a patient who acutely presented diplopia, unsteady gait, delusion, and marked fluctuation of body temperature following massive alcohol intake. The MRI shows abnormal signal around the third ventricle and in the mammillary bodies, suggestive of Wernicke encephalopathy.

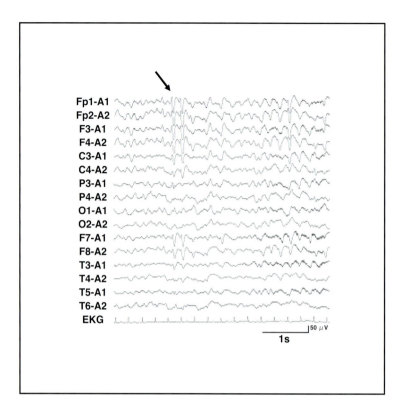

Figure 22-2 EEG of a patient with hepatic encephalopathy, showing lack of the posterior dominant rhythm and diffuse slow waves with frequent burst-like occurrence of high amplitude slow waves and occasional triphasic waves (arrow).

and limbic encephalitis (see Box 95). In these conditions, the patients commonly show emotional abnormalities, character change, and frivolous, unreliable personality. If this condition is further accompanied by abnormal behaviors like oral tendency and hypersexuality, it is called **Klüver-Bucy syndrome**. The latter syndrome is seen in association

with bilateral lesions of the mesial temporal lobes like herpes simplex encephalitis, limbic encephalitis, and postanoxic encephalopathy.

The neural circuit related to memory function has been known as the Papez circuit (Jang & Kwon, 2014, for review) (Figure 22-3). This circuit starts from the hippocampus and uncus, then goes through the fornix, septal nucleus, and mammillary body, **mammillothalamic tract of Vicq d'Azyr**, anterior nucleus of thalamus, and cingulum in this order, and finally returns to the hippocampus. In this circuit, a part of fibers from the septal nucleus is considered to enter the cingulate gyrus directly without going through the anterior nucleus of thalamus. This pathway, together with the **medial dorsal nucleus of the thalamus** (see Chapter 27-4), is known to play an important role in memory (Danet et al, 2015), and it is well known that bilateral lesions of the medial thalamus cause marked amnesia (Figure 22-4).

C. CALCULATION

For testing mental calculation, serial subtraction of 7 from 100 is commonly used. If the patient is suddenly given this order, he/she may be too upset to respond correctly. Therefore, it is important to judge by taking into account the patient's character and circumstances. In view of the fact that this task requires working memory and attention, if the patient has difficulty in responding verbally, it may be useful to give the same test in a written form. If the patient has any difficulty in calculation, it is important to judge whether it is a part of generalized cognitive

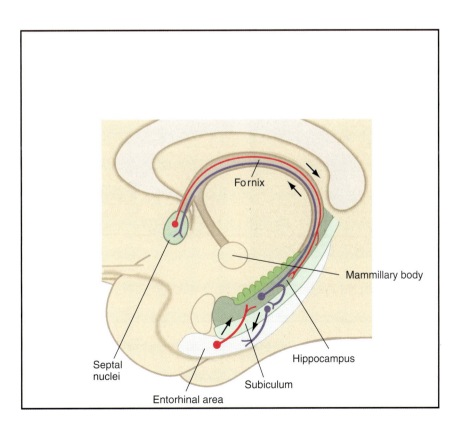

Figure 22-3 Schematic diagram showing the neuronal circuit related to memory. (Reproduced with minor modification from Brodal, 2010, with permission)

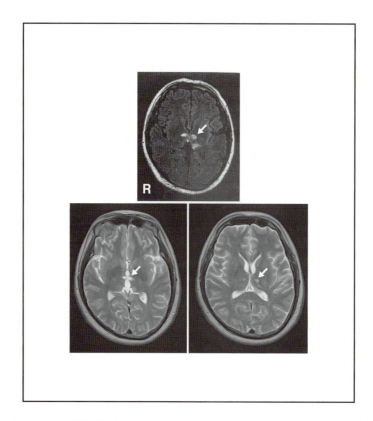

Figure 22-4 Diffusion MRI (top) and T2-weighted MRI (bottom) of a patient who presented marked amnesia following bilateral medial thalamic infarction (arrows). There was consciousness disturbance and abnormal sensation on the right half of the body at the clinical onset.

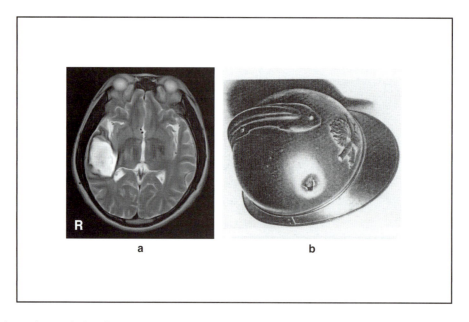

a   b

Figure 22-5 Character change due to a lesion of the right temporal lobe. (a) MRI of a patient who showed marked character change and left inferior quadrantanopsia following acute attack of severe headache and consciousness disturbance. A large hemorrhage is seen in the right temporal and parietal lobes. (b) Helmet used by the French poet Apollinaire during the war. His character changed dramatically after the head injury. (Reproduced from Bogousslavsky, 2005, with permission)

impairment or **acalculia**, which is a focal cortical sign due to a lesion of the left supramarginal gyrus and an important component of Gerstmann syndrome in the right-handed subject. This distinction is usually possible by taking other mental functions into consideration, but it is believed that the patients with acalculia tend to make more errors in the position of digits on the vertically written calculation. By contrast, patients with generalized cognitive impairment find it easier to make the written calculation than the mental calculation.

D. COMMON KNOWLEDGE AND JUDGMENT

Judgment is divided into two categories: cognitive judgment and social judgment. The cognitive judgment is directly related to the perception and recognition of external stimulus and internal milieu, whereas social judgment involves interpersonal relationship. For cognitive judgment of general sensory information, the primary as well as secondary sensory center for each modality plays a role. For special sensory modalities, special receptive areas in the parietal and temporal cortex are important (see Chapter 23-2C). Regarding social judgment, the orbitofrontal cortex and the dorsolateral prefrontal area play an important role for judgment based on visual information, and the amygdala is related to the judgment of face emotion (Mah et al, 2004). For moral judgment, the mesial prefrontal area is considered to be important (Avram et al, 2014).

Common knowledge and judgment can be evaluated during the history taking, by talking to the patient about topics of common interest, depending on the patient's educational level and occupation. The topics may include the recent news about society, sports, arts, and hobbies. It is also possible to evaluate the process of thinking and judgment by asking the patient about how he/she feels about that particular topic.

E. EMOTION AND CHARACTER

These features can also be estimated by observing facial expression and behavior of the patient during the history taking. It may also be judged by observing emotional reaction of the patient by presenting some jokes. Information obtained from the patient's family as to whether or not there has been any recent change in the patient's character is very useful (Box 76).

BOX 76 CHANGE OF EMOTION AND CHARACTER BY A LESION OF THE RIGHT TEMPORAL LOBE

A 35-year-old man developed severe headache, and 12 hours later he lost consciousness. After recovery from the acute episode, he often got angry at home and showed marked character change. The patient was found to be in a state of abulia with little facial expression and slow motor initiation and execution. There was also left homonymous inferior quadrantanopsia. A large hemorrhage was found in the right temporoparietal lobe (Figure 22-5a). In relation to this case, the French poet Apollinaire, after having sustained a war injury to the right temporal head (Figure 22-5b), became unable to control emotion and stopped writing to his fiancée, to whom he used to write almost every day before the injury (Bogouslavsky, 2005).

F. ILLUSION, HALLUCINATION, AND DELUSION

These are a group of positive psychiatric symptoms (see Chapter 1-1). In **illusion**, a given stimulus is sensed as different from what is expected to be sensed. In contrast, **hallucination** is a phenomenon of seeing or hearing what is not there to be seen or heard, respectively. A typical example of **visual hallucination** is seeing insects that are not actually present, and the patient often reacts to the image either verbally or behaviorally. Visual hallucination is commonly seen in **delirious states (delirium)** such as those due to alcohol intoxication, other toxic encephalopathies, and metabolic encephalopathies. Visual hallucination also occurs in patients with Parkinson disease during L-dopa treatment or in patients with diffuse Lewy body disease, especially at night.

Patients with **auditory hallucination** may hear voices of other people who are not there and may even respond to them by speaking or acting. **Delusion** is defined as abnormal belief of false ideas such as delusion of persecution and grandiose delusion. Auditory hallucination and delusion are often seen in patients with psychosis, schizophrenia among others, but they may also be seen in patients with intractable temporal lobe epilepsy during the interictal phase and other organic brain diseases.

G. STATE OF DAILY LIVING

Information about the patient's daily life obtained from the patient's family and housemates is most useful for evaluating mental functions. In case of women who work in the home, for example, information as to whether she makes any mistakes in shopping, cooking, cleaning and washing may disclose abnormalities, if any. Especially in Alzheimer disease, questions as to whether or not the patient has any difficulty in finding the way to his/her own house may provide useful information in relation to topographical abilities, which are commonly impaired in this disease.

2. DEMENTIA

Dementia is a condition in which all or some of the above-described mental/cognitive functions are impaired to various degrees and which, in the advanced stage, causes severe disability in social life. It is often accompanied by impairment of focal cortical functions (see Chapter 23), and in the very early stage, focal cortical dysfunction may predominate the clinical picture. It is known that the prevalence of dementia increases with aging between 65 and 85. In a study of 911 subjects above age 90 in California, 45% of women were diagnosed to have dementia versus 28% of men (Corrada et al, 2008). It was further shown that, in women of age over 90, the prevalence of dementia doubled every 5 years.

When examining patients with dementia, it is of utmost importance to consider treatable medical conditions before making diagnosis of neurodegenerative diseases and vascular dementia. Treatable conditions include nutritional disorders such as vitamin B12 deficiency and niacin deficiency (pellagra), chronic hepatic diseases, kidney failure, hypothyroidism, poor cerebral perfusion due to cardiac failure, hypoxia due to chronic lung diseases, and long-standing drug use.

A. ALZHEIMER DISEASE AND RELATED DISORDERS

Alzheimer Disease

This is the commonest cause of dementia involving the elderly population. The disease affects both sexes, but is more common in women than in men. The commonest initial symptom is memory disturbance, and disorientation to time is also commonly seen. At the advanced stage, it causes severe disability in social life. Compared with dementia due to multiple cerebral infarctions, the patients tend to lose insight into the disease.

Pathologically, neurodegeneration involves the hippocampus, amygdala, and parietal and temporal cortices. Histologically, it is characterized by neuronal degeneration and loss associated with neurofibrillary tangles and senile plaques. The neurofibrillary tangles are formed by deposit of tau protein, and the senile plaques are formed by deposit of amyloid.

Lewy Body Dementia and Parkinson Disease

Dementia characterized by accumulation of Lewy bodies is called **dementia with Lewy bodies (DLB)** or **diffuse Lewy body disease**, which clinically manifests progressive cognitive disorders and parkinsonism. Pathologically, Lewy bodies are seen diffusely in the cerebral cortex. Visual hallucination is commonly seen at night, and functional abnormalities of the occipital lobe have been suggested by EEG and functional neuroimaging studies.

As cognitive impairment is seen in more than half of patients with idiopathic Parkinson disease at the advanced stage (**Parkinson disease with dementia**), this might be distinguished from DLB. Two possibilities have been proposed for the cause of dementia in Parkinson disease: DLB and coexistence of Alzheimer disease (Compta et al, 2011). In a prospective, neuropathological study from Norway on 22 cases of Parkinson disease, the presence of Lewy bodies was the only finding that was positively correlated with the degree of dementia, and it was proposed that dementia in Parkinson disease was mostly due to DLB (Aarsland et al, 2005). Another study, using chemical imaging with PET looking for L-dopa uptake, acetylcholine metabolism, and glucose metabolism, found common abnormalities between patients with Parkinson disease with dementia and those with DLB (Klein et al, 2010). A recent neuropathological study of many cases of a spectrum of parkinsonian disorders disclosed concomitant pathologies, especially between DLB and Alzheimer disease (Dugger et al, 2014; Walker et al, 2015).

In relation to visual hallucination in DLB, it should be kept in mind that hallucination is also seen as a side effect of L-dopa treatment. The cholinesterase inhibitor donepezil may improve cognitive function and behavior in patients with DLB (Mori et al, 2012).

Basal Ganglia and Cognitive Functions

Degenerative disorders of the basal ganglia are often accompanied by dementia. Sawamoto et al. (2002, 2007) studied patients with Parkinson disease by presenting a day of the week and asking the patient to advance 1 to 3 days as quickly as possible; the patients showed poor performance (bradyphrenia) and lower blood flow activation in the basal ganglia in association with the task compared with the age-matched healthy control subjects. As the above study did not require a motor response, it was claimed that the results were not affected by bradykinesia.

B. FRONTOTEMPORAL LOBAR DEGENERATION

A group of neurodegenerative disorders characterized clinically by progressive behavioral abnormality and language impairment and pathologically by degeneration of the prefrontal cortex and the anterior temporal neocortex is referred to as **frontotemporal lobar degeneration (FTLD)**. This condition affects adults of age between 45 and 65, and there is no sex predilection. It often seems sporadic, but familial cases have been reported, and now genetic abnormalities are often etiologic. Some cases of FTLD are also accompanied by motor neuron diseases and parkinsonism.

Various clinical forms are known in FTLD, including **frontotemporal dementia (FTD)**, **semantic dementia**, **progressive nonfluent aphasia**, and **FTD/Pick complex** (Kertesz et al, 2005; Neary et al, 2005, and Lashley et al, 2015, for review). There is also the **behavioral variant of FTD**, which is characterized by progressive impairment of personality, social behavior, and cognitive functions (Rascovsky et al, 2011). Each of these categories shows characteristic clinical pictures at the initial stage, but at the advanced stage, they may show other abnormalities and become indistinguishable from each other.

Pathologically, FTLD is largely classified into two groups, a group with tau inclusions (tauopathies) and another group without tau but with ubiquitin-positive inclusions (FTLD-U). Neuropathological studies of patients who presented clinically with FTLD showed tauopathies in 46%, FTLD-U in 29%, Alzheimer disease in 17%, and others including DLB (Forman et al, 2006). In fact, there is some overlap between cases of FTLD and familial cases of Alzheimer disease in terms of phenotype, inclusion protein, and genotypes (van der Zee et al, 2008). In the second group (FLTD-U), there is a mutation of the progranulin gene (Beck et al, 2008).

It is also known that the autosomal dominant form of FTD and amyotrophic lateral sclerosis (ALS) occur in the same family, and these two conditions share common genetic risk loci on chromosome 9p21.2 and 19p13.11, suggesting a possible common pathogenesis in the two conditions (DeJesus-Hernandez et al, 2011; Renton et al, 2011; Hodges, 2012 for review; Diekstra et al, 2014). In fact, C9orf72 (chromosome 9 open reading frame 72) hexanucleotide repeat expansions are the most common cause of familial FTD and familial ALS, although patients with ALS with these expansions more frequently show behavioral and cognitive symptoms than those with classical ALS (Rohrer et al, 2015, for review) (Boxes 77, 78 and 79).

The familial occurrence of **ALS/parkinsonism-dementia complex** has been reported in Chamorro of Guam, the Kii peninsula of Japan, and in Western New Guinea. Clinical, pathological, and genetic studies have been extensively carried out in those cases, but so far

> **BOX 77** DEMENTIA PUGILISTICA (CHRONIC TRAUMATIC ENCEPHALOPATHY)
>
> It has been reported that boxers who have repeatedly received a punch on the head tend to develop memory disturbance, behavioral abnormality, character change, and motor disturbance later (dementia pugilistica, punch-drunk encephalopathy). It is also known that the similar condition occurs in players of other sports such as American football, hockey, soccer, and professional wrestling (**chronic traumatic encephalopathy, or CTE**). Various pathological abnormalities such as brain atrophy, abnormality of the cavum septi pellucidi, atrophy of the mammillary body, diffuse deposit of tau inclusion and amyloid, and inflammatory change with microglia have been reported. Although there are no diagnostic criteria either clinically or pathologically for this condition, it is considered to be different from Alzheimer disease (Gavett et al, 2011; Saing et al, 2012). However, based on neuropathological studies of a large number of cases of CTE, McKee et al. (2013) reported frequent association with other neurodegenerative disorders and found hyperphosphorylated tau (p-tau) throughout the brain in severely affected cases of CTE (McKee et al, 2015, for review). By using β-amyloid PET, increased β-amyloid burden was demonstrated in long-term survivors of traumatic brain injury (Scott et al, 2016).

In **acquired immunodeficiency syndrome (AIDS)** due to infection with the human immunodeficiency virus (HIV), a number of neurological complications are known to occur, involving the central and peripheral nervous system and muscles. Brain pathology is mediated by two different mechanisms: activation of microorganisms that were latent as a result of opportunistic infection on one hand and direct infection of the brain with HIV on the other. The microorganisms of the first group include toxoplasma, cryptococcus, cytomegalovirus, JC virus (Box 82), and syphilis. In the second group, a diffuse inflammatory change in the brain due to HIV infection causes dementia, depression, and parkinsonism (HIV-associated dementia, HIV-associated neurocognitive disorders) (Arendt & Nolting, 2008, and Gannon et al, 2011, for review). By recent introduction of the highly active antiretroviral therapy (HAART), the prevalence and severity of these neurological complications have decreased.

BOX 79 PROGRESSIVE SUPRANUCLEAR PALSY AND CORTICOBASAL DEGENERATION

Among neurodegenerative disorders presenting with progressive frontal dementia and parkinsonism, progressive supranuclear palsy (PSP, Steele-Richardson-Olszewski syndrome) and corticobasal degeneration (CBD) are most commonly encountered. CBD is clinically referred to as corticobasal syndrome (CBS) due to ambiguity about the pathology. These two conditions commonly occur in adults over age 60. It is generally believed that PSP is characterized by supranuclear vertical gaze palsy (see Chapter 9-2), retrocollis, postural reflex abnormality and parkinsonian gait disturbance, whereas CBS is characterized by asymmetric rigidity and bradykinesia, tremulous myoclonus, ideomotor apraxia, primitive reflexes, and cortical sensory loss. In clinical practice, however, distinction of these two conditions is not infrequently difficult, and in fact some cases show clinical features of both conditions. In fact, pathological studies of clinically diagnosed cases of CBS revealed either of the four conditions; CBD, Alzheimer disease, PSP, or FTLD (Lee et al, 2011). Furthermore, a recent retrospective multicenter study of 100 cases of autopsy-confirmed cases of PSP revealed remarkable phenotypic heterogeneity (Respondek et al, 2014).

heterogeneous results have been reported (Kokubo et al, 2012; Steele et al, 2015).

C. LEUKOENCEPHALOPATHY

Diffuse lesions of the cerebral white matter are divided into congenital or hereditary leukodystrophy and acquired leukoencephalopathy. The most common form of the latter group is a diffuse ischemic lesion of the cerebral white matter causing **vascular dementia**. The cerebral lesions causing vascular dementia are classified into three groups; a large cerebral infarction, multiple small infarctions, and diffuse white matter lesion. White matter hyperintensities in the brain are the consequence of cerebral small vessel disease, and can easily be detected on MRI (Prins & Scheltens, 2015, for review). **Binswanger disease**, previously known as progressive subcortical encephalopathy, occurs in hypertensive patients and is clinically characterized by progressive dementia and gait disturbance. An MRI of this condition reveals diffuse abnormalities in the periventricular white matter (**leukoaraiosis**), but it is often accompanied by multiple small infarctions in the basal ganglia. The autosomal dominant hereditary form of Binswanger disease is called cerebral autosomal dominant arteriopathy with subcortical infarcts and leukoencephalopathy (**CADASIL**). This disease occurs in adults of age mainly between 40 and 60 with progressive dementia and gait disturbance, and also convulsion in some cases. Mutation of the notch 3 gene has been identified in this condition. Families of autosomal recessive inheritance are also known as **CARASIL**, in which mutation of the HTRA1 gene was identified. This form is accompanied by alopecia and lumbago due to lumbar spondylosis, and is common among Asians (Fukutake, 2011, for review; Nozaki et al, 2015).

Hereditary leukodystrophy usually occurs in infants and children, but some forms may occur in adults. Adrenomyeloneuropathy is an adult form of adrenoleukodystrophy (see Box 38). **Alexander disease** due to mutations in the glial fibrillary acidic protein (GFAP) gene is pathologically characterized by the presence of Rosenthal fibers. Its infantile and juvenile forms are characterized by mental deterioration, but its adult form also presents with spastic paraparesis, cerebellar ataxia, and palatal tremor (Graff-Radford et al, 2014). **Hereditary diffuse leukoencephalopathy with spheroids** (HDLS) is characterized by progressive cognitive and behavioral dysfunction

This is an autosomal recessive hereditary leukoencephalopathy that occurs in children with cerebellar ataxia. This disease is characterized by acute worsening of symptoms in association with infection and head trauma. Characteristically, the follow-up studies with proton or FLAIR MRI reveal vanishing white matter. Mutation of the EIF2B genes 1 to 5 was found in this condition, and its phenotype is heterogeneous (Matsui et al, 2007; van der Lei et al, 2010).

followed by motor impairment such as gait disturbance and bradykinesia in adults below the age 60. This is an autosomal dominant disease, and recently a gene encoding the colony stimulating factor 1 receptor (CSF-1R) has been identified as a causative gene (Konno et al, 2014). In patients with **vanishing white matter disease** (Box 80) and **membranous lipodystrophy (Nasu-Hakola disease)** (Box 81), symptoms may first appear in childhood, but the patients may visit the adult neurology clinic at a later age.

Acquired diffuse white matter lesions are also caused by anticancer drugs such as fluorouracil and as a late effect of acute carbon monoxide poisoning (**interval form of acute carbon monoxide poisoning**). Furthermore, leukoencephalopathy might occur after whole-brain irradiation (**chronic postradiation leukoencephalopathy**), and some

This is an autosomal recessive hereditary disease characterized by multiple fractures since puberty, progressive memory disturbance, and psychiatric symptoms such as character change, euphoria and indifference, finally resulting in akinetic mutism. This disease was first reported by Nasu et al. from Japan in 1970, and later Hakola et al. coined the term "osteodysplasia polycystica hereditaria combined with sclerosing leucoencephalopathy" (Kaneko et al, 2010, for review). The main pathological abnormality of cerebral hemispheres is sudanophilic leukodystrophy, and systemically there are membranocystic lesions in the bones and fatty tissues. Diagnosis is made by finding cystic lesions in the epiphysis of long bones on X-ray examination. Mutation of TREM2 or DAP12 gene was identified in the families of this disease.

This is a progressive demyelinating disease of the cerebral white matter due to destruction of oligodendroglia via reactivation of latent **JC virus**. Clinically, the disease starts with focal cortical symptoms of the unilateral parietal lobe, and rapidly progresses to dementia and motor paralysis associated with MRI findings revealing fusion of multiple small white matter lesions to form diffuse leukoencephalopathy. It is usually associated with immunodeficiency states such as **malignant lymphoma** and **AIDS**, but more recently, its occurrence during **immunosuppressive treatment** of the relapsing and exacerbating form of multiple sclerosis (MS), especially with natalizumab, and in the immune deficient state following **organ transplantation** has drawn particular attention. Incidence of PML during the natalizumab treatment increases in proportion to the total number of its infusions, but PML in this condition is less severe than the ones caused by other etiologies, if discovered at the early stage (Vermersch et al, 2011; Chalkias et al, 2014). Recently, it was reported that anti-JC virus antibody index was higher in serum or plasma of MS patients who developed PML even before the natalizumab treatment, suggesting a possibility of predicting the risk of developing PML (Plavina et al, 2014). After organ transplantation PML may occur irrespective of the kind of transplanted organs, and is more severe compared with other causes (Mateen et al, 2011). The latent period from transplantation to clinical onset varies from 1 month to more than 20 years. Treatment of PML is aimed at the underlying systemic diseases and improvement of immune deficiency state. If PML is associated with AIDS, it is treated by the highly active antiretroviral therapy (HAART), which prevents the incidence of PML and suppresses its progression.

cases might show acute transient episodes of impaired consciousness and neurological deficits several years after the irradiation (Di Stefano et al, 2013). In relation to leukoencephalopathy, it should be kept in mind that the primary malignant lymphoma of the central nervous system may show progressive white matter lesion on MRI (Box 82).

BIBLIOGRAPHY

Aarsland D, Perry R, Brown A, Larsen JP, Ballard C. Neuropathology of dementia in Parkinson's disease: a prospective, community-based study. Ann Neurol 58;773–776, 2005.

Arendt G, Nolting T. Neurologische Komplikationen der HIV-Infektion. Nervenarzt 79:1449–1463, 2008. (review)

Avram M, Hennig-Fast K, Bao Y, Pöppel E, Reiser M, Blautzik J, et al. Neural correlates of moral judgments in first– and third-person perspectives: implications for neuroethics and beyond. BMC Neuroscience 15:1–11, 2014.

Bartsch T, Alfke K, Deuschl G, Jansen O. Evolution of hippocampal CA–1 diffusion lesions in transient global amnesia. Ann Neurol 62:475–480, 2007.

Bartsch T, Schönfeld R, Müller FJ, Alfke K, Leplow B, Aldenhoff J, et al. Focal lesions of human hippocampal CA1 neurons in transient global amnesia impair place memory. Science 328:1412–1415, 2010.

Beck J, Rohrer JD, Campbell T, Isaacs A, Morrison KE, Goodall EF, et al. A distinct clinical, neuropsychological and radiological phenotype is associated with progranulin gene mutations in a large UK series. Brain 131:706–720, 2008.

Bogousslavsky J. L'amour perdu de Gui et Madeleine. Rev Neurol 159:171–179, 2003.

Chalkias S, Dang X, Bord E, Stein MC, Kinkel RP, Sloane JA, et al. JC virus reactivation during prolonged natalizumab monotherapy for multiple sclerosis. Ann Neurol 75:925–934, 2014.

Chiti G, Pantoni L. Use of Montreal Cognitive Assessment in patients with stroke. Stroke 45:3135–3140, 2014. (review)

Compta Y, Parkkinen L, O'Sullivan SS, Vandrovcova J, Holton JL, Collins C, et al. Lewy- and Alzheimer-type pathologies in Parkinson's disease dementia: which is more important? Brain 134:1493–1505, 2011.

Corrada MM, Brookmeyer R, Berlau D, Paganini-Hill A, Kawas CH. Prevalence of dementia after age 90: results from the 90+ study. Neurology 71:337–343, 2008.

Daffner KR, Gale SA, Barrett AM, Boeve BF, Chatterjee A, Coslett HB, et al. Improving clinical cognitive testing. Report of the AAN Behavioral Neurology Section Workgroup. Neurology 85:910–918, 2015.

Danet L, Barbeau EJ, Eustache P, Planton M, Raposo N, Sibon I, et al. Thalamic amnesia after infarct. The role of the mammillothalamic tract and mediodorsal nucleus. Neurology 85:2107–2115, 2015.

DeJesus-Hernandez M, Mackenzie IR, Boeve BF, Boxer AL, Baker M, Rutherford NJ, et al. Expanded GGGGCC hexanucleotide repeat in noncoding region of C9ORF72 causes chromosome 9p-linked FTD and ALS. Neuron 72:245–256, 2011.

Diekstra FP, Van Deerlin VM, van Swieten JC, Al-Chalabi A, Ludolph AC, Weishaupt JH, et al. C9orf72 and UNC13A are shared risk loci for amyotrophic lateral sclerosis and frontotemporal dementia: a genome-wide meta-analysis. Ann Neurol 76:120–133, 2014.

Di Stefano AL, Berzero G, Vitali P, Galimberti CA, Ducray F, Ceroni M, et al. Acute late-onset encephalopathy after radiotherapy: an unusual life-threatening complication. Neurology 81:1014–1017, 2013.

Dugger BN, Adler CH, Shill HA, Caviness J, Jacobson S, Driver-Dunckley E, et al. Concomitant pathologies among a spectrum of parkinsonian disorders. Parkinsonism Relat Disord 20:525–529, 2014.

Folstein MF, Folstein SE, McHugh PR. Mini-Mental State: a practical method for grading the cognitive state of patients for the clinician. J Psychiat Res 12:189–198, 1975.

Forman MS, Farmer J, Johnson JK, Clark CM, Arnold SE, Coslett HB, et al. Frontotemporal dementia: clinicopathological correlations. Ann Neurol 59;952–962, 2006.

Fukutake T. Cerebral autosomal recessive arteriopathy with subcortical infarcts and leukoencephalopathy (CARASIL): from discovery to gene identification. J Stroke Cerebrovasc Dis 20:85–93, 2011. (review)

Gannon P, Khan MZ, Kolson DL. Current understanding of HIV-associated neurocognitive disorders pathogenesis. Curr Opin Neurol 24:275–283, 2011. (review)

Gavett BE, Stern RA, McKee AC. Chronic traumatic encephalopathy: a potential late effect of sport-related concussive and subconcussive head trauma. Clin Sports Med 30:179–188, 2011.

Graff-Radford J, Schwartz K, Gavrilova RH, Lachance DH, Kumar N. Neuroimaging and clinical features in type II (late-onset) Alexander disease. Neurology 82:49–56, 2014.

Hodges J. Familial frontotemporal dementia and amyotrophic lateral sclerosis associated with the C9ORF72 hexanucleotide repeat. Brain 135:652–655, 2012. (review)

Jang SH, Kwon HG. Perspectives on the neural connectivity of the fornix in the human brain. Neural Regen Res 9:1434–1436, 2014. (review)

Kaneko M, Sano K, Nakayama J, Amano N. Nasu-Hakola disease: The first case reported by Nasu and review. Neuropathology 30:463–470, 2010. (review)

Kertesz A, McMonagle P, Blair M, Davidson W, Munoz DG. The evolution and pathology of frontotemporal dementia. Brain 128:1996–2005, 2005.

Klein JC, Eggers C, Kalbe E, Weisenbach S, Hohmann C, Vollmar S, et al. Neurotransmitter changes in dementia with Lewy bodies and Parkinson disease dementia in vivo. Neurology 74:885–892, 2010.

Kokubo Y, Taniguchi A, Hasegawa M, Hayakawa Y, Morimoto S, Yoneda M, et al. α-synuclein pathology in the amyotrophic lateral sclerosis/parkinsonism dementia complex in the Kii peninsula, Japan. J Neuropathol Exp Neurol 71:625–630, 2012.

Konno T, Tada M, Tada M, Koyama A, Nozaki H, Harigaya Y, et al. Haploinsufficiency of CSF-1R and clinicopathologic characterization in patients with HDLS. Neurology 82:139–148, 2014.

Lashley T, Rohrer JD, Mead S, Revesz T. Review: an update on clinical, genetic and pathological aspects of frontotemporal lobar degenerations. Neuropathol Appl Neurobiol 41:858–881, 2015. (review)

Lee SE, Rabinovici GD, Mayo MC, Wilson SM, Seeley WW, DeArmond SJ, et al. Clinicopathological correlations in corticobasal degeneration. Ann Neurol 70:327–340, 2011.

Mah L, Arnold MC, Grafman J. Impairment of social perception associated with lesions of the prefrontal cortex. Am J Psychiatry 161:1247–1255, 2004.

Mateen FJ, Muralidharan RN, Carone M, van de Beek D, Harrison DM, Aksamit AJ, et al. Progressive multifocal leukoencephalopathy in transplant recipients. Ann Neurol 70:305–322, 2011.

Matsui M, Mizutani, K, Ohtake H, Miki Y, Ishizu K, Fukuyama H, et al. Novel mutation in EIF2B gene in a case of adult-onset leukoencephalopathy with vanishing white matter. Eur Neurol 57:57–58, 2007.

McKee AC, Stern RA, Nowinski CJ, Stein TD, Alvarez VE, Daneshvar DH, et al. The spectrum of disease in chronic traumatic encephalopathy. Brain 136:43–64, 2013.

McKee AC, Stein TD, Kierman PT, Alvarez VE. The neuropathology of chronic traumatic encephalopathy. Brain Pathol 25:350–364, 2015. (review)

Mori E, Ikeda M, Kosaka K. Donepezil for dementia with Lewy bodies: a randomized, placebo-controlled trial. Arch Neurol 72:41–52, 2012.

Neary D, Snowden J, Mann D. Frontotemporal dementia. Lancet Neurol 4:771–780, 2005. (review)

Nozaki H, Sekine Y, Fukutake T, Nishimoto Y, Shimoe Y, Shirata A, et al. Characteristic features and progression of abnormalities on MRI for CARASIL. Neurology 85:459–463, 2015.

Plavina T, Subramanyam M, Bloomgren G, Richman S, Pace A, Lee S, et al. Anti-JC virus antibody levels in serum or plasma further define risk of natalizumab-associated progressive multifocal leukoencephalopathy. Neurology 76:802–812, 2014.

Prins ND, Scheltens P. White matter hyperintensities, cognitive impairment and dementia: an update. Nature Rev Neurology 11:157–165, 2015. (review)

Rascovsky K, Hodges JR, Knopman D, Mendez MF, Kramer JH, Neuhaus J, et al. Sensitivity of revised diagnostic criteria for the behavioural variant of frontotemporal dementia. Brain 134:2456–2477, 2011.

Renton AE, Majounie E, Waite A, Simon-Sanchez J, Rollinson S, Gibbs JR, et al. A hexanucleotide repeat expansion in C9ORF72 is the cause of chromosome 9p21–linked ALS-FTD. Neuron 72:257–268, 2011.

Respondek G, Stamelou M, Kurz C, Ferguson LW, Rajput A, Chiu WZ, et al. The phenotypic spectrum of progressive supranuclear palsy: a retrospective multicenter study of 100 definite cases. Mov Disord 29:1758–1766, 2014.

Rohrer JD, Isaacs AM, Mizielinska S, Mead S, Lashley T, Wray S, et al. C9orf72 expansions in frontotemporal dementia and amyotrophic lateral sclerosis. Lancet Neurol 14:291–301, 2015. (review)

Saing T, Dick M, Nelson PT, Kim RC, Cribbs DH, Head E. Frontal cortex neuropathology in dementia pugilistica. J Neurotrauma 29:1054–1070, 2012.

Sawamoto N, Honda M, Hanakawa T, Fukuyama H, Shibasaki H. Cognitive slowing in Parkinson's disease: a behavioral evaluation independent of motor slowing. J Neurosci 22:5198–5203, 2002.

Sawamoto N, Honda M, Hanakawa T, Aso T, Inoue M, Toyoda H, et al. Cognitive slowing in Parkinson disease is accompanied by hypofunctioning of the striatum. Neurology 68:1062–1068, 2007.

Scott G, Ramlackhansingh AF, Edison P, Hellyer P, Cole J, Veronese M, et al. Amyloid pathology and axonal injury after brain trauma. Neurology 86:821–828, 2016.

Steele JC, Guella I, Szu-Tu C, Lin MK, Thompson C, Evans DM, et al. Defining neurodegeneration on Guam by targeted genomic sequencing. Ann Neurol 77:458–468, 2015.

van der Lei HDW, van Berkel CGM, van Wieringen WN, Brenner C, Feigenbaum A, Mercimek-Mahmutoglu S, et al. Genotype-phenotype correlation in vanishing white matter disease. Neurology 75:1555–1559, 2010.

van der Zee J, Sleegers K, Van Broeckhoven C. The Alzheimer disease-frontotemporal lobar degeneration spectrum. Neurology 71:1191–1197, 2008.

Vermersch P, Kappos L, Gold R, Foley JF, Olsson T, Cadavid D, et al. Clinical outcomes of natalizumab-associated progressive multifocal leukoencephalopathy. Neurology 76:1697–1704, 2011.

Walker L, McAleese KE, Thomas AJ, Johnson M, Martin-Ruiz C, Parker C, et al. Neuropathologically mixed Alzheimer's and Lewy body disease: burden of pathological protein aggregates differs between clinical phenotypes. Acta Neuropathol 129:729–748, 2015.

23.

APHASIA, APRAXIA, AND AGNOSIA

1. NEURAL CIRCUITS RELATED TO LANGUAGE, PRAXIS, AND RECOGNITION

Several hypotheses have been proposed for the neural circuits related to language, praxis, and recognition based on the correlation between clinical symptoms/ signs and pathological findings of patients who died of head trauma or vascular brain lesions, and more recently based on the correlation with neuroimaging data in clinical cases (Figure 23-1). Moreover, as a consequence of the recent advance in various noninvasive techniques for studying brain functions in healthy subjects (Shibasaki, 2008, for review), and as the result of presurgical evaluation of patients with medically intractable partial epilepsy by intracranial recording, further information on the **functional localization (specialization)** as well as **inter-areal functional coupling** has been accumulated.

Functions of the nervous system are generally symmetric, but the hemispheric language dominance is of utmost importance for evaluating these higher cortical functions. Although there seems to be some racial difference in the language dominance, it is believed that about 95% of the population is right-handed, and the left cerebral hemisphere is dominant in the majority of those right-handed subjects. The remaining 5% of population may be left-handed, but about half of left-handed subjects are also believed to have dominance in the left hemisphere. Thus, only a very small proportion of population has dominance in the right hemisphere.

An exception to the above rule is the occurrence of aphasia in right-handed subjects with a lesion of the right hemisphere, although it is extremely rare. This phenomenon is called **crossed aphasia**. In this chapter, higher cortical functions are discussed for right-handed subjects who have language dominance in the left hemisphere.

Focal Neurologic Deficit and Disconnection Syndrome

It is considered that higher cortical functions are impaired either by a focal lesion of the association cortex (**focal neurological deficit**) or by interruption of the functional connection among different cortical areas (**disconnection syndrome**). The concept of disconnection syndrome was brought into prominence in modern times by Geschwind (Geschwind, 1965a, 1965b; Hallett, 2015, for book review). As a consequence of recent advances in electrophysiological and neuroimaging techniques, functional connectivity has been documented in healthy subjects, and the notion of disconnection syndrome is drawing increasing attention (Catani & ffytche, 2005, for review). In the clinical setting, it is reasonable and practical to consider the two concepts in combination.

A. LANGUAGE

When evaluating language function, it is important to consider both **spoken language** and **written language**. Anatomically, in addition to the **anterior language area** in the left inferior frontal gyrus and the **posterior language area** in the left superior temporal gyrus, it is useful to consider a third language area in the left parietal lobe (Figure 23-2). These areas cover a large region along the left sylvian fissure and receive blood supply from the left middle cerebral artery (see Figures 7-4 and 7-7). In addition, participation of the left basal temporal lobe in language function was proposed by Lüders et al. (1986), and the **basal temporal language area** has been demonstrated electrophysiologically (Matsumoto et al, 2004b; Usui et al, 2009).

Regarding spoken language, an auditory input is received by the auditory cortex located in the bilateral superior temporal gyri and is transmitted to **Wernicke's area** in the posterior part of the left superior temporal

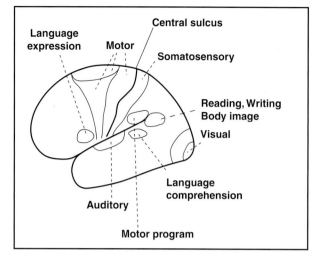

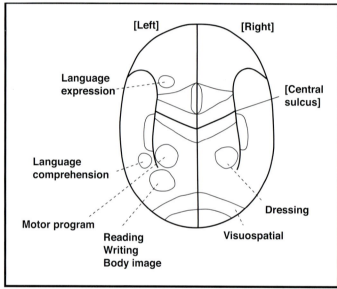

Figure 23-1 Schematic diagram showing functional localization in the cerebral cortex in right-handed subjects. (a) Lateral view of the left hemisphere. (b) Axial view.

gyrus (Figure 23-3-a). This information has been obtained primarily from the observation of patients with stroke, but in neurodegenerative diseases presenting with primary progressive aphasia, it has been shown that word comprehension is actually located in the left anterior temporal lobe and sentence comprehension is distributed widely throughout the language network (Mesulam et al, 2015). In Wernicke's area, words are understood with the aid of functional connectivity with other related cortical areas, and it plays a critical role in speech production (Binder, 2015 for review). For repeating orally presented words (**repetition**), the information is conducted from Wernicke's area through the **arcuate fasciculus** (Figure 23-3-b) to **Broca's area** in the left inferior frontal gyrus (Figure 23-3-c). From there, the words are pronounced through the bilateral motor cortices. For speaking spontaneously, Broca's area receives the relevant information from other related cortical areas, and from there the words are pronounced through the bilateral motor cortices.

For written language, the information is transmitted from the visual center in the bilateral occipital cortices to the reading center in the **left angular gyrus** (Figure 23-3-e), where the written words are understood with the aid of functional connectivity with other related cortical areas. For copying the written words, the information from the left angular gyrus is transmitted through the arcuate fasciculus to the **writing center** (Exner's area) in the left middle frontal gyrus (Figure 23-3-g). Then, the words are written with the right hand through the corticospinal tract from the left motor cortex. For writing spontaneously, the above pathway from the left angular gyrus to the frontal writing center plays a part. For this reason, patients with a lesion

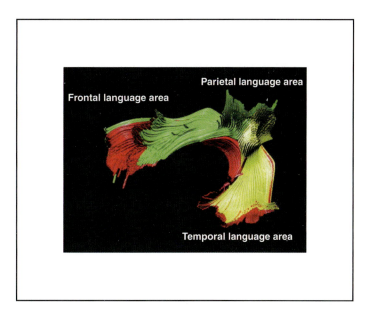

Figure 23-2 Functional connectivity related to language, reconstructed based on the diffusion tensor tractography (DTT). (Reproduced from Catani & ffytche, 2005, with permission)

in the left occipital white matter and the splenium of the corpus callosum interrupting the input of visual information to the left angular gyrus can write, but cannot read the words written by him-/herself (**alexia without agraphia, pure alexia**) (Figure 23-3-d). The most common cause of this typical disconnection syndrome is an infarction in the left medial occipital white matter.

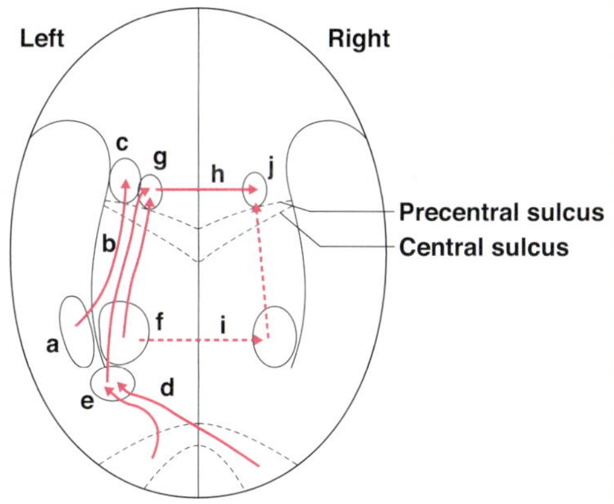

Figure 23-3 Schematic diagram showing the neural circuits related to language, praxis and gnosis in right-handed subjects. View from the top of head. a. Wernicke's area, b. arcuate fasciculus, c. Broca's area, d. corpus callosum related to visual function, e. left angular gyrus, f. left supramarginal gyrus, g. left premotor area (Exner's area), h and i: corpus callosum, j. right premotor area.

By intraoperative stimulation studies in patients as well as functional MRI studies in healthy subjects, Exner's writing area was identified in a cortical area just anterior to the hand area of the left primary motor cortex (Roux et al, 2009).

Classification of Aphasia

Impairment or loss of acquired language function is called **aphasia**. If Wernicke's area is damaged, the patient is unable to understand spoken language and also unable to repeat spoken words. This condition is called **sensory aphasia** or **Wernicke aphasia**. In this case, the patient is rather talkative and speaks incomprehensible language (**jargon aphasia**), because he/she is unable to understand his/her own spoken words. This condition is often called fluent aphasia, but the use of the term "fluent" here is rather misleading in this situation.

In contrast, the patient with a lesion of Broca's area is neither able to speak spontaneously nor to repeat given words (**motor aphasia**, **Broca aphasia**). In this case, the patient does not try to speak much or even becomes mute, because he/she can understand his/her own mistakes. Speech in this condition is characterized by abnormal intonation (**dysprosody**) and abnormal sentence construction, which sounds like a telegraph (**telegraphic speech**). When repeating given words, a syllable might be replaced by another different and yet similar syllable (**literal paraphasia**), and a word might be replaced by another different and yet similar word (**verbal paraphasia**).

Spoken Language and Written Language

In most cases of sensory aphasia, comprehension is impaired not only for spoken language but also for written language. This might be explained by postulating either that Wernicke's area is involved in the comprehension of both spoken and written languages, or that the angular gyrus situated just posterior to Wernicke's area is also affected by the same lesion (Figure 23-3-e). Likewise, in most cases of Broca aphasia, both speaking and writing are impaired. This might also be explained by postulating either that Broca's area is engaged in speaking as well as writing, or that Exner's area situated just dorsal to Broca's area is also affected by the same lesion (Figure 23-3-g).

Some patients can understand written words but cannot understand spoken words (**pure word deafness**). In this condition, the patient usually can hear and understand the meaning of nonverbal sounds. Likewise, the condition in which the patient can write but cannot speak is called **pure word dumbness**. Some patients with Broca aphasia are unable to stick out their tongue in response to verbal command. This condition can be called verbal apraxia or apraxia of speech, but "lingual apraxia" might be the better terminology for this condition, because Broca aphasia itself might be considered as "apraxia of language."

In contrast, some patients can speak and understand the spoken language but can neither read nor write. This condition is called **alexia with agraphia** and is due to a lesion of the left angular gyrus (see comparison with alexia without agraphia) (Box 83; Figures 23-4 and 23-5).

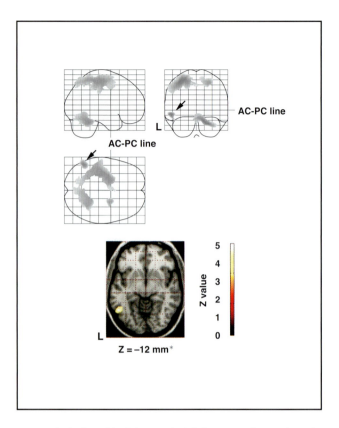

Figure 23-4 Activation of the left posterior inferior temporal cortex (arrow) associated with reading and writing of kanji (morphogram) of Japanese language, demonstrated by a functional MRI study. The transverse MRI on the bottom was obtained at 12 mm below the anterior commissure (AC)–posterior commissure (PC) line on the Talairach coordinate. (Reproduced from Nakamura et al, 2000, with permission)

If the arcuate fasciculus is selectively affected while Broca's area and Wernicke's area are preserved, the patient cannot repeat verbally given words in spite of the fact that he/she can understand the spoken language and speak relatively well. This phenomenon called **conduction aphasia** is another typical example of a disconnection syndrome. If the perisylvian area is widely affected, the patient shows features of all types of aphasia (**total aphasia**). Furthermore, in contrast with the ordinary Wernicke aphasia in which repetition is also impaired, some patients with sensory aphasia may be able to repeat although he/she cannot understand the spoken words. This is called **transcortical sensory aphasia**. Likewise, some patients with motor aphasia may be able to repeat given words although he/she cannot speak spontaneously. This condition is called **transcortical motor aphasia**. These phenomena may be explained by postulating lesions in the language areas but without directly interrupting the neural circuits necessary for repetition (Figure 23-3-a, b, c).

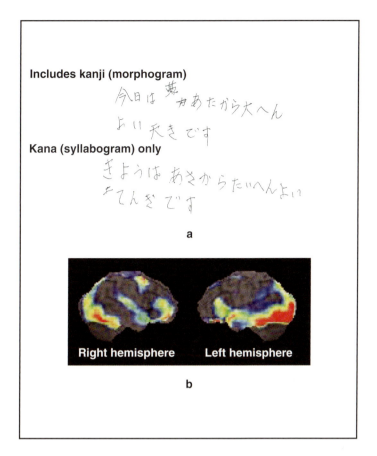

Includes kanji (morphogram)

今日は 燕 力あたがら大へん
より天きです

Kana (syllabogram) only

きようは あさから たいへんよい
Ｆてんぎ です

a

Right hemisphere **Left hemisphere**

b

Figure 23-5 Disturbance of kanji (morphogram) writing seen with a dictation task in a Japanese patient with clinical diagnosis of Alzheimer disease. (a) The patient can write kana (syllabogram) relatively well but can write only simple kanji (morphogram). (b) The blood flow study by three-dimensional stereotactic surface projections (3D-SSP) analysis of SPECT data in this patient revealed hypoperfusion in the left posterior inferior temporal region (shown in red).

B. PRAXIS

Based on clinical and experimental data, it is believed that the left parietal lobe, especially the supramarginal gyrus, plays a main role in programming daily activities like tool use and gesture (Figure 23-3-f). The fibers from there project anteriorly through the arcuate fasciculus to the premotor area of the left middle frontal gyrus (Wheaton et al, 2005; Hattori et al, 2009; Matsumoto et al, 2012). The information from the left premotor area is conducted to the right premotor area through the corpus callosum, and the primary motor cortex is activated by the premotor area on each side, so that actual movements are executed.

Classification of Apraxia

If the left parietal lobe including the supramarginal gyrus is damaged, the patient is unable to program a motor task, and finds it difficult to use given tools in an appropriate sequence. For example, if a set of cup, kettle and coffee is presented, the patient may put coffee directly into the kettle instead of the cup. This phenomenon is called **ideational apraxia**, and is often accompanied by difficulty in copying geometric forms of any complexity (**constructional apraxia**). In this condition, the patient may be able to draw individual shapes, but unable to synthesize them into a complex figure. This phenomenon can be also tested by asking the patient to imitate given forms by hands such as the posture of the examiner's fingers.

For daily living, reaching and grasping are important tasks in which the left inferior parietal lobule takes part (Figure 23-6) (Hattori et al, 2009). Furthermore, a lesion of the fiber tracts projecting from the left parietal cortex to the left frontal cortex causes difficulty in using tools or making gestures (**ideomotor apraxia**). In contrast, a lesion of the premotor area makes the movement of the contralateral hand clumsy (**limb-kinetic apraxia**). In this case, however, it is a prerequisite that there is no spastic paresis, rigidity, or motor ataxia in the corresponding hand.

It is considered that the right premotor area is activated only through the left premotor area. Therefore, a lesion of the left premotor area makes not only the right hand movement clumsy but also the left hand movement. In this case,

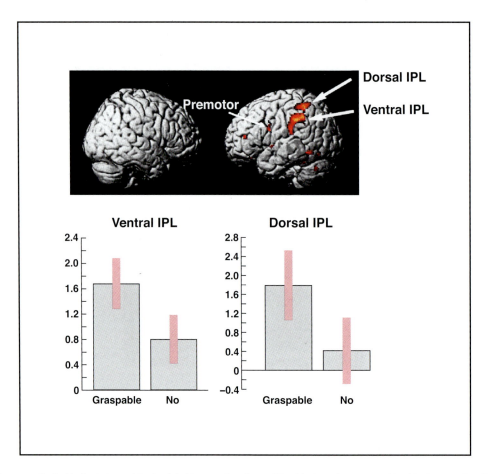

Figure 23-6 Cortical areas activated in the judgment task related to grasping. Graspable objects and nongraspable objects were visually presented to healthy subjects in a random sequence in an event-related functional MRI study. Greater activation was seen in the dorsal and ventral inferior parietal lobule (IPL) of the left parietal lobe and in the left premotor area in the graspable objects (Graspable) compared with the nongraspable objects (No). (Reproduced from Hattori et al, 2009, with permission).

however, the right hand may be paralyzed at least to a certain degree due to involvement of the hand area of the left primary motor cortex. Limb-kinetic apraxia seen in the left hand due to a lesion of the left premotor area is called **sympathetic apraxia**. If the corpus callosum connecting the left and right premotor areas is damaged by an ischemic lesion in the anterior cerebral artery territory, the information from the left to the right premotor area is interrupted, so that the limb-kinetic apraxia occurs only in the left hand. This disconnection syndrome is called **callosal apraxia**. Some patients with a subcortical lesion in the ventral part of the left postcentral gyrus may present with apraxia in both hands, because the fiber tract projecting from the left parietal cortex to the left premotor area is damaged just before reaching the left premotor area.

Among neurodegenerative diseases, ideomotor apraxia and limb-kinetic apraxia are commonly seen in patients with corticobasal degeneration. In this condition, other motor abnormalities such as alien hand sign, utilization behavior, and diagonistic apraxia may also be seen. **Alien hand sign** is a goal-directed but unintended action of one hand which the patient cannot control. If the affected hand interferes with action of the other hand, it is called **diagonistic apraxia**. Patients with **utilization behavior** cannot resist grabbing and using presented objects. Utilization behavior is commonly seen in association with frontal lobe lesions, and may be categorized into the primitive reflexes in the broad sense (see Chapter 10-2E) (Schott & Rossor, 2003, for review).

Task-Specific Apraxia

Some cortical areas are known to be related to performance of specific tasks. The area including the supramarginal gyrus of the right parietal lobe shows specific apraxia for dressing if damaged (Figure 23-1). In **dressing apraxia**, the patient is unable to figure out how to put on given clothes. There seems to be an area in the left parietal cortex that is engaged in calculation. Acalculia, finger agnosia, left-right disorientation, and agraphia form **Gerstmann syndrome** due to a lesion of the left parietal lobe. In **acalculia**, patients tend to have greater difficulty in written calculation than in mental calculation (see Chapter 22-1C). In particular, patients make mistakes in the position of digits in vertically written calculation.

Mirror Neuron

Rizzolatti and his group found neurons in area 44 (F5 in monkey) of the inferior frontal gyrus that recognize actions of other people, and coined the term "mirror neuron." These neurons are believed to recognize not just movement itself but to recognize the goal of action, and even the intention and emotion of others (Rizzolatti & Fogassi, 2014, for review). The unique function of these neurons has drawn special attention in relation to social communication. In fact, functional abnormality of mirror neurons has been proposed in children with autism such as Asperger syndrome, who have behavioral abnormalities because of difficulty in understanding actions and emotions of other people. It has been also reported that similar neurons are also present in the primary motor cortex, but only 30% of those neurons in the primary motor cortex are oriented to the action goal, whereas almost all neurons in area 44 are goal-oriented (Rizzolatti & Craighero, 2004, for review).

C. RECOGNITION

Recognition of each sensory modality is believed to be primarily processed in the secondary sensory area that is located adjacent to each primary sensory area. For the somatosensory modality, areas 5 and 7 of the parietal cortex and the secondary somatosensory areas in the upper bank of the sylvian fissure are involved in somesthetic recognition. As for nociceptive recognition, however, other structures including the insula, amygdala, and anterior cingulate gyrus are also involved in particular relation to the emotional response (see Figure 19-4; see Chapter 19-1; Box 84).

Disturbance of Auditory Recognition

The secondary auditory cortex is not clearly defined, but it is considered to be around the primary auditory cortex in the **Heschl gyrus** (see Figure 12-2). From the results of evoked magnetoencephalographic studies, it is known that sounds of different pitch are received in different areas of the primary auditory cortex (**tonotopic organization**) (see Chapter 12-1). Qualitative recognition of sounds seems to take place in the secondary auditory cortex. Clinically,

some patients can hear a sound but cannot tell what the sound is (**auditory agnosia**). Judgment of the spatial source of sounds, as to where the sound came from, is believed to be recognized based on a subtle difference in the arrival time of sound at each ear and by processing of the time lag in the auditory cortex (Boxes 85, 86 and 87).

Higher Visual Functions and Their Disturbance

Processing of visual information has been extensively investigated. The primary visual area is area 17 (V1) located in

SAVANT SYNDROME

It is well known that some persons with diffuse cerebral disturbance have an extraordinarily good ability in a special field. The special ability is not just preserved undamaged, but it is outstanding like a genius. This condition was named "savant," which means a great scholar, by Down in 1887. This unique condition is mainly seen in men who have congenital brain disorders or autism, but it is also seen in patients with an acquired brain lesion. Examples of the special ability are detailed knowledge about music and sports, absorption in and super memory of the number plate and maps (splinter skills), super ability and skill in music and arts (talented savant, prodigious savant), and so forth. Regardless of the kind of ability, the savant is especially good at memory. The underlying mechanism of this condition has not been clarified yet, although a plastic change is believed to play a primary role (Treffert, 2009 for review). Application of various noninvasive techniques may help elucidate the mechanism.

the calcarine sulcus and the adjacent area. There is a precise topographic interrelationship between the retina and V1 (**retinotopic organization**). The secondary visual area (V2) is in areas 18 and 19. Projection from V2 is divided into two pathways: the ventral pathway, which goes to the temporal cortex and is primarily engaged in the processing of the shape of objects, and the dorsal pathway, which goes to the parietal cortex and primarily takes part in the processing of spatial information. Thus, the ventral pathway is called the "what" pathway, and the dorsal pathway is called the "where" pathway (see Chapter 7-1F).

If V1 is bilaterally damaged by an acute insult, the patient cannot see at all. This condition is called **cortical blindness**, and is distinguished from bilateral optic neuritis by an intact light reflex (see Chapter 8-2). However, visual evoked responses may not be helpful in the distinction because they are expected to be absent in both conditions. In the recovery phase from cortical blindness, the patient can see objects but cannot recognize what they are unless he/she touches them. This condition is called **visual object agnosia**. Furthermore, the object may look deformed to the patient (**metamorphopsia**).

Face recognition is processed in the fusiform gyrus at the mesial basal temporal cortex bilaterally, and a lesion of this structure causes inability to recognize familiar faces (**prosopagnosia**). In this condition, the patient can recognize who the person is as soon as he/she hears the voice. As for the hemispheric dominance, the right hemisphere used to be claimed to be dominant for this function, but it is still controversial. **Color recognition** is believed to be processed also in a region similar to that for face recognition. Recognition of movement (**visual motion**) is known to be processed in the posterior part of the superior temporal sulcus (V5, MT in monkey) (Matsumoto et al, 2004a) (Box 88).

VENTRILOQUIST EFFECT AND COCKTAIL PARTY EFFECT

It is easier to understand what another person is talking about if one watches his/her mouth. This phenomenon is known as the **ventriloquist effect**, and is considered to be a result of integrative recognition of sensory input of different modalities—auditory and visual input in the above case. In relation to this, **polysensory areas** are known to exist; for example in the temporoparietal junction, where evoked responses are recorded in response to all stimuli of somatosensory, visual, and auditory modalities (Matsuhashi et al, 2004).

In a noisy place like cocktail party, one can still hear what a particular person is talking about if one attends to his/her voice. This **cocktail party effect** is considered to be mediated by a mechanism of **selective attention**. Where in the brain the selective attention takes place differs, depending on the kind of sensation. For the somesthetic modality, the selective attention is considered to take place in the secondary somatosensory cortex, while the primary auditory cortex is important for the auditory modality.

WILLIAMS SYNDROME

This developmental abnormality of higher brain functions has drawn increasing attention in relation to the genetics of brain development. It involves infants before the age of 1 year with disturbance of visuospatial recognition, excessive emotional reaction (unusually sociable with a person whom he/she has never met before), stereotypy, auditory hypersensitivity, and phobia about a certain sound. It is a unique condition in which the patient is above average or even superior in language development, face recognition, interest and talent in music, and sociability. Physically, the child often has cardiovascular abnormality, among others aortic stenosis, and facial deformity like elfin. Microdeletion of a gene on chromosome 7q11.23 was shown in this condition. A neuroimaging study in this condition reported a smaller volume of the parietal and occipital lobes but a larger volume of the face area of the fusiform gyrus than controls (Golarai et al, 2010).

In relation to face recognition, the amygdala is believed to play an important role in the **recognition of facial emotion**. Impairment of this function was reported in a unilateral lesion of the amygdala on either side (Cristinzio et al, 2010). In this relation, the ventromedial prefrontal cortex was shown to mediate visual attention during facial emotion recognition (Wolf et al, 2014).

Visuospatial Agnosia

In processing visual spatial information, the secondary visual area in the right hemisphere is believed to be dominant, because **visuospatial agnosia** commonly occurs in patients with right parieto-occipital lesions. For example, the patient is unable to count the number of visual targets presented simultaneously (**agnosia of optic counting**), to read a clock (**agnosia of clock reading**), to distinguish between near and far (**agnosia of distance**), or to understand what is going on by looking at a complex visual scene (**simultanagnosia**). It is known that area 31 in the mesial parietal cortex is related to the processing of geographic information, and its damage causes a disturbance of heading in the correct direction (**topographic disorientation**) (Takahashi et al, 1997; Baumann & Mattingley, 2010).

Gerstmann Syndrome

The left supramarginal gyrus is engaged in various important functions. In addition to writing and calculation as described above, it seems to be engaged in recognition of the left and right and that of fingers. Thus, its lesion causes **left-right disorientation**, **finger agnosia**, agraphia and acalculia; this condition is called **Gerstmann syndrome**. Furthermore, this condition is often accompanied by ideational apraxia and constructional apraxia. There seems to be also a center related to the body image or body schema in the left parietal lobe, and its lesion causes inability to identify parts of one's own body (**autotopagnosia**).

A question as to whether Gerstmann syndrome is due to a loss of focal cortical functions or disconnection of intercortical connectivity has long been controversial, but Rusconi et al. (2010), based on the results of functional neuroimaging studies, proposed that the syndrome might be primarily caused by subcortical disconnection in the parietal lobe.

Positive Symptoms of Higher Visual Functions

Some abnormalities of higher visual functions are thought to be positive symptoms. For example, a single object might look as if there is more than one (**polyopia**). Short presentation of an object might be followed by its repeated appearance (**palinopsia**). On the contrary, a patient may be unable to recall an image that has been just shown (**Charcot-Wilbrand syndrome**), although this does not belong to the positive symptoms.

A given sensory stimulus might be accompanied by sensation of another modality in addition to its original sensation. This phenomenon is called **synesthesia**. For example, about 2% of healthy population sees color when they read characters (grapheme-color synesthetes) (Weiss & Fink, 2009).

As locations of the primary sensory areas for the olfactory, gustatory, and vestibular sensations are not well defined, the distinction from each secondary sensory area is not precisely understood. As described in each respective chapter (Chapter 6-1, Chapter 11-1C, and Chapter 13-1, respectively), the limbic system including the mesial temporal cortex and insula is considered to be important for these functions.

2. EXAMINATION OF LANGUAGE, PRAXIS, AND RECOGNITION

As for the patient's state of language, praxis, and recognition, general information is usually obtained during the history taking. If any deficit in these functions is confirmed to be present, it provides an important clue to the anatomical diagnosis. Information about the patient's handedness is important before evaluating these higher cortical functions. In order to assess these cortical functions correctly, it is a prerequisite that the patient does not have any general cognitive impairment or dementia, but in some patients focal cortical symptoms such as aphasia, apraxia, and agnosia might be superimposed on general cognitive impairment. Furthermore, in the early clinical stage of Alzheimer disease or frontotemporal lobar degeneration, the patient may present solely with progressive aphasia, apraxia, or agnosia (**primary progressive aphasia**), and the general cognitive decline might appear later in the clinical course (Mesulam et al, 2014). Therefore, this possibility should be kept in mind when the patient presents with any focal cortical symptom with progressive course.

A. EXAMINATION OF LANGUAGE AND APHASIA

Language abnormality, if any, is usually noticed of during the history taking. When spontaneous speech is found abnormal, first whether it is due to dysarthria or aphasia should be distinguished (see Chapter 14-7). If the speech is difficult to understand but grammatically correct, it is more likely to be dysarthria than aphasia. In contrast, if there are grammatical errors, it is more likely to be aphasia. It is also useful to ask the patient whether he/she finds it difficult to pronounce the words that he/she has in mind or to compose a sentence. In general, the patients with aphasia can sing songs that they have learned before or can make an exclamation like "ouch," whereas those with dysarthria has difficulty also in singing or exclaiming because it involves the final common pathway for speaking.

Motor Aphasia

The patient with motor aphasia hesitates to talk because he is aware of his own mistakes. This condition is sometime called nonfluent aphasia. If the patient is asked to repeat a given syllable, word, or sentence, the syllable or word is replaced by a different syllable or word, respectively (**paraphasia**). Motor aphasia is caused by a lesion of Broca's area or adjacent structures in the left inferior frontal gyrus. As patients with motor aphasia also have difficulty in writing, it is important to test not only spoken language but also written language.

Sensory Aphasia

In order to test the ability to understand spoken language, it is useful to give a verbal instruction to perform a complex motor task. If the patient is unable to do as instructed, it is useful to see how he/she can imitate a motor task that is visually demonstrated by the examiner. If the patient can imitate, it suggests a problem in verbal comprehension (sensory aphasia), but if he/she cannot imitate, it might suggest a problem in motor execution (apraxia). The instruction to imitate the given motor task is usually understood even by the patient with sensory aphasia, if the instruction is given by the examiner's gesture. If the patient is severely demented, however, this test is not possible.

Patients with typical sensory aphasia are usually talkative, but their speech is totally incomprehensible, because they do not understand what they are saying. This condition is called **jargon aphasia**. Repetition of spoken words is also impaired in sensory aphasia. It is also important to test understanding of the written language (reading). Alexia with agraphia is caused by a lesion of the area including the angular gyrus of the left parietal lobe. If the supramarginal

gyrus is also damaged, agraphia is seen together with the left-right disorientation, finger agnosia, and acalculia (Gerstmann syndrome).

Conduction Aphasia

In patients who are suspected of suffering from language disturbance and yet showing apparently normal performance in the tests of understanding and spontaneous speech, it is necessary to test **repetition**. If the arcuate fasciculus connecting Wernicke's area and Broca's area is disconnected, a difficulty in repeating verbally presented words might predominate the clinical picture (conduction aphasia). In this case, literal paraphasia and verbal paraphasia are commonly seen (Box 89).

While testing the naming of objects by presenting a series of different pictures, some patients might answer the name of the object just presented on the preceding test. This phenomenon is called **verbal perseveration**. However, perseveration is also seen for motor tasks, and may be seen in patients with dementia like Alzheimer disease.

B. EXAMINATION OF PRAXIS AND APRAXIA

Limb-kinetic apraxia can be noticed while carrying out the physical examination. In contrast, **ideomotor apraxia** might be detected for the first time by specifically asking the patient to make a gesture or pantomime tool use. For example, the patient is asked to salute with his hand, or to use a toothbrush, comb, or scissors or to imitate the use of those tools. The patient with ideomotor apraxia is unable or clumsy in doing these motor tasks. For testing the presence

---

BOX 89 LANDAU-KLEFFNER SYNDROME

A child with epilepsy may develop difficulty in understanding the spoken language that he/she has already learned (verbal auditory agnosia), and may become progressively aphasic. This condition is called Landau-Kleffner syndrome. In this condition, the type of epilepsy varies among patients, including simple partial motor seizure, atypical absence, and generalized convulsion. As a result of magnetoencephalographic studies, spikes have been shown to arise near the sylvian fissure on either side. It is postulated that involvement of the language area by epileptogenic activities might cause progressive aphasia (Castillo et al, 2008).

THE NEUROLOGIC EXAMINATION

or absence of **ideational apraxia**, it is useful to adopt a motor task that uses two or more kinds of tools in combination. For example, the patient is given a piece of paper and a pair of scissors and asked to cut the paper in half, or to brush his teeth with a toothbrush and toothpaste. For detecting **dressing apraxia**, it is important to ask the patient to actually put on a folded piece of clothing.

Inability to continue a motor task in spite of the absence of sensorimotor disturbance might be called **motor impersistence**. However, a similar condition might also be seen in association with poor motivation or lack of motor attention. Some investigators include inability to perform two different motor tasks simultaneously (**simultanapraxia**) in the concept of motor impersistence. Simultanapraxia is believed to occur with right frontal lobe lesions (Sakai et al, 2000).

While examining a series of different motor tasks, the patient might repeat the motor task that he/she did just before. Just as in the case of language, this phenomenon is called **perseveration**.

Gait Apraxia and Freezing of Gait

Gait apraxia is defined as inability to start walking in patients with no bradykinesia or rigidity in the supine position. In most cases of so-called gait apraxia, the disturbance is due to **freezing of gait** or akinesia, because the patient has difficulty in moving legs also in the supine position. Paradoxical kinesia (see Box 70) is seen in association with both gait apraxia and freezing of gait.

C. EXAMINATION OF RECOGNITION AND AGNOSIA

Recognition related to the somatosensory system includes stereognosis, graphesthesia, two-point discrimination, baroesthesia, and touch localization (see Chapter 19-1 and Table 19-1). For the auditory sense, identification and spatial localization of the source of sound are tested as necessary.

Visual Recognition

Presented with objects or their pictures, the patient is asked to answer the name, size, and color of the objects. However, if the patient has difficulty in naming, then presented with two or more objects or their pictures of different quality (for example of different color or shape), the patient is asked whether they are the same or different. Likewise, presented with two visual targets at different distances from the patient's eyes, the patient is asked to judge which is near and which is far. For testing visuospatial recognition, presented with a picture of clock without digits, the patient is asked to read the time (if impaired, **agnosia of clock reading**). Likewise, shown different numbers of fingers on the examiner's two hands, the patient is asked to tell how many fingers are seen in total. Alternatively, presented with two large circles containing different numbers of small dots in them, the patient is asked to tell the total number of small dots (if impaired, **disturbance of optic counting**). Furthermore, presented with a cartoon scene, the patient may be asked to tell what is going on in the scene. Inability to judge the situation is called **simultanagnosia**.

Hemispatial Neglect

When disturbance of visual attention or visual recognition is limited to the left or right side, it is called hemispatial neglect. To test this, the patient may be asked to divide a straight line into two or three equal parts. Alternatively, presented with a large number of small marks drawn on a sheet of paper, the patient is asked to cross out all the signals with a pencil. In this test, the signals on the neglected side may remain uncrossed. Furthermore, the patient with hemispatial neglect may neglect a half of his/her own body, like forgetting to shave one side of the face. As visual attention is primarily controlled by the right hemisphere, hemispatial neglect is commonly seen on the left half. To confirm the presence of hemispatial neglect, it is important to exclude hemianopsia. In practice, however, as the visual field test is often difficult to carry out in this situation because of poor visual attention, it may have to be judged by the confrontation test (see Chapter 7-2B) (Box 90).

Patients with a gross vascular lesion in the right hemisphere might deny the presence of left hemiplegia, which is called **anosognosia** (Orfei et al, 2007).

D. USE OF SIMPLE TEST BATTERY

As the time spent for the whole neurologic examination might be limited in the daily clinical setting, it is useful to prepare a simple battery of tests covering most of the important aspects of higher brain functions. An example battery is shown in Figure 23-9. Of course, this is just for a screening test, and a detailed evaluation has to be done as necessary.

BALINT SYNDROME

This unique syndrome is characterized by disturbance of visual attention and visually guided praxis. This condition had been described since the end of the 19th century, but in 1909 Balint coined the term "optische Ataxie." A triad of this syndrome is formed by optic ataxia (difficulty in grasping a visually presented target), psychic paralysis of gaze, and disorder of spatial attention (Pisella et al, 2008). The patient with this syndrome keeps fixating his/her gaze on a spot in space and is unable to direct his visual attention to the approaching examiner. If the patient is asked to grasp an object, his/her hand misses the target by far (Figure 23-7). There is no clear hemianopsia, but the patient tends to neglect one side. This condition is caused by bilateral ischemic lesions of the parieto-occipital junction, which is a watershed area between the middle and posterior cerebral arteries, as a result of hemodynamic change with hypoperfusion (see Chapter 2-4) (Figure 23-8). In most cases, the predominant lesion is on the right hemisphere, but the original case reported by Balint was on the left.

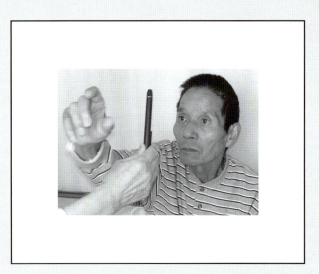

Figure 23-7 Inability to grasp a visual target seen in a patient with Balint syndrome. (With the patient's permission)

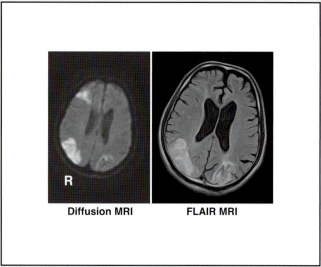

Diffusion MRI   FLAIR MRI

Figure 23-8 MR images of the patient shown in Figure 23-7, showing infarctions in the bilateral parieto-occipital junction areas, predominantly affecting the right.

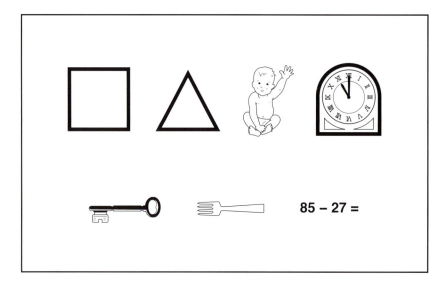

Figure 23-9 A simple battery for testing language, praxis and recognition in the bedside examination, which was used in the University of Minnesota Hospital when one of the authors (HS) was a neurology resident there. The two figures on the top left are for testing recognition of the shape and naming. The picture of a baby is for testing naming and judgment of the left and right. The picture of clock is used for testing naming and visuopatial recognition, and two pictures on the bottom left are for naming and praxis pantomime.

BIBLIOGRAPHY

Alossa N, Castelli L. Amusia and musical functioning. Eur Neurol 61:269–277, 2009. (review)

Baumann O, Mattingley JB. Medial parietal cortex encodes perceived heading direction in humans. J Neurosi 30:12897–12901, 2010.

Bayen E, de Langavant LC, Fenelon G. Le syndrome d'Alice au pays des merveilles: une aura migraineuse inhabituelle. Rev Neurol 168:457–459, 2012.

Binder JR. The Wernicke area. Modern evidence and a reinterpretation. Neurology 85:2170–2175, 2015.

Castillo EM, Butler IJ, Baumgartner JE, Passaro A, Papanicolaou AC. When epilepsy interferes with word comprehension: findings in Landau-Kleffner syndrome. J Child Neurol 23:97–101, 2008.

Catani M, ffytche DH. The rises and falls of disconnection syndromes. Brain 128:2224–2239, 2005. (review)

Cristinzio C, N'Diaye K, Seeck M, Vuilleumier P, Sander D. Integration of gaze direction and facial expression in patients with unilateral amygdala damage. Brain 133:248–261, 2010.

Geschwind N. Disconnexion syndromes in animals and man. I. Brain 88:237–294, 1965a.

Geschwind N. Disconnexion syndromes in animals and man. II. Brain 88:585–644, 1965b.

Golarai G, Hong S, Haas BW, Galaburda AM, Mills DL, Bellugi U, et al. The fusiform face area is enlarged in Williams syndrome. J Neurosi 30:6700–6712, 2010.

Hallett M. Apraxia: the rise, fall and resurrection of diagrams to explain how the brain works. Brain 138:229–231, 2015. (Book review)

Hattori N, Shibasaki H, Wheaton L, Wu T, Matsuhashi M, Hallett M. Discrete parieto-frontal functional connectivity related to grasping. J Neurophysiol 101:1267–1282, 2009.

Iwata M. Kanji versus Kana: neuropsychological correlates of the Japanese writing system. Trends Neurosci 7:290–293, 1984.

Lüders H, Lesser RP, Hahn J, Dinner DS, Morris H, Resor S, et al. Basal temporal language area demonstrated by electrical stimulation. Neurology 36:505–510, 1986.

Matsuhashi M, Ikeda A, Ohara S, Matsumoto R, Yamamoto J, Takayama M, et al. Multisensory convergence at human temporo-parietal junction—epicortical recording of evoked responses. Clin Neurophysiol 115:1145–1160, 2004.

Matsumoto R, Ikeda A, Nagamine T, Matsuhashi M, Ohara S, Yamamoto J, et al. Subregions of human MT complex revealed by comparative MEG and direct electrocorticographic recordings. Clin Neurophysiol 115:2056–2065, 2004a.

Matsumoto R, Nair DR, LaPresto E, Najm I, Bingaman W, Shibasaki H, et al. Functional connectivity in the human language system: a cortico-cortical evoked potential study. Brain 127:2316–2330, 2004b.

Matsumoto R, Nair DR, Ikeda A, Fumuro T, Lapresto E, Mikuni N, et al. Parieto-frontal network in humans studied by cortico-cortical evoked potential. Human Brain Map 33:2856–2872, 2012.

Mesulam M-M, Weintraub S, Rogalski EJ, Wieneke C, Geula C, Bigio EH. Asymmetry and heterogeneity of Alzheimer's and frontotemporal pathology in primary progressive aphasia. Brain 137:1176–1192, 2014.

Mesulam M-M, Thompson CK, Weintraub S, Rogalsky EJ. The Wernicke conundrum and the anatomy of language comprehension in primary progressive aphasia. Brain 138:2423–2437, 2015.

Nakamura K, Honda M, Osaka T, Hanakawa Y, Toma K, Fukuyama H, et al. Participation of the left posterior inferior temporal cortex in writing and mental recall of kanji orthography: a functional MRI study. Brain 123:954–967, 2000.

Orfei MD, Robinson RG, Prigatano GP, Starkstein S, Rüsch N, Bria P, et al. Anosognosia for hemiplegia after stroke is a multifaceted phenomenon: a systematic review of the literature. Brain 130:3075–3090, 2007.

Pisella L, Ota H, Vighetto A, Rossetti Y. Optic ataxia and Balint's syndrome: neuropsychological and neurophysiological prospects. Handb Clin Neurol, 88:393–415, 2008.

Rizzolatti G, Craighero L. The mirror-neuron system. Annu Rev Neurosci 27:169–192, 2004. (review)

Rizzolatti G, Fogassi L. The mirror mechanism: recent findings and perspectives. Philos Trans R Soc Lond B Biol Sci 369 (1644): 20130420. doi: 10.1098/rstb.2013.0420. Print 2014. (review)

Roux F-E, Dufor O, Giussani C, Wamain Y, Draper L, Longcamp M, et al. The graphemic/motor frontal area Exner's area revisited. Ann Neurol 66:537–545, 2009.

Rusconi E, Pinel P, Dehaene S, Kleinschmidt A. The enigma of Gerstmann's syndrome revisited: a telling tale of the vicissitudes of neuropsychology. Brain 133:320–332, 2010. (review)

Sakai Y, Nakamura T, Sakurai A, Yamaguchi H, Hirai S. Right frontal areas 6 and 8 are associated with simultanapraxia, a subset of motor impersistence. Neurology 54:522–524, 2000.

Schott JM, Rossor MN. The grasp and other primitive reflexes. J Neurol Neurosurg Psychiatry 74:558–560. 2003. (review)

Shibasaki H. Human brain mapping: hemodynamic response and electrophysiology. Clin Neurophysiol 119:731–743, 2008. (review)

Takahashi N, Kawamura M, Shiota J, Kasahata N, Hirayama K. Pure topographic disorientation due to right retrosplenial lesion. Neurology 49:464–469, 1997.

Treffert DA. The savant syndrome: an extraordinary condition. A synopsis: past, present, future. Philos Trans R Soc Lond B Biol Soc 364:1351–1357, 2009. (review)

Ueki Y, Mima T, Nakamura K, Oga T, Shibasaki H, Nagamine T, et al. Transient functional suppression and facilitation of Japanese ideogram writing induced by repetitive transcranial magnetic stimulation of posterior inferior temporal cortex. J Neurosci 26:8523–8530, 2006.

Usui K, Ikeda A, Nagamine T, Matsuhashi M, Kinoshita M, Mikuni N, et al. Temporal dynamics of Japanese morphogram and syllabogram processing in the left basal temporal area studied by event-related potentials. J Clin Neurophysiol 26:160–166, 2009.

Weiss PH, Fink GR. Grapheme-colour synaesthetes show increased grey matter volumes of parietal and fusiform cortex. Brain 132:65–70, 2009.

Wheaton LA, Shibasaki H, Hallett M. Temporal activation pattern of parietal and premotor areas related to praxis movements. Clin Neurophysiol 116:1201–1212, 2005.

Wolf RC, Philippi CL, Motzkin JC, Baskaya MK, Koenigs M. Ventromedial prefrontal cortex mediates visual attention during facial emotion recognition. Brain 137:1772–1780, 2014.

24.

PAROXYSMAL AND FUNCTIONAL DISORDERS

Epileptic seizures, migraine, and sleep disorders might eventually be classified into organic diseases at the histological, cellular, or molecular level, but in this book, these disorders are described in a category of paroxysmal or functional disorders. In most cases of these disorders, patients may not show any neurologic abnormality during the physical examination. Therefore, the history taking and laboratory examinations are quite important for diagnosis of these conditions. The term "functional" has a variety of meanings, and is now often used as a synonym for "psychogenic." Here it refers to a disorder of function in an episode without a constant abnormality.

1. EPILEPSY AND CONVULSION

Epileptic seizure is defined as "transient occurrence of symptoms and/or signs due to abnormal excessive or synchronous neuronal activity in the brain." It is currently considered that most cases of epileptic seizures are based on organic cerebral lesions. The prevalence of epilepsy is believed to be as high as 0.5% of the population.

A. CLASSIFICATION OF EPILEPTIC SEIZURES

Classification of epileptic seizures was proposed by the International League Against Epilepsy (ILAE) in 1981, and then it was revised twice, first in 1989 and then in 2010. In this book, classification of epileptic seizures is explained by using the 2010 classification of the ILAE (Berg et al, 2010).

Epileptic seizures are largely classified into three groups: generalized seizures, focal seizures, and unknown, and the first two groups are further classified into subgroups mainly based on the clinical manifestations (Table 24-1). **Generalized epileptic seizures** are defined as

TABLE 24-1 CLASSIFICATION OF EPILEPTIC SEIZURES BY ILAE COMMISSION

I. Generalized seizures
A. Tonic-clonic (in any combination)
B. Absence
1. Typical
2. Atypical
3. Absence with special features
Myoclonic absence
Eyelid myoclonia
C. Myoclonic
1. Myoclonic
2. Myoclonic atonic
3. Myoclonic tonic
D. Clonic
E. Tonic
F. Atonic
II. Focal seizures
A. Without impairment of consciousness or awareness.
1. With observable motor or autonomic components. This roughly corresponds to the concept of "simple partial seizure."
2. Involving subjective sensory or psychic phenomena only.
B. With impairment of consciousness or awareness. This roughly corresponds to the concept of "complex partial seizure."
C. Evolving to a bilateral, convulsive seizure (involving tonic, clonic, or tonic and clonic components). This expression replaces the term "secondarily generalized seizure."
III. Unknown
A. Epileptic spasms

SOURCE: Berg et al, 2010.

seizures occurring in and rapidly engaging bilaterally distributed networks, and **focal epileptic seizures** are seizures occurring within networks limited to one hemisphere and either discretely localized or more widely distributed (Berg et al, 2010). Theoretically, generalized epileptic seizures in the strict sense are considered to be extremely rare, because even generalized tonic-clonic seizures may actually start focally and be secondarily generalized. In this case, an epileptogenic focus, if any, may not be detected by the routine laboratory examination. In contrast, typical absence seizure (**petit mal**), which is characterized by a short lapse of consciousness and an EEG burst of bilaterally synchronous high amplitude 3-Hz rhythmic spike-and-wave discharges (Figure 24-1) may be considered as a typical example of generalized epilepsy.

1) Focal Epileptic Seizures

Focal seizures are classified into three groups: group A without impairment of consciousness or awareness, group B with impairment of consciousness or awareness, and group C evolving to a bilateral, convulsive seizure. Group A is further classified into group A1, with observable motor or autonomic components, and group A2, involving subjective sensory or psychic phenomena only. Group A1 roughly corresponds to **simple partial seizure** of the 1981 ILAE classification (Commission on Classification and Terminology of the International League Against Epilepsy,

1981). Group B roughly corresponds to **complex partial seizure**, and group C corresponds to **secondarily generalized seizure** of the 1981 classification. Group A1 (simple partial seizure) may be further divided into neocortical epilepsy and mesial temporal lobe epilepsy depending on the source of epileptogenic focus.

A representative form of neocortical focal seizure is **focal motor seizure**, which originates from the primary motor cortex (MI) and manifests itself as tonic and/or clonic convulsion in the corresponding part of the body. A form of focal motor seizure characterized by marching of the convulsion according to the MI somatotopy is called **Jacksonian seizure**. Focal motor seizure is commonly followed by transient weakness of the involved extremity (**postictal paralysis**, **Todd paralysis**). Seizures arising from the supplementary motor area (SMA) might show bilateral dystonic posturing and bizarre movements (Figure 24-2).

Simple partial seizure originating from the primary somatosensory cortex (SI) manifests itself with abnormal sensation on the corresponding part of skin, which might spread according to the SI somatotopy just as in the case of motor seizure. In the focal seizure originating from supplementary motor area (SMA) or insular cortex, pain might be one of the ictal symptoms. **Painful somatosensory seizures** often originate in the operculo-insular cortex (Montavont et al, 2015). A focal seizure arising from the occipital cortex may present with a flash of light. In many cases of neocortical partial epilepsy, **cortical dysplasia** is found by detailed

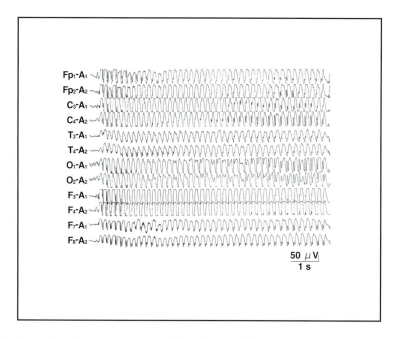

Figure 24-1 EEG of a 13-year-old patient with petit mal during hyperventilation. A burst of bilaterally synchronous rhythmic high amplitude 3 Hz spike-and-wave discharges is seen.

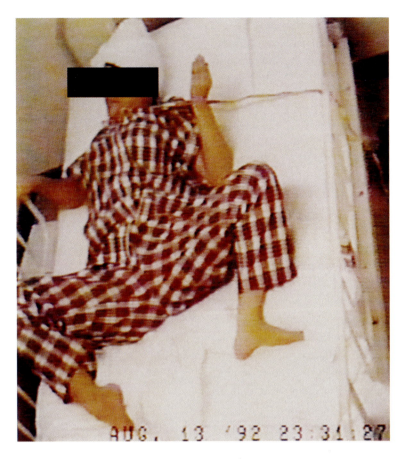

Figure 24-2 Bilateral dystonic posturing seen in a 21-year-old patient with SMA seizure. (Courtesy of Dr. Akio Ikeda of Kyoto University)

neuroimaging studies, which may be a candidate for surgical treatment (Kim et al, 2009).

Mesial Temporal Lobe Epilepsy

Epilepsy originating from the mesial temporal cortex (**mesial temporal lobe epilepsy, MTLE**) is the commonest form of epilepsy in adults. Clinically, MTLE presents with various neurologic symptoms: sensory symptoms, autonomic symptoms, abnormal emotion, and abnormal thought or behavior. Sensory symptoms of mesial temporal lobe origin include sensation of abnormal smell (**uncinate fit**), abnormal taste (**gustatory seizure**), and vertigo (**vertiginous seizure**, **epileptic vertigo**) (Tarnutzer et al, 2015). The most common autonomic symptom is a sensation of nausea ascending from the epigastrium (**epigastric rising sensation**). Other autonomic ictal symptoms include bradycardia, facial pallor, flushing, sweating, and mydriasis. Cardiac or autonomic involvement might lead to sudden unexpected death in epilepsy (SUDEP), especially in patients with longstanding and medication refractory epilepsy (Bermeo-Ovalle et al, 2015, for review). Apnea might

also be an ictal symptom, although its origin has not been confirmed (**ictal apnea**) (Tezer et al, 2009).

Emotional symptoms include sudden attacks of feeling of fear, anxiety, or pleasure. Sudden attacks of hallucination might be a manifestation of MTLE (**hallucinatory seizure**). In a hallucinatory seizure, the patient always sees the same concrete landscape or situation during the attacks. Furthermore, the patient may feel as if a totally new situation has already been seen before (**déjà vu**), or to the contrary, the patient may feel as if the familiar situation has never been seen before (**jamais vu**).

Attacks characterized by abnormal behavior or actions are called **automatism** or **psychomotor seizure**. Consciousness is impaired in most cases. Typically, the patient first feels an epigastric rising sensation, followed by loss of consciousness, and may show chewing movement of the mouth or rubbing movement of the hands, but does not respond to a verbal call. The patient may even walk or move about during the ictal episode, but the patient does not recall the abnormal behavior at all after the episode. Dystonic posture may be seen in the upper limb contralateral to the epileptic focus and may evolve to a generalized convulsion. After the generalized convulsion, the patient appears obtunded for a short time. The EEG often shows spikes in the temporal region even during the intervals (Figure 24-3) (Box 91).

2) Generalized Epileptic Seizures

Most of the above-described simple partial seizures may evolve to generalized seizures. Those prodromal symptoms and/or signs occurring before the generalization are called **aura**. Focal seizure symptoms are common in idiopathic generalized epileptic seizures (Seneviratne et al, 2015).

Generalized tonic-clonic seizures are characterized by bilateral tonic extension of the trunk and limbs followed by synchronous muscle jerking associated with loss of consciousness. There may be a loud vocalization during the attacks. Postictally, patients are often lethargic and confused for various lengths of time. Ictal and interictal EEG shows a burst of generalized high-amplitude spike-and-waves, but the burst may not start synchronously and often starts with focal paroxysmal abnormalities.

A typical **absence seizure (petit mal)** is an attack of lapse lasting about 5 seconds. For example, a child suddenly stops moving while eating and cannot respond to the surroundings. Frequent blinks might be seen during the episode. Ictal as well as interictal EEG shows a burst of bilaterally synchronous high amplitude 3 Hz rhythmic spike-and-wave discharges (Figure 24-1). The EEG burst is characteristically induced or enhanced by hyperventilation.

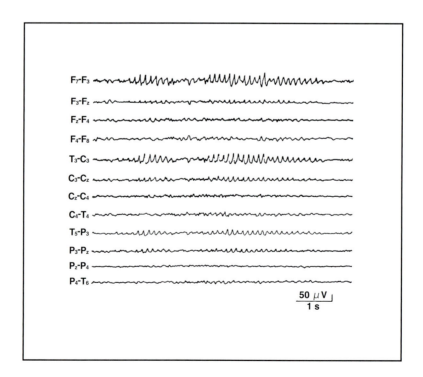

Figure 24-3 Interictal EEG of a patient with psychomotor seizure. Rhythmic spikes are seen at the left temporal leads (F7, T3).

Stimulus-Sensitive and Task-Specific Epilepsy

Most epileptic seizures occur spontaneously without any precipitating factor, but some seizures are sensitive to a specific stimulus or occur during performance of a certain task. A typical example of stimulus-sensitive epilepsy is **photosensitive epilepsy**, such as TV anime-induced (animation) epilepsy. In this case, EEG spikes are often induced by photic stimulation, and sensitivity to the kind of visual stimulus differs among patients (Takahashi, 2008). Task-specific epilepsy occurs during performance of a specific task or game such as playing chess, calculating, and listening to a special kind of music. In the latter case, the attack tends to occur while listening to a particular piece of music composed by a specific composer.

Autosomal dominant lateral temporal lobe epilepsy is induced by auditory stimulus in children or young adults. Several point mutations of the LGI1 (leucine-rich glioma inactivated-1) gene have been identified, and phenotypes are also different among families (Kawamata et al, 2010). Following auditory or visual hallucination as an aura, marked psychiatric symptoms appear and in some cases may evolve to generalized convulsion. **Autosomal dominant nocturnal frontal lobe epilepsy** is considered to be an ion channel disorder of the acetylcholine receptor (see Chapter 25-1A). Recently, genetic epilepsy has drawn increasing attention. Even focal epilepsy could be genetically inherited, like glucose transporter type 1 (Glut1) defects (Wolking et al, 2014).

B. DIAGNOSIS OF EPILEPSY

As it is rare to encounter the ictal episode in the clinic, its clinical diagnosis primarily depends on the information obtained from the patient or the witnesses. Since an epileptic attack is caused by pathological hyperexcitation of a certain neuronal group, an important feature of epilepsy is a repeated occurrence of the same symptomatology in all ictal episodes. The kind of ictal symptoms depends on which part of the cerebral cortex is involved by the epileptogenic activity. Although some patients might have more than one epileptogenic focus, the ictal pattern is expected to be stereotyped for each focus. It has to be kept in mind, however, that the attacks originating from the same epileptogenic focus might differ among attacks in its severity ranging from a mild attack to a severe one. In MTLE, it ranges from aura to psychomotor seizure.

When examining the paroxysmal disorders, it is important to obtain information about when and in which circumstances the attacks occur, and about the presence of any precipitating factor. For example, the periodicity of seizure recurrence might be associated with the menstrual cycle (catamenial epilepsy). Furthermore, in patients who are taking antiepileptic drugs, it is important to know whether the patient is taking the medication as prescribed or not. When there is any possibility about **psychogenic nonepileptic seizure (PNES) (pseudoseizure)**, it is useful to carry out long-term video-EEG monitoring in the hospital. In patients with epileptic seizures, EEG and neuroimaging study are always indicated.

Furthermore, since an epileptic seizure might be a manifestation of systemic diseases, a possibility of **symptomatic epilepsy** has to be taken into account. Brain tumors commonly cause convulsive seizures. Systemic lupus erythematosus (SLE) might start with generalized convulsion, and metabolic abnormalities such as electrolyte abnormalities and endocrine disorders might underlie epileptic seizures. In children, in addition to general physical examination, careful observation of skin for congenital lesions (nevus) is important. Among others, angiofibroma on the face suggests tuberous sclerosis as an underlying cause of seizure (see Figure 3-1).

Generalized convulsion may occur in the acute phase of severe head injury, but the first seizure may occur several months after the head trauma (**posttraumatic epilepsy**). Its underlying mechanism might differ among cases, but scar formation following cerebral contusion is considered to be an important factor. In elderly people, epileptic attacks related to strokes are not rare (Box 92).

Evaluation of Medically Intractable Epileptic Seizures

Medically intractable epileptic seizures are defined as epileptic attacks that occur more than once a month in patients who are taking the appropriate dose of appropriate kinds of antiepileptic drugs. In this case, it is useful to admit the patient in a hospital where the epilepsy specialist is available and to confirm the presence of epileptic seizures, to classify the seizure and to look for the presence of any organic brain lesion (American Clinical Neurophysiology Society, 2008; Kanazawa et al, 2015; Usui et al, 2015). If an organic lesion is discovered or if a single epileptogenic focus is detected, it might be possible to treat the patient surgically after carefully evaluating functions of the brain areas surrounding the epileptogenic focus (Shibasaki et al, 2007, for review). In MTLE, which is the most common form of epileptic seizures in adults, partial resection of anterior part of the temporal lobe or selective resection of the amygdala and hippocampus

The most common cause of the first seizure in elderly people is cerebrovascular disease. A seizure in the acute phase of the first stroke is not rare, although the prevalence varies among reports. A survey of 714 cases of strokes in Italy showed occurrence of seizures during the acute phase in 6.3% of all cases. Among those cases with seizures, 16.2% had intracerebral hemorrhage, 12.5% had cerebral infarction evolving to hemorrhage, and 4.2% had cerebral infarction (Beghi et al, 2011). Regardless of the kind or location of the stroke, epilepsy was particularly common in those cases with strokes involving the cerebral cortex. In contrast, the prevalence of **post-stroke seizures** varies among different reports, but according to the study by Myint et al. (2006), about 10% of the patients with stroke develop seizures within 5 years. Risk factors for cerebral infarction to cause post-stroke seizures include severity of acute phase, severity of residual symptoms, number and size of infarctions, degree of cortical damage, and involvement of the hippocampus. A long-term follow-up study of a large number of patients with subarachnoid hemorrhage (SAH) from saccular intracranial aneurysm in Finland showed a cumulative incidence of epilepsy of 12% at 5 years (Huttunen et al, 2015). It was especially common in those patients with SAH associated with intracerebral hemorrhage.

is effective in about two-thirds of cases (Engel et al, 2003). In epileptic seizures of neocortical origin, however, there is no definitive conclusion as to the effect of surgical intervention (Jeha et al, 2007; Cho et al, 2014).

Psychogenic Nonepileptic Seizures

Some seizures may look like epileptic seizures but are not associated with any epileptic discharge of cerebral neurons. Psychogenic nonepileptic seizures (PNES) often present a diagnostic problem. Generally speaking, during convulsive seizures associated with impairment of consciousness, the patient's eyes are open. Therefore, if the eyes are kept closed during the convulsive seizures, it is more likely to be psychogenic. Furthermore, if a convulsion seen during the attack looks unusual for the ordinary convulsive seizure, it may make the examiner suspect a possibility of PNES. However, autosomal dominant nocturnal frontal lobe epilepsy may manifest itself as extremely bizarre movements. If there is any doubt about the diagnosis, long-term video-EEG monitoring is indicated.

2. HEADACHE AND MIGRAINE

A. CLASSIFICATION OF HEADACHE

Headache is one of the most common symptoms presenting in the neurology clinic, and it is caused by a variety of mechanisms. Among the cranial structures, pain receptors are present only in the scalp, its subcutaneous tissue, skull bones, meninges, walls of blood vessels, and cranial nerves possessing somatosensory fibers. There is no pain receptor in the brain parenchyma. That is why stereotactic surgery can be done without general anesthesia. Headache is classified by the International Headache Society into three groups: **the primary headaches, the secondary headaches**, and painful cranial neuropathies, other facial pains, and other headaches (Table 24-2) (Headache Classification Subcommittee of the International Headache Society [IHS], 2013).

When a patient with headache is seen in the clinic, it is most important not to overlook the secondary or symptomatic headache due to organic lesion of intra- as well as extracranial structures. Headache due to intracranial hemorrhage or tumor used to be called traction

TABLE 24-2 INTERNATIONAL CLASSIFICATION OF HEADACHE

The primary headaches
1. Migraine
2. Tension-type headache
3. Trigeminal autonomic cephalalgias
4. Other primary headache disorders
The secondary headaches
5. Headache attributed to trauma or injury to the head and/or neck
6. Headache attributed to cranial or cervical vascular disorder
7. Headache attributed to nonvascular intracranial disorder
8. Headache attributed to a substance or its withdrawal
9. Headache attributed to infection
10. Headache attributed to disorder of homoeostasis
11. Headache or facial pain attributed to disorder of the cranium, neck, eyes, ears, nose, sinuses, teeth, mouth, or other facial or cervical structures
12. Headache attributed to psychiatric disorder
Painful cranial neuropathies, other facial pains, and other headaches
13. Painful cranial neuropathies and other facial pains
14. Other headache disorders

Source: Headache Classification Subcommittee of the International Headache Society, 2013.

headache, and nowadays its diagnosis is relatively easy with the aid of neuroimaging techniques. It is especially important to keep in mind that headache is often caused by ophthalmological disorders; diseases of ear, nose, and pharynx; dental and oral diseases; and disorders of cervical spine. Headache due to cerebrovascular diseases, fever, and hypertension is common and used to be called nonmigrainous vascular headache. Headache due to intracranial hypertension is commonly accompanied by nausea and vomiting and is characterized by its aggravation when awake in the morning (**morning headache**, **morning vomiting**). This is considered to be due to an increase in the blood carbon monoxide level as a result of nocturnal hypoventilation, which causes an increase in intracranial arterial perfusion, resulting in intracranial hypertension in the morning.

Intracranial hypertension with no causative space-occupying lesion (**idiopathic intracranial hypertension**) used to be called pseudotumor cerebri. It is commonly associated with endocrine/metabolic abnormalities, drugs, and high protein concentration in the cerebrospinal fluid, and some investigators include intracranial venous sinus thrombosis in this category.

Severe headache may occur due to a sudden decrease in intracranial pressure. A typical example is **post-lumbar puncture headache**, which occurs after traumatic lesion of the dura mater by lumbar puncture for the purpose of examination or anesthesia (Box 93). Headache may be also caused by a spontaneous drop in intracranial pressure with no preceding lumbar puncture (**spontaneous intracranial hypotension**). Spontaneous leakage of the cerebrospinal fluid is considered to be its main cause (Schievink et al, 2015). In this condition, the T1-weighted MR image with gadolinium characteristically shows diffuse enhancement of the dura mater.

B. MIGRAINE AND RELATED DISORDERS

In contrast with the secondary (symptomatic) headaches, the primary headaches may be called functional headaches, and migraine and tension headache are two representative forms of this category. **Migraine** is characterized by repetition of paroxysmal headaches with no symptom during the intervals. Migraine is often inherited in autosomal dominant transmission. Many attacks of migraine are preceded by **aura**, most commonly a flashing light in a hemifield or in the rim of a hemifield in a crescent shape (**scintillating scotoma**). Aura is believed to be caused by enhanced susceptibility to cortical spreading depression, which increases sensitivity to focal cerebral ischemia (Ferrari et al, 2015, for

---

BOX 93 POST-LUMBAR PUNCTURE HEADACHE

This is a typical example of headache due to a sudden drop in intracranial pressure. The headache begins several seconds after standing up from the lying position, reaches its peak within 1 minute, and disappears within 20 seconds after returning to the lying position. The kind and degree of headache differs greatly among subjects. It is relatively more common in young women. Although the mechanism of post-lumbar puncture headache is not precisely known, it is believed that intracranial pain receptors are pulled downward because of a decreased amount of cerebrospinal fluid (CSF). On the other hand, based on the fact that extradural blood patch is effective, it is postulated that the split injury caused by dural puncture persists and the CSF leaks out through the split in the upright position. In order to prevent this headache, it is important to use as small a puncture needle as possible, to match the slant of the needle tip to the direction of dural fibers, to not rotate the needle after puncture, and to keep the patient supine for at least 2 hours after the puncture. The headache will improve spontaneously with water supplementation and by keeping the lying position, but when it is severe, epidural patch of the split with the patient's own blood is effective (Bezov et al, 2010).

---

review). It may present a positive symptom like scintillating scotoma or a negative symptom like hemianopsia. In the following phase, the corresponding artery dilates and activates pain receptors in the arterial wall, which is felt as a throbbing headache. Thus, the kind of aura depends on which artery is involved by the migraine, namely, scintillating scotoma or hemianopsia in the territory of posterior cerebral artery, blindness of one eye in the ophthalmic artery (**retinal migraine**), and brainstem symptoms in the vertebrobasilar artery (**basilar artery migraine**).

In some attacks of migraine, a neurologic deficit seen as an aura might continue during or even after the migraine attack, like **hemiplegic migraine** and **ophthalmoplegic migraine**. These forms of migraine are usually inherited in autosomal dominant transmission. **Familial hemiplegic migraine** is often associated with spinocerebellar ataxia 6 (SCA6) or episodic ataxia, or both, and is considered to be a calcium channel disorder (see Chapter 25-1A).

When examining patients with headache, it is of utmost importance to obtain detailed information about the nature of the headache, including the presence or absence of any precipitating factor such as food and action, time of the day, and relationship to menstruation in case of women. If the headache fluctuates in its severity in synchrony with the arterial pulsation, it is called **throbbing headache** or **pulsating headache**. The pathological mechanism of migraine has not been fully clarified yet, but pharmacologically a decrease in blood serotonin level is believed to play a primary role. Drugs acting on the serotonin receptor are effective in many cases. For the treatment of migraine, subcutaneous injection of sumatriptan succinate 6 mg, or oral administration of zolmitriptan 2.5 ~ 5.0 mg or ergotamine tartrate 1 ~ 2 mg is usually effective. If the above initial dose of ergotamine tartrate is not effective, it may be repeated every 30 minutes, but it should not exceed 6 mg in total for one attack.

A migraine attack might be complicated by cerebral infarction (**migrainous cerebral infarction**), although this is rare. This condition is relatively common in young women with migraine starting with aura in the posterior cerebral artery territory. If neurological deficits continue after the migraine attack, it is necessary to examine the patient with diffusion MRI (Wolf et al, 2011).

Cluster Headache

This type of paroxysmal headache begins with severe pain in the deep orbit and is associated with autonomic symptoms such as conjunctival hyperemia, lacrimation, nasal obstruction, nasal discharge, facial sweating, miosis, ptosis, and palpebral edema. This kind of migraine used to be called histamine headache or Horton's headache, but now it is called **cluster headache** or **trigeminal autonomic cephalalgia**. It is common in young men and induced by ethanol and nitroglycerin. An attack lasts 15 minutes to 3 hours, and it tends to occur in repeated clusters over a period of several days to more than a month. Subcutaneous injection of sumatriptan is effective in some cases.

Reversible Cerebral Vasoconstriction Syndrome

This condition is clinically similar to migraine because of repeated attacks of severe headaches over a period of about a week, and because it may be associated with focal neurologic symptoms (Chen et al, 2015). It is characterized by angiographic finding of bead-like appearance of arteries (Ducros et al, 2007). Some cases of this condition may develop subarachnoid hemorrhage or **reversible posterior leukoencephalopathy** as complications.

C. TENSION-TYPE HEADACHE

This type of headache is as common as migraine, and is considered to be due to abnormal contraction of the muscles surrounding the cranium. It used to be called **muscle contraction headache**, and is characterized by a feeling of the head tightened by a headband. It is often influenced by weather and the patient's mood. In clinical practice, it is common to see a combination of tension-type headache and migraine in the same patient.

3. SLEEP DISORDERS

Sleep disorders are an important topic of clinical neurology because they are much more common than thought, and they may be results of functional or organic brain disorders. Based on the EEG and behavioral characteristics, sleep is divided into two stages: **rapid eye movement sleep (REM sleep)** and **non-REM sleep (NREM sleep, slow wave sleep)**. Non-REM sleep is further divided into three stages: N1, N2, and N3, corresponding to NREM stage 1, stage 2, and stage 3 plus 4 of the Rechtschaffen and Kales classification, respectively (Table 24-3) (Silber et al, 2007). In the REM stage, the EEG is similar to the waking EEG, but it is characterized by the occurrence of rapid eye movements and a decrease or loss of muscle discharge in the jaw muscles. The subject usually dreams during REM sleep. The mechanism of sleep stages has been extensively investigated physiologically as well as pharmacologically.

Sleep disorders are classified into insomnias, sleep-related breathing disorders, hypersomnias, circadian rhythm sleep disorders, parasomnias, and sleep-related movement disorders. As most patients with sleep disorders are not aware of their trouble at night, it is important to obtain information from their family or persons who live with them. The patients often visit the clinic with the chief complaint of daytime sleepiness. The most useful test for sleep disorders is **polysomnography (PSG)** in which EEG, surface EMG, electrocardiogram, electrooculogram, respiration, and blood oxygen saturation are simultaneously monitored throughout the nocturnal sleep.

A. OBSTRUCTIVE SLEEP APNEA-HYPOPNEA SYNDROME

Transient arrest or decrease of breathing during sleep is believed to be relatively common in adults. In this condition, breathing suddenly stops and recovers spontaneously in 10 ~ 15 seconds, during which time the blood oxygen saturation is also decreased. The PSG during this episode shows loss of nasal airflow in spite of the presence of the thoracic

TABLE 24-3 SLEEP STAGES OF ADULTS BASED ON EEG

Stage R & K	Features of EEG	EEG waveforms	Stage AASM
Waking	Waking	C ‿‿‿‿ O ∿∿∿∿	Stage W
Stage 1	Relatively low voltage, 2 ~ 7 Hz activities. Vertex sharp wave (V wave) may appear in the late phase.	C ‿‿⋀‿ O ‿‿⋁‿‿	Stage N1
Stage 2	Sleep spindles and K complex are seen. Slow waves are seen in less than 20% of the time.	C ‿⋀⋀⋀⋀↑‿ O ‿‿‿‿	Stage N2
Stage 3	Slow waves seen 20 ~ 50% of the time. Spindles are seen.	C ‿⋀⋀⋀‿ O ‿⋀‿⋀‿	Stage N3
Stage 4	Slow waves seen more than 50% of the time. Spindles are seen.	C ⋀⋀⋀⋁⋀⋀ O ⋀‿⋀⋀‿	
Stage REM	The same as stage 1. Rapid eye movements are seen. Tone of jaw muscles lost or decreased.	C ‿‿⋀‿ O ‿‿⋁‿‿	Stage R

R & K: Rechtschaffen & Kales, AASM: American Academy of Sleep Medicine

Slow waves: less than 2 Hz and higher than 75 μV.

C: central EEG, O: occipital EEG.

Source: Modified from Silber et al, 2007.

and abdominal excursion. This syndrome is commonly seen in markedly obese persons and is also called **pickwickian syndrome**. **Daytime sleepiness** is common because the patient wakes up frequently at night. Lying in the recumbent position and the use of a mouthpiece during nocturnal sleep might help to some extent, but positive pressure ventilation is effective in severe cases. As the patients with obstructive diseases of upper airway might present with a similar sleep disorder, the laryngological examination is mandatory.

B. CENTRAL SLEEP APNEA-HYPOPNEA SYNDROME

In this type of sleep apnea-hypopnea syndrome, the respiratory excursion of the thorax and abdomen is also lost or decreased on PSG during the episode. This phenomenon is commonly seen in patients with various neurodegenerative diseases, and it is especially common in those diseases affecting the brainstem reticular formation. A typical example is **multiple system atrophy**, in which sudden death may occur during sleep (Nishizawa & Shimohata, 2009). This condition is also seen in association with a vascular lesion of the brainstem, and a combined occurrence of central and obstructive types is not infrequent (Box 94).

C. REM SLEEP BEHAVIOR DISORDERS

This condition, REM sleep behavior disorders (RBD), is characterized by episodes of behavioral abnormalities during REM sleep. Patients with RBD may get up and behave violently during REM sleep. The PSG is also abnormal during the episode. For example, rapid eye movements may be present, but the jaw muscles maintain their discharges (lack of muscle atonia), and periodic movements may be seen in the lower limbs. Patients with Parkinson disease tend to suffer from insomnia and daytime sleepiness, and it has been shown that RBD is common in Parkinson disease (Arnulf

---

BOX 94 COULD SLEEP APNEA SYNDROME CAUSE COGNITIVE DISTURBANCE?

It might be questioned whether repeated drops of blood oxygen saturation might cause dementia in the future or not. In a multi-institutional study in the United States, 298 women over age 65, who had no dementia and were studied with polysomnography (PSG), were followed up for 3.2 ~ 6.2 years. Results showed that mild cognitive impairment (MCI) was more common in those women with sleep apnea syndrome at the time of PSG study than those without (44.8% vs. 31.1%) (Yaffe et al, 2011). Another cross-sectional analysis of a large population also reported an association of sleep apnea with worse neurocognitive function (Ramos et al, 2015). A recent analysis of a large number of participants from the Alzheimer's Disease Neuroimaging Initiative (ADNI) showed that the presence of sleep-disordered breathing was associated with an earlier age at cognitive decline and the use of continuous positive airway pressure (CPAP) was associated with delayed onset of cognitive decline (Osorio et al, 2015). In these kinds of studies, it is expected to be difficult to match various other factors including the past medical history and the environmental factors between the two groups, and further studies might be warranted to answer this important question.

et al, 2008a; Hu et al, 2015). In a report from Germany, 46% of 467 patients with Parkinson disease complaining of sleep disturbance had RBD (Sixel-Doring et al, 2011). In relation to this, it is known that, in Parkinson disease, the Lewy bodies appear also in the locus coeruleus and hypothalamus, which are important for REM sleep (Braak & Del Tredici, 2008, for review) (see Box 26).

Since patients with Parkinson disease having RBD commonly develop cognitive impairment and hallucination, there has been some controversy as to whether or not those patients might have dementia with Lewy bodies (DLB) (see Chapter 22-2A). A prospective study of 234 cases of dementia in the United States, who were followed up and whose diagnosis was pathologically confirmed, revealed that 76% of DLB cases had RBD versus only 4% of other cases (Ferman et al, 2011). Postuma et al. (2009) followed up a number of cases with idiopathic RBD and reported that, after 12 years, about a half of those cases developed neurodegenerative diseases such as Parkinson disease and DLB.

D. NARCOLEPSY AND RELATED DISORDERS

Narcolepsy is characterized by four cardinal symptoms: irresistible desire to sleep during the day, hypnagogic hallucination, sleep paralysis, and cataplexy. The symptoms usually start to occur in puberty, and the disease is strongly associated with the major histocompatibility complex HLA-DR2 and HLA-DQB1*0602. The patient with narcolepsy becomes excessively sleepy during the day (**irresistible desire to sleep during the day**). In contrast with normal sleep, which starts from the light non-REM sleep progressing to deep non-REM sleep and then to REM sleep, the sleep of narcoleptic patients begins with REM sleep. Therefore, the patient dreams from the transition to sleep, which corresponds to the **hypnagogic hallucination**. Furthermore, the patient becomes unable to move, as if being firmly bound during the transmission between wakefulness and sleep (**sleep paralysis**). **Cataplexy** manifests itself as sudden falling as soon as the patient starts laughing, which is believed to be due to generalized reflex atonia. In this type of cataplexy, **hypocretin (orexin),** which is produced in the hypothalamus, is decreased in the cerebrospinal fluid. For the pathogenesis of this condition, autoimmune damage of hypocretin-producing cells in the hypothalamus has drawn special attention (Fontana et al, 2010).

It should be kept in mind that daytime sleepiness can occur as a side effect of drugs. For example, patients with Parkinson disease who are taking dopamine agonists may suddenly become sleepy. However, these patients may also have excessive daytime sleepiness as a part of their disorder (see Chapter 16-2B).

E. PERIODIC LIMB MOVEMENT IN SLEEP

Periodic limb movement in sleep (PLMS) is a series of periodic movements of unilateral or bilateral lower limbs during sleep at a regular interval; usually once in about 20 seconds. It has drawn special attention because many cases of PLMS also suffer from **restless legs syndrome** (see Chapter 18-10). Patients with restless legs syndrome have unpleasant sensation in legs while resting at night and develop a strong urge to move the legs. Once they move the legs, the symptom is temporarily released. As dopamine agonists were found to be effective for this condition, its relationship with Parkinson disease has drawn particular attention. However, there is no pathological evidence suggestive of Parkinson disease in the autopsied cases of restless legs syndrome, and there are no data suggesting progression of this condition to Parkinson disease, although the co-occurrence is greater than chance. The prevalence of PLMS is not precisely known because its diagnosis requires study with PSG, but it is believed to be high in the elderly population (Natarajan, 2010, for review). These conditions are mostly sporadic, but there are some familial cases, and the genetic studies of these two phenomena are under way (Stefansson et al, 2007).

F. KLEINE-LEVIN SYNDROME

This unique syndrome is characterized by repetitive episodes of severe hypersomnia, cognitive impairment, apathy, derealization, and behavioral disturbances such as hyperphagia and hypersexuality in male teens (Kas et al, 2014). Even during the intervals, the patients tend to be easily tired, need naps, fall asleep rapidly, and have high anxiety/depression scores (Lavault et al, 2015). As there are occasional familial cases and as it is common among Jews, some genetic factors are postulated, but it has not been clarified (Arnulf et al, 2008b).

G. FATAL FAMILIAL INSOMNIA

This disease was first reported by Lugaresi in 1986, and mutation of the prion protein gene was found later (see Box 62). It occurs in adults, and equally affects men and women, but the age of onset varies widely. Clinically it is characterized by intractable insomnia and progressive cognitive decline, but it lacks other symptoms seen in typical Creutzfeldt-Jakob disease, and its clinical course may be relatively long (Krasnianski et al, 2008).

BIBLIOGRAPHY

American Clinical Neurophysiology Society. Guidelines for long-term monitoring for epilepsy. J Clin Neurophysiol 25:170–180, 2008.

Arnulf I, Leu S, Oudiette D. Abnormal sleep and sleepiness in Parkinson's disease. Curr Opin Neurol 21:472–477, 2008a.

Arnulf I, Lin L, Gadoth N, File J, Lecendreux M, Franco P, et al. Kleine-Levin syndrome: a systematic study of 108 patients. Ann Neurol 63:482–493, 2008b.

Beghi E, D'Alessandro R, Beretta S, Consoli D, Crespi V, Delaj L, et al. Incidence and predictors of acute symptomatic seizures after stroke. Neurology 77:1785–1793, 2011.

Berg AT, Berkovic SF, Brodie MJ, Buchhalter J, Cross JH, van Emde Boas W, et al. Revised terminology and concepts for organization of seizures and epilepsies: report of the ILAE Commission on Classification and Terminology, 2005–2009. Epilepsia 51:676–685, 2010.

Bermeo-Ovalle AC, Kennedy JD, Schuele SU. Cardiac and autonomic mechanisms contributing to SUDEP. J Clin Neurophysiol 32:21–29, 2015. (review)

Bezov D, Ashina S, Lipton RB. Post-dural puncture headache: Part II—Prevention, management, and prognosis. Headache 50:1482–1498, 2010.

Braak H, Del Tredici K. Invited article: nervous system pathology in sporadic Parkinson disease. Neurology 70:1916–1925, 2008. (review)

Chen S-P, Fuh J-L, Lirng J-F, Wang Y-F, Wang Sh-J. Recurrence of reversible cerebral vasoconstriction syndrome: a long-term follow-up study. Neurology 84:1552–1558, 2015.

Cho JR, Koo DL, Joo EY, Seo DW, Hong SC, Jiruska P, et al. Resection of individually identified high-rate high-frequency oscillations region is associated with favorable outcome in neocortical epilepsy. Epilepsia 55:1872–1883, 2014.

Commission on Classification and Terminology of the International League Against Epilepsy. Proposal for revised clinical and electrographic classification of epileptic seizures. Epilepsia 22:489–501, 1981.

Ducros A, Boukobza M, Porcher R, Sarov M, Valade D, Bousser MG. The clinical and radiological spectrum of reversible cerebral vasoconstriction syndrome: a prospective series of 67 patients. Brain 130:3091–3101, 2007.

Engel JJr, Wiebe S, French J, Sperling M, Williamson P, Spencer D, et al. Practice parameter: temporal lobe and localized neocortical resections for epilepsy. Report of the Quality Standards Subcommittee of the American Academy of Neurology, in association with the American Epilepsy Society and the American Association of Neurological Surgeons. Neurology 60:538–547, 2003.

Ferman TJ, Boeve BF, Smith GE, Lin SC, Silber MH, Pedraza O, et al. Inclusion of RBD improves the diagnostic classification of dementia with Lewy bodies. Neurology 77:875–882, 2011.

Ferrari MD, Klever RR, Terwindt GM, Ayata C, van den Maagdenberg AM. Migraine pathophysiology: lessons from mouse models and human genetics. Lancet Neurol 14:65–80, 2015. (review)

Fontana A, Gast H, Reith W, Recher M, Birchler T, Bassetti CL. Narcolepsy: autoimmunity, effector T cell activation due to infection, or T cell independent, major histocompatibility complex class II induced neuronal loss? Brain 133:1300–1311, 2010.

Headache Classification Committee of the International Headache Society (IHS). The International Classification of Headache Disorders: 3rd edition (beta version). Cephalalgia 33:629–808, 2013.

Hu YH, Yu S-Y, Zuo L-J, Cao C-J, Wang F, Chen Z-J. et al. Parkinson disease with REM sleep behavior disorder: featured, α-synuclein, and inflammation. Neurology 84:888–894, 2015.

Huttunen J, Kurki MI, von und zu Fraunberg M, Koivisto, T, Ronka-inen A, Rinne J, et al. Epilepsy after aneurysmal subarachnoid hemorrhage: a population-based, long-term follow-up study. Neurology 84:2229–2237, 2015.

Jeha LE, Najm I, Bingaman W, Dinner D, Widdess-Walsh P, Lüders H. Surgical outcome and prognostic factor of frontal lobe epilepsy surgery. Brain 130:574–584, 2007.

Kanazawa K, Matsumoto R, Imamura H, Matsuhashi M, Kikuchi T, Kunieda T, et al. Intracranially recorded ictal direct current shifts may precede high frequency oscillations in human epilepsy. Clin Neurophysiol 126:47–59, 2015.

Kas A, Lavault S, Habert M-O, Arnulf I. Feeling unreal: a functional imaging study in patients with Kleine-Levin syndrome. Brain 137:2077–2087, 2014.

Kawamata J, Ikeda A, Fujita Y, Usui K, Shimohama S, Takahashi R. Mutations in LGI1 gene in Japanese families with autosomal dominant lateral temporal lobe epilepsy: the first report from Asian families. Epilepsia 51:690–693, 2010.

Kim DW, Lee SK, Chu K, Park KI, Lee CH, Chung CK, et al. Predictors of surgical outcome and pathologic considerations in focal cortical dysplasia. Neurology 72:211–216, 2009.

Krasnianski A, Bartl M, Sanchez Juan PJ, Heinemann U, Meissner B, Varges D, et al. Fatal familial insomnia: clinical features and early identification. Ann Neurol 63:658–661, 2008.

Lavault S, Golmard J-L, Groos E, Brion A, Dauvilliers Y, Lecendreux M, et al. Kleine-Levin syndrome in 120 patients: differential diagnosis and long episodes. Ann Neurol 77:529–540, 2015.

Montavont A, Mauguière F, Mazzola L, Garcia-Larrea L, Catenoix H, Ryvlin P, et al. On the origin of painful somatosensory seizures. Neurology 84: 594–601, 2015.

Natarajan R. Review of periodic limb movement and resltess leg syndrome. J Postgrad Med 56:157–162, 2010. (review)

Nishizawa M, Shimohata T. Clinical features of multiple system atrophy. Clin Neurol 49:249–253, 2009. (Review with abstract in English)

Myint PK, Staufenberg EFA, Sabanathan K. Post-stroke seizure and post-stroke epilepsy. Postgrad Med J 82:568–572, 2006.

Natarajan R. Review of periodic limb movement and restless leg syndrome. J Postgrad Med 56:157–162, 2010. (review)

Osorio RS, Gumb T, Pirraglia E, Varga AW, Lu S, Lim J, et al. Sleep-disordered breathing advances cognitive decline in the elderly. Neurology 84:1964–1971, 2015.

Parvizi J, Le S, Foster BL, Bourgeois B, Rriviello JJ, Prenger E, et al. Gelastic epilepsy and hypothalamic hamartomas: neuroanatomical analysis of brain lesions in 100 patients. Brain 134:2960–2968, 2011.

Postuma RB, Gagnon JF, Vendette M, Fantini ML, Massicotte-Marquez J, Montplaisir J. Quantifying the risk of neurodegenerative disease in idiopathic REM sleep behavior disorder. Neurology 72:1296–1300, 2009.

Postuma RB, Iranzo A, Hogl B, Arnulf I, Ferini-Strambi L, Manni R, et al. Risk factors for neurodegeneration in idiopathic rapid eye movement sleep behavior disorder: a multicenter study. Ann Neurol 77:830–839, 2015.

Ramos AR, Tarraf W, Rundek T, Redline S, Wohlgemuth WK, Loredo JS, et al. Obstructive sleep apnea and neurocognitive function in a Hispanic/Latino population. Neurology 84:391–398, 2015.

Schievink WI, Maya MM, Chu RM, Moser FG. False localizing sign of cervico-thoracic CSF leak in spontaneous intracranial hypotension. Neurology 84:2445–2448, 2015.

Seneviratne U, Woo JJ, Boston RC, Cook M, D'Souza W. Focal seizure symptoms in idiopathic generalized epilepsies. Neurology 85:589–595, 2015.

Shibasaki H, Ikeda A, Nagamine T. Use of magnetoencephalography in the presurgical evaluation of epilepsy patients. Clin Neurophysiol 118:1438–1448, 2007. (review)

Silber MH, Ancoli-Israel S, Bonnet MH, Chokroverty S, Grigg-Damberger MM, Hirshkowitz M, et al. The visual scoring of sleep in adults. J Clin Sleep Med 3:121–131, 2007.

Sixel-Döring F, Trautmann E, Mollenhauer B, Trenkwalder C. Associated factors for REM sleep behavior disorder in Parkinson disease. Neurology 77:1048–1054, 2011.

Stefansson H, Rye DB, Hicks A, Petursson H, Ingason A, Thorgeirsson TE, et al. A genetic risk factor for periodic limb movements in sleep. N Engl J Med 357:639–647, 2007.

Takahashi T. EEG Atlas of Photosensitive Epilepsy Studied Using Low-Luminance Visual Stimulation. Tohoku University Press, Sendai, 2008.

Tarnutzer AA, Lee S-H, Robinson KA, Kaplan PW, Newman-Toker DE. Clinical and electrographic findings in epileptic vertigo and dizziness: a systematic review. Neurology 84:1595–1604, 2015. (review)

Tezer FI, Remi J, Noachtar S. Ictal apnea of epileptic origin. Neurology 72:855–857, 2009.

Usui N, Terada K, Baba K, Matsuda K, Usui K, Tottori T, et al. Significance of very-high-frequency oscillations (over 1,000Hz) in epilepsy. Ann Neurol 78:295–302, 2015.

Wolf ME, Szabo K, Griebe M, Förster A, Gass A, Hennerici MG, et al. Clinical and MRI characteristics of acute migrainous infarction. Neurology 76:1911–1917, 2011.

Wolking S, Becker F, Bast T, Wiemer-Kruel A, Mayer T, Lerche H, et al. Focal epilepsy in glucose transporter type 1 (Glut1) defects: case reports and a review of literature. J Neurol 261:1881–1886, 2014.

Yaffe K, Laffan AM, Harrison SL, Redline S, Spira AP, Ensrud KE, et al. Sleep-disordered breathing, hypoxia, and risk of mild cognitive impairment and dementia in older women. JAMA 306:613–619, 2011.

25.

ION CHANNEL DISORDERS

Ion channels are transmembrane glycoprotein pores of the membrane of nerve fibers and muscles and are important for controlling the membrane permeability of ions. There are two kinds of ion channels: the **transmitter-gated (ligand-gated) ion channels**, which are controlled by neurotransmitters, and the **voltage-gated ion channels**, which are controlled depending on the amplitude of membrane potentials. Recently many diseases have been categorized into the ion channel disorders. Ion channel disorders (**channelopathies**) are either hereditary or autoimmune. Phenotypes of hereditary channelopathies are usually paroxysmal or episodic disorders such as hereditary epilepsies, familial hemiplegic migraine (see Chapter 24-2B), startle disease (see Chapter 18-8B), episodic ataxia, and periodic paralysis.

Hereditary channelopathies are characterized by **phenotypic heterogeneity**. Namely, mutation of a single gene may manifest different clinical phenomena (**phenotypic overlap**). For example, patients with spinocerebellar ataxia type 6 (SCA6) may also show episodic ataxia or familial hemiplegic migraine or both. In contrast, mutation of different genes may show a similar clinical phenomenon (**genetic heterogeneity**) (Bernard & Shevell, 2008, for review). Representative forms of hereditary ion channel disorders and autoimmune ion channel disorders of the central nervous system are shown in Table 25-1 and Table 25-2, respectively.

1. HEREDITARY CHANNELOPATHIES

Hereditary ion channel disorders may involve the central nervous system, the peripheral nervous system, or muscles, as follows.

A. HEREDITARY CHANNELOPATHIES OF THE CENTRAL NERVOUS SYSTEM

Representative forms of hereditary ion channel disorders of the central nervous system are shown in Table 25-1.

Familial Hemiplegic Migraine

In this form of migraine, hemiplegia or other motor paralysis appears as an aura or during the headache attack. It is usually transmitted with autosomal dominant inheritance, and three forms are known (Table 25-1). Of these forms, type I is due to mutation of a voltage-gated calcium channel gene (*CACNA1*), and is often overlapped with SCA6 and episodic ataxia type II (see Chapter 24-2B). For treatment, a carbonic anhydrase inhibitor, acetazolamide, is known to be effective.

Episodic Ataxia

This autosomal dominant hereditary disease is characterized by paroxysmal episodes of ataxia and dysarthria, and six forms are known. In an episode of type I, ataxia and dysarthria last several minutes and myokymia might be seen during the intervals. The episode occurs spontaneously, but it may be provoked by startle, emotional change, fatigue, illness, or motor action. It is due to mutation of a voltage-gated potassium channel gene (*KCNA1*). Type II occurs in children or young adults with episodes of ataxia and dysarthria lasting several hours to several days, and there might be interictal nystagmus. It is also provoked by stress, motor action, caffeine, alcohol, intake of carbohydrate-rich food, or fever. It is due to mutation of a voltage-gated calcium channel gene (*CACNA1*), and as described above, it may overlap with familial hemiplegic migraine type I and SCA6. Thus, SCA6 is a unique neurodegenerative disease associated with calcium channelopathy. These two types of episodic ataxia may be treated with anticonvulsants such as phenytoin, carbamazepine and sodium valproate, and acetazolamide and a potassium channel blocker, 4-aminopyridine. It is also prevented by avoiding the above provoking factors.

Hereditary Startle Disease, Hyperekplexia

As described in the section on myoclonus of brainstem origin (see Chapter 18-8B), this is an excessive startle reaction

Diseases	Inheritance	Ion channel	Chromosome	Gene mutation
Familial hemiplegic migraine	AD			
I		Cav 2.1α1	19p13	*CACNA1*
II		Na, K-ATPaseα2	1q23	*ATP1A2*
III		Nav 1.1	2q24	*SCN1A*
Episodic ataxia*1	AD			
I		Kv 1.1	12p13	*KCNA1*
II		Cav 2.1α1	19p13	*CACNA1*
Hereditary startle disease*2	AD, AR			
I		GlyR α1	5q33.1	*GLRA1*
II		GlyR β	4q32.1	*GLRB*
ADNFLE*3	AD			
I		AchR α4	20q13.2-13.3	*CHRNA4*
III		AchR β2	1q21.3	*CHRNB2*
IV		AchR α2	8p21	*CHRNA2*
Juvenile myoclonic epilepsy	Variable	GABAR, Ca, Cl		Multiple
BAFME	AD			
I			8q23.3-q24.11	
II			2p11.1-q12.2	
III			5p15.31-p15.1	
IV			3q26.32-q28	
Childhood absence seizure	Variable	GABAR, Cl, Ca		Multiple
Ring chromosome 20	Mostly sporadic		20	Unknown

AD: autosomal dominant, AR: autosomal recessive, R: receptor, v for ion channel: voltage-gated, Gly: glycine, Ach: acetylcholine, GABA: gamma-amino butyric acid, ADNFLE: autosomal dominant nocturnal frontal lobe epilepsy,

*1: only representative types are shown, *2: two other types are not shown, *3: type II is not shown.

SOURCE: Modified from Bernard & Shevell, 2008.

provoked by unexpected sudden stimulus, and is transmitted in either autosomal dominant or recessive inheritance. Patients with this disorder are noted to be excessively hypertonic in the newborn period. Four types are known, and all types are due to mutation of genes related to the receptor of an inhibitory transmitter, glycine. Mutation of the glycine receptor α1 subunit gene (*GLRAI*) is known for type I, and that of the glycine receptor β subunit gene (*GLRB*) is known for type II (Bode & Lynch, 2014, for review). Clonazepam is effective in most cases.

Epilepsies

Most cases of idiopathic epilepsy due to mutation of a single gene are related to a channel gene of a nicotinic acetylcholine receptor or GABA-A receptor, or a gene mutation

TABLE 25-2 HEREDITARY ION CHANNEL DISORDERS OF MUSCLES

Diseases	Inheritance	Ion channel	Chromosome	Gene mutation
Hypokalemic periodic paralysis	AD			
I		Cav α1	1q31–q32	CACNA1S*2
II		Nav α	17q23–q25	SCN4A*2
Hyperkalemic periodic paralysis	AD	Nav α	17q23-q25	SCN4A
Myotonia congenita		ClvC 1	7q35	CLCN1
Thomsen	AD			
Becker	AR			
Paramyotonia congenita	AD	Nav α	17q23–q25	SCN4A
Andersen-Tawil syndrome	AD	Kir2.1	17q23	KCNJ2
Malignant hyperthermia susceptibility*1	AD	Ryanodine receptor 1	19q13.1	RYR1
Central core disease	AD or AR	Ryanodine receptor 1		Multiple
Congenital myasthenic syndrome	AR	Ach receptors (multiple)		Multiple

ir: inward rectifier, otherwise the same designation as in Table 25-1.

*1: Only the representative type is shown, *2: Typical types are shown.

SOURCE: Modified from Lehmann-Horn & Jurkat-Rott, 2007. and Bernard & Shevell, 2008.

of the sodium, chloride, calcium, or potassium channel (Heron et al, 2007, for review).

Autosomal dominant nocturnal frontal lobe epilepsy (ADNFLE) is a unique seizure occurring in childhood at night (see Chapter 24-1A). The attack begins with groaning or vocalization, and shows abnormal movements such as vigorous or thrusting movements of legs and waist. It is rare to progress to generalized convulsion, but the attacks may occur several times per night. The interictal EEG is often normal, and the ictal EEG may show paroxysmal abnormalities at the midline frontal region, suggesting its origin in the supplementary motor area. Clinically, it is often difficult to distinguish from pseudoseizures (see Chapter 24-1B). Mutation of the gene related to the nicotinic acetylcholine receptor α4 subunit (*CHRNA4*) is known for type I, and likewise β2 subunit (*CHRNB2*) for type III, and α2 subunit (*CHRNA2*) for type IV. Carbamazepine is effective for these seizures.

Juvenile myoclonic epilepsy is a form of myoclonus epilepsy affecting persons of puberty, predominantly female, and it may be complicated by generalized tonic-clonic seizures and absence seizures in some cases. It is especially characterized by worsening upon awakening in the morning. Mutation of multiple genes related to the GABA receptor, calcium channel and chloride channel are known in this disorder.

Benign adult familial myoclonus epilepsy (BAFME) is a unique form of autosomal dominant hereditary myoclonus epilepsy reported from Japan and some European countries (see Box 56). Myoclonus of cortical origin begins in adults and its progression to generalized convulsion is rather rare. The mutation has been localized on chromosome 8q for type I, 2p for type II, 5p for type III, and 3q for type IV, but genes have not been discovered yet. This condition may also be a hereditary ion channel disorder.

Childhood absence seizure is characterized by frequent attacks of absence, each lasting several seconds affecting infants and children, and it is commonly called **petit mal** (see Chapter 24-1A). The EEG typically shows a burst of bilaterally synchronous high amplitude 3 Hz rhythmic spike-and-wave discharges (see Figure 24-1). Mutations of multiple genes related to the GABA receptor, chloride channel and calcium channel have been reported.

Patients with **ring chromosome 20** show mental retardation, behavioral abnormalities, and epileptic seizures. Seizures of various forms including nocturnal frontal lobe epilepsy, nonconvulsive status epilepticus, and prolonged confusion start at around 5 years of age, and tend to resist antiepileptic medication. This condition is also believed to be an ion channel disorder.

Type II of **congenital long QT syndrome** is due to mutation of the cardiac potassium channel gene, and is often complicated by epileptic seizures. The seizure in this condition is considered to be a primary ion channel disorder of the brain rather than seizure secondary to ventricular arrhythmia (Johnson et al, 2009).

B. HEREDITARY CHANNELOPATHIES OF THE PERIPHERAL NERVOUS SYSTEM

Mutations of the genes related to the voltage-gated sodium channel (*SCN9A*) in the dorsal root ganglion and in the sympathetic ganglion are known to cause several kinds of pain disorders. Among those disorders, **erythermalgia** (called **erythromelalgia** in acquired cases) and paroxysmal extreme pain disorder are known to be caused by gain of the channel function, and **congenital insensitivity to pain** is known as an example of loss of channel function (Drenth & Waxman, 2007, for review). Congenital insensitivity to pain is a rare condition transmitted in autosomal recessive inheritance. Patients with this disorder do not feel pain at all since birth, and they easily suffer from trauma and burn. Other somatosensory functions are normal, but autonomic disturbances such as anhidrosis are present in many cases (Norcliffe-Kaufmann et al, 2015).

C. HEREDITARY CHANNELOPATHIES OF MUSCLES

Periodic paralysis, a variety of nondystrophic myotonia, malignant hyperthermia, central core disease, and congenital myasthenic syndrome are known to belong to this category (Table 25-2).

Hypokalemic Periodic Paralysis

This is an autosomal dominant hereditary disease, starting in young age, affecting predominantly males. Generalized weakness usually occurs upon awakening in the morning and lasts for several hours. Any factor lowering the blood potassium level can provoke this episode, including excessive intake of carbohydrate-rich food or salt, stress, drugs, and heavy physical exercise on the preceding day. Mutations of multiple genes related to the voltage-gated calcium channel α1 subunit in the muscle are known for type I, and mutations of multiple genes related to the voltage-gated sodium channel α subunit are known for type II. Avoiding the above precipitating factors is important for preventing the attacks, but correction of serum potassium level and chronic administration of acetazolamide are effective for treatment. It is believed that acetazolamide causes metabolic acidosis, which helps move potassium into the muscle fibers. There is no symptom during the intervals. In Asian male patients, this condition is often accompanied by hyperthyroidism (Vijayakumar et al, 2014, for review).

Hyperkalemic Periodic Paralysis

This is an autosomal dominant hereditary disease that affects children before puberty with frequent episodes of generalized weakness, each attack lasting less than an hour. During the attack, the serum potassium level is either elevated or normal. During the intervals, myotonia is seen in the face, tongue, and hands and myopathy might develop in many cases. Mutation of the voltage-gated sodium channel gene on the chromosome 17q (*SCN4A*) is known in most cases. In some cases, physical exercise and sugar intake might ameliorate the attacks.

Myotonia Congenita

In this disease, stiffness due to disturbance of muscle relaxation (myotonia) (see Chapter 16-3F) occurs in childhood. Just as in the case of myotonic dystrophy, myotonia will improve by repeating contraction of the involved muscles (warm-up phenomenon). There are two types of this disorder: **Thomsen type**, which is transmitted in an autosomal dominant inheritance and is relatively mild, and **Becker type**, which is transmitted in an autosomal recessive inheritance and is severe. The first case was reported by Thomsen in 1876, and it is known that Thomsen himself suffered from this disease. For both types, mutations of multiple genes related to the voltage-gated chloride channel (*CLCN1*) in the skeletal muscles are known. It is believed that this gene abnormality impairs the chloride channel gating, which causes decreased chloride conductance and electrical instability of the sarcolemma, resulting in the repetitive continuous electrical discharges. Various drugs including mexiletine, quinine, lithium carbonate, procainamide, carbamazepine, phenytoin and acetazolamide have been found effective for this condition.

Paramyotonia Congenita

This autosomal dominant hereditary disease was first described by von Eulenburg in 1886. In this condition, in contrast with ordinary myotonia, in which muscle relaxation is most difficult after its first contraction and becomes easier with the increasing number of repetition (warm-up phenomenon), relaxation becomes increasingly difficult

26.

PSYCHOGENIC NEUROLOGIC DISEASES

Many neurologic symptoms may appear without organic lesions of the nervous system. Based on the underlying mechanisms, **psychogenic neurologic diseases** are classified into three categories: **conversion disorders**, **factitious disease**, and **malingering** (Hallett et al, 2012, for review). The term "functional" is beginning to replace "psychogenic" in many circumstances. Patients with conversion disorders are not aware of the psychogenic origin of their illnesses, whereas patients with the other two conditions are aware of the psychogenic origin at least to a certain extent. Malingering, in particular, might be purposeful for personal benefits such as financial reasons and escape from jail. In fact, these three conditions may not always be distinguishable from each other, and many cases of psychogenic neurologic diseases might have an overlap of these three components, and may be situated on a spectrum ranging from the completely unintended state, like conversion disorders, to the completely intended state, like malingering.

Negative neurologic symptoms like loss of consciousness, blindness, constriction of the visual field, motor paralysis, and loss of pain sense are commonly seen in psychogenic diseases, but positive symptoms like convulsion and involuntary movements are not uncommon. Among others, psychogenic movement disorders are not infrequent, and have drawn particular attention in the recent years (Fahn, 2007, Lang & Voon, 2011, and Czarnecki & Hallett, 2012, for review) (see Chapter 18-10).

1. PSYCHOGENIC MOTOR PARALYSIS

Motor paralysis due to conversion disorders is not infrequently encountered. It is characterized by being incongruous with ordinary paralysis, inconsistency in time, tendency to give-way during manual muscle testing (**give-way weakness**), and the presence of psychogenic factors in the background. Furthermore, muscle tone and tendon reflexes are usually normal in psychogenic paralysis.

In cases of asymmetric motor paralysis, it is possible to test how much the patient is cooperating with the muscle testing by taking advantage of the intact or less affected side. For example, in case of unilateral paralysis of the biceps brachii muscle, if the patient is cooperating with flexion of the paralyzed forearm, the contralateral triceps brachii muscle is expected to contract, thus extending the contralateral forearm. Likewise, in unilateral paralysis of the triceps brachii muscle, the patient's attempt to extend the paralyzed forearm is expected to flex the contralateral forearm. If there is no movement of the contralateral (intact) extremity, it might suggest poor cooperation of the patient. A similar principle can be applied to the psychogenic paralysis of lower extremities as far as it is asymmetric (**Hoover sign**) (Box 96).

Conversion disorders may present with complete paraplegia. In this case, muscle tone and tendon reflexes are expected to be entirely normal, and there are no pathological reflexes. Psychogenic inability to stand up and walk may be called **astasia-abasia**.

Electrophysiologically, the muscle potentials evoked by transcranial magnetic stimulation of the primary motor cortex (motor evoked potentials, MEP) are expected to be absent in the lower extremities if complete paraplegia is due to an organic lesion. Thus, normal MEP in patients with complete paraplegia might suggest psychogenic origin, but it should be kept in mind that, in mild paraplegia due to mild lesion of the corticospinal tract, MEP could be normal. In contrast, unilateral absence of MEP or delayed conduction of the corticospinal tract in patients with hemiplegia suggests that the hemiplegia is due to an organic lesion.

2. PSYCHOGENIC SENSORY LOSS

The most common sensory symptom in the psychogenic neurologic diseases is complete loss of nociceptive sensation on either half of the body (hemianalgesia). In this case, the nociceptive loss is seen on the whole hemibody from the top of the head to the toes, and there is no reaction to pain or back-off movement away from the nociceptive stimulus. In the thoracic and lumbar segments, the somatosensory innervation crosses the midline and overlaps between the two sides for 1.0 ~ 1.5 cm from the midline. Therefore, the borderline of the hemianesthesia due to an organic lesion is shifted toward the anesthetic side by 1.0 ~ 1.5 cm. Therefore, if the borderline of the intact and affected sides is found exactly on the midline of the chest or abdomen, it suggests a possibility of psychogenic origin, although the final judgment should not be based on this finding alone.

Furthermore, as the frontal skull bone and the sternum are formed each of a single bone, a vibratory stimulus is expected to be felt bilaterally. Therefore, if the vibration sense is unilaterally lost over those bones, it might serve as a clue to the diagnosis of psychogenic disorders.

Electrophysiologically, the somatosensory evoked potentials (SEP) are useful in some cases of psychogenic sensory loss. However, it should be kept in mind that electrical stimulation of the peripheral nerve activates only large fibers and it does not reflect the nociceptive conduction. For unilateral or asymmetric loss of nociceptive senses, SEP following laser stimulation is useful. If laser-evoked potential is normally recorded in patients with complete loss of pain sense, it might suggest its psychogenic origin. In order to avoid misinterpretation of the SEP results due to a technical failure, comparison of two sides is always important.

3. PSYCHOGENIC CONSTRICTION OF VISUAL FIELD

Constriction of the visual field due to conversion disorders is characterized by the fact that the visible angle does not change depending on the distance from the target (**tunnel vision, tubular vision**) (see Chapter 7-2B). In healthy subjects, the visible angle is expected to become larger as they move away from the target.

4. COMMON FEATURES OF PSYCHOGENIC NEUROLOGIC DISEASES

Clinical features common to all kinds of psychogenic neurologic disorders include **incongruity** with ordinary neurologic symptoms, **inconsistency** (variability) of nature, degree and distribution in time, and change due to **distraction** to other stimuli or other matters, and the presence of **psychogenic factors** in the social or family background. In case of rhythmic or periodic abnormal movements of a part of the body, if the patient is requested to repeat rhythmic or periodic movements of other parts of the body at a certain rate, the rate of abnormal movements might be entrained into that of the assigned movements (**entrainment**). Regarding the psychogenic positive neurologic symptoms, convulsion is described in Chapter 24-1B, and involuntary movements are explained in Chapter 18-10. Electrophysiological techniques are often useful for supplementing the clinical impression of psychogenic disorders.

BIBLIOGRAPHY

Czarnecki K, Hallett M. Functional (psychogenic) movement disorders. Curr Opin Neurol 25:507–512, 2012. (review)

Fahn S. Psychogenic movement disorders. In Jankovic J, Tolosa E. (eds). Parkinson's Disease & Movement Disorders. 5th ed. Lippincott Williams & Wilkins, Philadelphia, 2007, pp. 562–566. (review)

Hallett M, Weiner WJ, Kompoliti K. Psychogenic movement disorders. Parkinsonism Relat Disord 18S1:S155–S157, 2012. (review)

Lang AE, Voon V. Psychogenic movement disorders: past developments, current status, and future directions. Mov Disord 26:1175–1182, 2011. (review)

27.

THALAMUS

Although this book is organized according to the functional anatomy of the nervous system, this chapter is arranged with respect to the anatomy because the thalamus is the relay center for all kinds of ascending pathways to the cerebral cortex, and also because it is commonly involved by the cerebrovascular diseases.

1. GENERAL STRUCTURE OF THE THALAMUS

The thalamus is a relatively large, egg-shaped structure situated deep in each cerebral hemisphere. It borders medially on the third ventricle, laterally on the internal capsule, and inferiorly on the hypothalamus and midbrain. Each thalamus is divided by the Y-shaped internal medullary lamina into four divisions: the lateral, medial, and anterior nuclear groups and the posterior nucleus (pulvinar) (Figure 27-1). The left and right thalami are connected by transverse fibers (**massa intermedia**). Furthermore, lateral to the pulvinar, there are the lateral geniculate body and the medical geniculate body, which are the relay nuclei for the visual and auditory pathways, respectively (see Chapter 7 and Chapter 12, respectively).

In the **lateral nuclear group** are the relay nuclei important for sensory functions and motor control. The relay nuclei for the somatosensory, vestibular, and taste senses are situated in the ventral posterior nuclei, and the motor-related relay nuclei from the basal ganglia and cerebellum are in the lateral nucleus. The main nucleus of the **medial nuclear group** is the medial dorsal nucleus, which is involved in the higher mental functions by projecting to the prefrontal cortex and cingulate gyrus. The **anterior thalamic nucleus** is a relay nucleus of the Papez circuit (see Chapter 22-1B and Figure 22-3), and it is involved in memory function. The **internal medullary lamina** is primarily formed of white matter, but it contains a number of neuronal groups that receive input from the brainstem reticular formation and activate the cerebral cortex via the ascending reticular activating system (see Figure 4-1). The

posterior nucleus called the **pulvinar** is closely connected with the parietal cortex and is primarily engaged in the visual cognitive functions.

In addition to the above-described roles as the relay center of the ascending projection to the cerebral cortex, the thalamus also receives strong input from the cerebral cortex. It is noteworthy that there are bidirectional fiber connections between each area of the thalamus and the corresponding area of the cerebral cortex. The thalamus is also believed to be involved in cognitive and language functions. Aphasia has been reported in patients with a lesion of the left thalamus (de Witte et al, 2011, for review).

The most common cause of thalamic lesion is infarction or hemorrhage. Clinical symptoms caused by a **thalamic infarction** are quite variable, because there is great interindividual variability in the arterial supply of thalamic nuclei, a single artery supplies multiple thalamic nuclei, and an ischemic lesion might occur in the territory of multiple arteries (Schmahmann, 2003, for review). In a **thalamic hemorrhage**, although clinical symptoms vary depending on the size of the hemorrhage, motor paralysis and sensory loss develop in the contralateral extremities in the acute stage, and soon thereafter it is accompanied by consciousness disturbance of various degrees. If the lesion extends to affect the hypothalamus and midbrain, pupillary abnormalities and downward medial deviation of the eyes are also seen. If the hemorrhage ruptures into the third ventricle, the patient may fall into coma.

2. VENTRAL POSTERIOR NUCLEUS AS THE SENSORY RELAY CENTER

The tertiary neurons of the somatosensory pathway are located in the ventral posterior nucleus of thalamus and receive afferent projection from the secondary neurons for both nociceptive and proprioceptive senscs. Inputs from the spinal nerve territories are received in the **ventral**

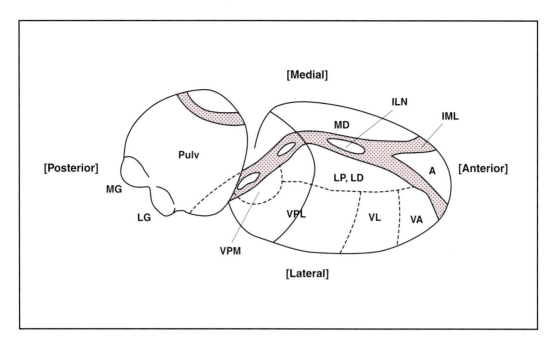

Figure 27-1 Schematic diagram of the thalamus, showing its main nuclei. Lateral upper view of the right thalamus. A: anterior nucleus, ILN: intralaminar nucleus, IML: internal medullary lamina, LD: lateral dorsal nucleus, LG: lateral geniculate body, LP: lateral posterior nucleus, MD: medial dorsal nucleus, MG: medial geniculate body, Pulv: pulvinar, VA: ventral anterior nucleus, VL: ventral lateral (ventrolateral) nucleus, VPL: ventral posterolateral nucleus, VPM: ventral posteromedial nucleus. A complex of VA and VL is also named Voa, Vop, and Vim from anterior to posterior. (Modified from Brodal, 2004, with permission)

posterolateral nucleus (VPL), and those from the trigeminal nerve territory reach the ventral posteromedial nucleus (VPM) (Figure 27-1). Thus, the lateral spinothalamic tract and the medial lemniscus project to the VPL (see Figure 19-2), and the trigeminothalamic tract and the fibers from the main sensory nucleus of trigeminus project to the VPM (see Figure 10-1). There is somatotopic organization in the VPL. Afferents arising from the caudal part of the body project to the lateral part of the VPL, while those from the rostral part of the body project to the medial part of the VPL, so that its most medial part borders on the VPM. Therefore, as for the somatosensory system, there is somatotopy in all the related nuclei from the spinal cord to the primary sensory cortex.

While the tactile and deep/proprioceptive afferents project solely to the VPL and VPM, the nociceptive afferents project to wider areas of the thalamus. Namely, in addition to VPL and VPM, the medial ventral nucleus, the intralaminar nucleus and the medial dorsal nucleus also receive the nociceptive input.

The tertiary neurons from VPL and VPM project to each corresponding area of the primary somatosensory cortex (SI) in the postcentral gyrus and partially to the second somatosensory cortex (SII) in the upper bank of the sylvian fissure. Nociceptive inputs from multiple thalamic nuclei (see above) project not only to the SI and SII but also to the amygdala, insula, and cingulate gyrus, which are related to the emotional aspect of nociception (see Figure 19-4).

It is known that the ventral posterior nucleus also receives afferents of sense of equilibrium and taste sense. The vestibular afferents originating from the vestibular nuclei reach the VPL, and the tertiary neurons project to the area just posterior to the S1 face area in the postcentral gyrus and the parietal insular vestibular cortex located at the parieto-insular junction (see Chapter 13-1). The gustatory afferents originating from the solitary nucleus project to the VPM, and the tertiary neurons project to the SI tongue area and anterior insula like the olfactory sense (see Chapter 11-1C).

There is considerable interindividual variability in the arterial perfusion of the thalamus. The VPL and VPM receive perfusion from the thalamogeniculate artery, which is a branch of the posterior cerebral artery (see Figure 9-3). Therefore, if this artery is occluded by infarction, the somatosensory symptoms predominate. In this case, all the somesthetic modalities are lost or impaired on the contralateral side, but especially the deep/proprioception and stereognosis (ability to recognize the shape of an object by touching) are completely lost. In contrast, the superficial modalities often become hypersensitive with unpleasant sensation induced by pin prick, which is felt over a wider area of the skin and lasts longer than expected.

It is also characterized by intolerable pain that might occur spontaneously or is induced by stimuli. Spontaneous pain is often associated with unpleasant dysesthesia and hyperalgesia to stimulus, and this condition is called **central pain**. In this case, even a soft breeze presented to the skin might cause unpleasant pain (**hyperpathia**) (see Chapter 19-2B and Box 65).

The central pain following a stroke (**central post-stroke pain**) is commonly seen in an infarction involving the posterior lateral thalamus, but it also occurs in brainstem infarction involving the spinothalamic tract. The central post-stroke pain usually involves the whole aspect of the contralateral body, but it may be especially severe on the face and the upper limb. In most cases, the pain starts sometime after the stroke, ranging from two weeks to even a few years after the stroke. This kind of pain is usually intractable to medical treatment, but some benefit of electrical stimulation of the motor cortex by subdurally placed electrodes was reported (Hosomi et al, 2015, for review; Sokal et al, 2015).

In infarction of the posterior cerebral artery territory involving the posterior lateral thalamus, ataxia and involuntary movements might be seen in addition to the above sensory symptoms. This condition is called **thalamic syndrome** or **Dejerine-Roussy syndrome** (see Box 65). In this case, ataxia is considered to be primarily caused by a partial lesion of the cerebellar relay center (see Section 3 of this chapter), but it may also be explained as sensory ataxia due to interruption of the proprioceptive input to the VPL. Any kind of involuntary movements may appear in the thalamic lesion, but chorea, dystonia, and slow rhythmic movements (myorhythmia) are especially common in the infarction of the posterior lateral thalamus (Lera et al, 2000).

3. VENTRAL ANTERIOR NUCLEUS AND VENTROLATERAL NUCLEUS AS THE MOTOR THALAMUS

The thalamic nuclei related to motor control (motor thalamus) are located in the ventral anterior part of the lateral nuclear group (Figure 27-1). There is some confusion about the terminology of these motor nuclei. The terms VA and VL are used in the Jones classification, while the Hassler classification (Voa, Vop, and Vim) is used for deep brain stimulation, though there is no precise correlation between these two classifications (Krack et al, 2002, for review; Molnar et al, 2005).

GABAergic fibers originating from the internal segment of the globus pallidus project to the ventral anterior nucleus (VA) and a part of the ventrolateral nucleus (VL) of the ipsilateral thalamus, which correspond to the anterior oral ventral nucleus (Voa) and the posterior oral ventral nucleus (Vop) in the Hassler classification (see Chapter 16-2B).

Glutamatergic fibers originating from the cerebellar dentate nucleus project through the superior cerebellar peduncle mainly to the VL or the **ventral intermediate nucleus (Vim)** of the contralateral thalamus (Krack et al, 2002, for review; Molnar et al, 2005) (see Chapter 16-2C). However, as a result of recording from the thalamic nuclei during the treatment of tremor with deep brain stimulation, the local field potentials recorded from both Vop and Vim show correlation with the tremor of the contralateral hand at the tremor frequency (Marsden et al, 2000; Katayama et al, 2005; Kane et al, 2009).

The motor thalamus receives its blood supply from the **tuberothalamic artery**, which bifurcates from the posterior communicating artery (see Figure 9-3). If the projection fibers from the basal ganglia to the motor thalamus are affected by infarction, a variety of symptoms such as hypokinesia, thalamic hand, dystonic posture, chorea and athetosis might appear in the contralateral upper extremity. In contrast, with a lesion of the cerebellar projection to the motor thalamus, the contralateral hand shows ataxia, which may be combined with action tremor and myoclonus. Negative motor symptoms like ataxia appear from the time of stroke, but involuntary movements commonly develop sometime after the stroke (Lera et al, 2000; Lehericy et al, 2001).

Abnormal posture of the hand consisting of flexion of the metacarpophalangeal joints and extension of the interphalangeal joints may appear in a vascular lesion of the thalamus (**thalamic hand**). However, as it is often associated with somatosensory abnormalities, dystonic posture, and other involuntary movements (see above), the thalamic hand may be modified in various ways.

4. MEDIAL DORSAL NUCLEUS AS A RELAY CENTER TO THE PREFRONTAL CORTEX

The medial dorsal (mediodorsal) nucleus (MD) is situated at the most medial part of thalamus. It receives input from the hypothalamus, amygdala, ventral pallidum, and nucleus accumbens, and sends projections to the prefrontal cortex. It is believed that there is some functional localization in the MD and its projection to the prefrontal cortex is relatively localized. The prefrontal cortex receives inputs of all sensory modalities, and under the influence of will and emotion, it plays an important role in higher brain functions such as attention, selection of behavior and its planning, execution and inhibition, learning, working memory, and long-term memory. Among others, the MD and the mammillothalamic tract compose an important memory circuit (see Chapter 22-1B). As the MD is closely connected to the hypothalamus, its lesion may cause sleep disturbance, autonomic dysfunction, and endocrine abnormalities (see Chapter 28).

The MD receives its blood supply from the **paramedian thalamic artery**, which bifurcates from the proximal part of the posterior cerebral artery. As ischemia in the territory of that artery tends to affect the MD bilaterally, consciousness is impaired in the acute stage, and loss of initiative and emotional reaction and marked memory disturbance remain in the chronic stage (see Chapter 22-1B and Figure 22-4). Furthermore, it often involves the rostral midbrain and causes extraocular muscle paralysis and abnormalities of ocular movements.

5. ANTERIOR NUCLEUS AND MEMORY

The anterior thalamic nucleus forms the Papez circuit as its important constituent and is related to memory (see Chapter 22-1B). The information arising from the hippocampus is transmitted through the fornix to the mammillary body, and then through the mammillothalamic tract to the cingulate gyrus. As for the blood supply, the mammillothalamic tract is supplied by either the tuberothalamic artery or the paramedian thalamic artery, and the anterior thalamic nucleus is mainly supplied by the paramedian thalamic artery. Thus, as the anterior nucleus and MD receive the blood supply from the same artery, infarction of that artery affects both structures and causes consciousness disturbance in the acute stage and marked memory disturbance in the recovery phase.

6. PULVINAR AS A RELAY CENTER TO THE PARIETAL LOBE

The pulvinar is a relatively large structure situated in the posterior thalamus, and is connected to the parietal and temporal lobes. In monkey, the inferior part of the pulvinar receives input from the superior colliculus and projects to the MT area (see Chapter 7-1F). As a result of functional MRI studies in human, it is believed that the pulvinar is involved in visual attention, ocular movement, recognition of facial expression, and language (Benarroch, 2015, for

review). The pulvinar receives its blood supply from the posterior choroidal artery, thalamogeniculate artery, and paramedian thalamic artery. The pulvinar is known to be affected especially in **variant Creutzfeldt-Jakob disease** (mad cow disease), which is revealed as an abnormal signal on MRI (see Box 62) (Shinde et al, 2009).

Aphasia is known to occur in a lesion of the left thalamus, most likely by affecting the functional connection between the pulvinar and the cortex. Among others, naming, writing, and comprehension of spoken language are impaired in a left thalamic lesion (de Witte et al, 2011, for review).

7. INTRALAMINAR NUCLEUS AS A RELAY CENTER OF THE ASCENDING RETICULAR ACTIVATING SYSTEM

The intralaminar nucleus (ILN) is formed of scattered neuronal groups in the internal medullary lamina. It receives input from the brainstem reticular formation and sends projections to the cerebral cortex. There is some somatotopic organization in the ILN, but each subgroup projects to a wider area of the cortex than the specific sensory relay nucleus. For example, the centrolateral nucleus of the ILN is known to project to the parietal cortex. The main function of the ILN is considered to increase the excitability of the sensory cortex and to facilitate the cortical reception at each specific receptive area. Electrical stimulation of the ILN is known to produce an arousal pattern on EEG. Multiple neurotransmitters are involved in the reticular activating system (see Chapter 4-1).

The ILN also sends a powerful projection to the striatum. Among others the **centromedian parafascicular nucleus complex (CM-Pf complex)** projects to the putamen and caudate nucleus. It is postulated that the CM-Pf complex is related to pain information processing and motor control, although its functions have not been clarified in detail (Benabid, 2009, for review).

As the ILN is distributed widely in the thalamus, it receives blood supply from multiple arteries including the posterior choroidal artery, thalamogeniculate artery, and paramedian thalamic artery.

8. RELAY NUCLEUS FOR THE VISUAL AND AUDITORY SYSTEM

The lateral geniculate body (LGB) and the medial geniculate body (MGB) are situated in the posterior lateral part of the thalamus, partially surrounded by the pulvinar. The LGB and MGB are important relay centers for the visual and auditory system, respectively. The LGB projects to the primary visual cortex in the calcarine fissure by maintaining the retinotopic organization (Chapter 7-1C). The MGB projects to the auditory cortex in the Heschl gyrus by maintaining the tonotopic organization (Chapter 12-1). These two nuclei receive blood supply from the posterior choroidal artery, but the LGB is also supplied by the anterior choroidal artery (see Figure 7-4).

As all visual inputs from a hemifield cross at the optic chiasm and reach the contralateral LGB, its lesion causes the contralateral hemianopsia (see Figure 7-5). In contrast, as the MGB receives inputs from both ears, its unilateral lesion cannot be detected by an ordinary hearing test (see Figure 12-2). However, as the proportion of crossed fibers is known to be larger than that of uncrossed fibers, auditory abnormality due to the MGB lesion might be detected by testing the auditory spatial recognition or by recording the auditory evoked response with magnetoencephalogram (MEG).

BIBLIOGRAPHY

Benabid AL. Targeting the caudal intralaminar nuclei for functional neurosurgery of movement disorders. Brain Res Bull 78:109–112, 2009. (review)

Benarroch EE. Pulvinar. Associative role in cortical function and clinical correlations. Neurology 84:738–747, 2015. (review)

Brodal P. The Central Nervous System: Structure and Function. 3rd ed. Oxford University Press, New York, 2004.

de Witte L, Brouns R, Kavadias D, Engelborghs S, De Deyn PP, Marien P. Cognitive, affective and behavioral disturbances following vascular thalamic lesions: a review. Cortex 47:273–319, 2011. (review)

Hosomi K, Seymour B, Saitoh Y. Modulating the pain network—neurostimulation for central poststroke pain. Nat Rev Neurol 11:290–299, 2015. (review)

Kane A, Hutchison WD, Hodaie M, Lozano AM, Dostrovsky JO. Enhanced synchronization of thalamic theta band local field potentials in patients with essential tremor. Exp Neurol 217:171–176, 2009.

Katayama Y, Kano T, Kobayashi K, Oshima H, Fukaya C, Yamamoto T. Difference in surgical strategies between thalamotomy and thalamic deep brain stimulation for tremor control. J Neurol 252 (Suppl 4):IV17–IV22, 2005.

Krack P, Dostrovsky J, Ilinsky I, Kultas-Ilinsky K, Lenz F, Lozano A, et al. Surgery of the motor thalamus: problems with the present nomenclatures. Mov Disord 17 (Suppl 3): S2–S8, 2002. (review)

Lehéricy S, Grand S, Pollak P, Poupon F, Le Bas JF, Limousin P, et al. Clinical characteristics and topography of lesions in movement disorders due to thalamic lesions. Neurology 57:1055–1066, 2001.

Lera G, Scipioni O, Garcia S, Cammarota A, Fischbein G, Gershanik O. A combined pattern of movement disorders resulting from posterolateral thalamic lesions of a vascular nature: a syndrome with clinico-radiologic correlation. Mov Disord 15:120–126, 2000.

Marsden JF, Ashby P, Limousin-Dowsey P, Rothwell JC, Brown P. Coherence between cerebellar thalamus, cortex and muscle in man: cerebellar thalamus interactions. Brain 123:1459–1470, 2000.

Molnar GF, Pilliar A, Lozano AM, Dostrovsky JO. Differences in neuronal firing rates in pallidal and cerebellar receiving areas of thalamus in patients with Parkinson's disease, essential tremor, and pain. J Neurophysiol 93:3094–3101, 2005.

Schmahmann JD. Vascular syndromes of the thalamus. Stroke 34:2264–2278, 2003. (review)

Shinde A, Kunieda T, Kinoshita Y, Wate R, Nakano S, Ito H, et al. The first Japanese patient with variant Creutzfeldt-Jakob disease (vCJD). Neuropathology 29:713–719, 2009.

Sokal P, Harat M, Zieliński P, Furtak J, Paczkowski D, Rusinek M. Motor cortex stimulation in patients with chronic central pain. Adv Clin Exp Med 24:289–296, 2015.

HYPOTHALAMUS AND NEUROENDOCRINOLOGY

The hypothalamus is a center for controlling important functions necessary for living, in close relation to the autonomic nervous system, endocrine system, sleep and circadian rhythm, emotion and its related behavior, control of internal milieu necessary for adjusting to the external environment, and above all, integration of all those functions.

1. STRUCTURE AND FUNCTION OF THE HYPOTHALAMUS

The hypothalamus is largely divided into the medial part and the lateral part. In the **medial part**, there are the paraventricular nucleus, supraoptic nucleus, and suprachiasmatic nucleus anteriorly, the dorsomedial nucleus, ventromedial nucleus and infundibular nucleus in the middle, and the posterior nucleus posteriorly (Figure 28-1). Furthermore, the mammillary nucleus is in the mammillary body, which is located at the base of the third ventricle.

In the **lateral part**, there are no distinct nuclear divisions, and it is called **lateral hypothalamic area** en bloc. The lateral hypothalamic area is penetrated by poorly demarcated fiber tracts called the **medial forebrain bundle**, which projects to the frontal lobe and amygdala.

The paraventicular nucleus, suprachiasmatic nucleus, and mammillary body are clearly distinguishable, but other nuclei are not clearly demarcated, and many of those nuclei are connected to each other. The hypothalamus as a whole receives inputs from many brain areas and sends projections to many areas. In addition to multiple neurotransmitters including acetylcholine, norepinephrine, dopamine, serotonin, histamine, and neuropeptides, the hypothalamus is characterized by the fact that multiple hormones participate in information transmission.

As for the autonomic functions, the sympathetic nervous system and the parasympathetic nervous system are clearly distinguishable in the brainstem and spinal cord, but the distinction between the two systems is not clear in the hypothalamus (see Chapter 20-1). The autonomic system in the hypothalamus is rather arranged in terms of specific functions.

2. NEUROENDOCRINOLOGY

The hypothalamus is the highest center for controlling the endocrine system. Information from the hypothalamus is transmitted to each endocrine organ via the **pituitary gland (hypophysis)**. The pituitary gland is divided into the anterior lobe and posterior lobe.

A. ANTERIOR LOBE OF THE PITUITARY GLAND (ADENOHYPOPHYSIS)

The anterior lobe of the pituitary gland, also called the adenohypophysis, receives releasing hormones from the hypothalamus via the **hypophysial portal vascular system**, and the pituitary epithelial cells secrete growth hormone, thyroid stimulation hormone (TSH), adrenocorticotropic hormone (ACTH), gonadotropic hormone, and prolactin. These hormones stimulate the respective target organs to produce hormones. There are two kinds of gonadotropic hormone: follicle-stimulating hormone and luteinizing hormone.

There are three kinds of epithelial cells in the anterior lobe of hypothalamus: eosinophilic, basophilic, and chromophobe cells. It is known that the eosinophilic cells produce growth hormone and prolactin, but other hormones are postulated to be produced by basophilic cells. **Eosinophilic pituitary adenoma** causes **gigantism** in children and **acromegaly** in adults as a result of excessive production of growth hormone. Furthermore, excessive production of prolactin may cause **galactorrhea** or **galactorrhea-amenorrhea syndrome** in women.

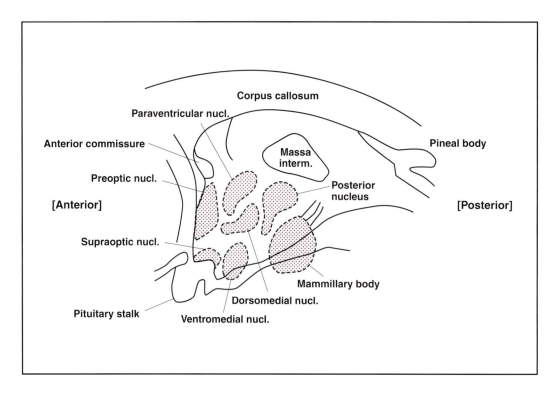

Figure 28-1 Schematic diagram showing main nuclei of the hypothalamus. Sagittal view. nucl.: nucleus, interm.: intermedia. (Modified from Brodal, 2004, with permission)

ACTH-producing pituitary adenoma, as a result of excessive production of glucocorticoid, causes central obesity, moon face, buffalo hump, striae and plethora of the skin, hypertension, proximal muscle weakness, and hypokalemia. This condition, called **Cushing disease**, is more common in women than in men. A similar clinical picture may be seen in patients who are receiving corticosteroid treatment, or in association with adrenal tumor and aberrant ACTH-producing tumor. This condition is called **Cushing syndrome**.

The releasing hormones produced in the hypothalamus are also known to be transmitted to brain regions other than the pituitary gland through the nerve fiber connection. Those examples are thyrotropin-releasing hormone (TRH), corticotropin-releasing hormone (CRH), and somatostatin.

B. POSTERIOR LOBE OF THE PITUITARY GLAND (NEUROHYPOPHYSIS)

The posterior lobe of pituitary gland, also called the neurohypophysis, is directly innervated by the hypothalamus via the **hypothalamohypophysial tract**. The related hormones are **antidiuretic hormone (ADH)**, also called **vasopression**, and **oxytocin**. These two hormones are produced in the paraventricular nucleus and the supraoptic nucleus, and they are examples of quite unique hormones that are transmitted to the posterior lobe via the axonal flow of the tract. Thus, cells of these two nuclei are called **neurosecretory cells**. Among these nuclei, ADH is primarily produced in the supraoptic nucleus, and oxytocin is mainly produced in the paraventricular nucleus. ADH acts on the water channel, aquaporin in the kidney, and promotes reabsorption of water, so that it suppresses urinary excretion. Cells of the supraoptic nucleus and other hypothalamic areas are considered to be equipped with receptors sensitive to the osmotic pressure of blood, thus controlling the water content. Furthermore, ADH is known to act on the blood vessels to contract their smooth muscles. That is why it is also called vasopressin.

If ADH secretion is impaired due to a hypothalamic lesion, its antidiuretic action is lost, causing **diabetes insipidus**. In contrast, if ADH is excessively produced by various etiologies, the osmotic pressure and sodium level of blood are decreased because urinary excretion is decreased, and the osmotic pressure of urine is increased. This condition is called **syndrome of inappropriate secretion of ADH**

(**SIADH**), and should be kept in mind when dealing with hyponatremia of unknown etiology. The SIADH is not infrequently seen in patients with neuromyelitis optica who have positive antibody against aquaporin-4 (see Box 35), and it may even appear as the initial symptom of neuromyelitis optica (Iorio et al, 2011).

Wolfram syndrome is characterized by familial occurrence of diabetes insipidus. This disease is transmitted in autosomal recessive inheritance and affects young people with diabetes insipidus, diabetes mellitus, optic atrophy, and deafness (DIDMOAD). Multiple mutations of *WFS1* gene are known, and some cases might also show cognitive disturbance and epileptic seizures (Chaussenot et al, 2011).

Oxytocin is produced mainly in the paraventricular nucleus. As it provokes contraction of the uterine smooth muscles, it plays an important role in obstetric deliveries. Furthermore, oxytocin promotes milk secretion by increasing contraction of the mammary smooth muscles. It is considered that sucking of mammary papilla by the newborn sends somatosensory input to the paraventricular nucleus, which activates the secretory cells to promote oxytocin and increases milk secretion.

The pituitary gland may be affected by congenital tumors, especially **craniopharyngioma**, which is more common in children and may present with various endocrine disorders such as small stature, hypothyroidism and diabetes insipidus, and visual disturbance associated with signs of increased intracranial pressure.

3. ADJUSTMENT TO THE EXTERNAL ENVIRONMENT AND CONTROL OF THE INTERNAL MILIEU

The hypothalamus is important for the control of body temperature, feeding and nutrition, circadian rhythm, and sexual functions. Functional localization within the hypothalamus is not clearly known, but it is often named by attaching "center" to each function.

A. CONTROL OF CIRCADIAN RHYTHM

For this function, the **suprachiasmatic nucleus**, located just above the optic chiasm, receives impulses generated by light through a branch of the optic tract (see Chapter 7-1B) and activates the pineal gland to promote secretion of melatonin, which is important for controlling the circadian rhythm.

B. CONTROL OF FEEDING

Based on experimental stimulation of hypothalamus in animals, it is postulated that the lateral part of hypothalamus promotes feeding (**feeding center**) and the medial part, especially the ventromedial nucleus, suppresses feeding (**satiety center**). Lesion of the satiety center causes **hyperphagia**. Episodes of abnormal behavior characterized by hyperphagia and hypersomnia is known as **Kleine-Levin syndrome** (see Chapter 24-3F). This syndrome is considered to be caused by disturbed control mechanism of both circadian rhythm and feeding.

C. CONTROL OF BODY TEMPERATURE

As a result of experimental studies in animals, the anterior part of the hypothalamus is activated when the core temperature is excessively elevated, and it lowers the temperature by dilating the subcutaneous blood vessels and by increasing sweating. In contrast, the posterior part becomes active when the core temperature is excessively low, and it elevates the temperature by promoting shivering and voluntary muscle contraction. Thus, these parts of the hypothalamus are considered to serve as a thermostat. As the hypothalamus is commonly affected by a necrotic lesion associated with small hemorrhages in **Wernicke encephalopathy**, the control mechanism of body temperature is severely impaired, resulting in marked fluctuation of the body temperature (**poikilothermia**) (see Box 74).

As the **mammillary nucleus** is an important component of memory circuits, its lesion causes marked memory loss and confabulation (**Korsakoff syndrome**) (see Chapter 22-1B). Furthermore, although the functional localization is not clear, the hypothalamus is known to control sexual behavior via the gonadotropic hormones and the autonomic nervous system.

D. HOMEOSTASIS

As described above, the hypothalamus plays an important role in integrating the control mechanisms of the autonomic nervous system, endocrine system and behaviors, and it is the control center indispensable for the maintenance and control of living. The hypothalamus is also considered to be involved in the control of the immunological system. Control of the interaction between psychological function and the somatic activities is another important function of hypothalamus. Thus, a lesion of the hypothalamus causes psychosomatic diseases, and that is why the hypothalamus is a target organ for the research of psychosomatic medicine.

BIBLIOGRAPHY

Brodal P. The Central Nervous System: Structure and Function. 3rd ed. Oxford University Press, New York, 2004.

Chaussenot A, Bannwarth S, Rouzier C, Vialettes B, Mkadem SA, Chabrol B, et al. Neurologic features and genotype-phenotype correlation in Wolfram syndrome. Ann Neurol 69:501–508, 2011.

Iorio R, Lucchinetti CF, Lennon VA, Costanzi C, Hinson S, Weinshenker BG, et al. Syndrome of inappropriate antidiuresis may herald or accompany neuromyelitis optica. Neurology 77:1644–1646, 2011.

29.

NEUROLOGIC EMERGENCY

A neurologic emergency is defined as a condition that is life-threatening or in which the patient is faced with poor functional recovery unless treated promptly. Among others, respiratory paralysis and disturbance of consciousness are life-threatening (Table 29-1). Regarding disturbance of consciousness, diagnosis and treatment of coma are described in Section 5 of this chapter.

1. DISORDERS WITH RESPIRATORY PARALYSIS

When faced with patients who cannot breathe, it is important to exclude mechanical suffocation such as aspiration before considering paralysis of respiratory muscles due to neurologic disorders. Among neurologic disorders, myasthenia gravis, Guillain-Barré syndrome, acute anterior poliomyelitis, brainstem encephalitis, and acute intoxication with puffer poison (tetrodotoxin) and botulinum toxin are important causes of respiratory paralysis (Box 97). It is noteworthy that motor neuron diseases, although they are chronic progressive conditions, may cause respiratory paralysis rather acutely.

A. CRISIS OF MYASTHENIA GRAVIS

Symptoms of myasthenia gravis may become suddenly worse (crisis). There are two kinds of crisis: myasthenic crisis and cholinergic crisis. In **myasthenic crisis**, nicotinic acetylcholine is insufficient at the neuromuscular junction due to worsening of myasthenia in association with upper respiratory infection, insufficient dose of cholinesterase inhibitors, or reduced effectiveness of drugs. Clinically, excretion of airway discharge becomes difficult because of weakness of respiratory as well as bulbar muscles. **Cholinergic crisis** is caused by excessive doses

of cholinesterase inhibitors. Clinically, airway secretion is increased due to increased muscarinic transmission, which worsens respiration. For either type of crisis, the first procedure to be taken is to aspirate the airway, and if necessary, the airway should be managed by intubation. Differentiation between the two types of crisis can be estimated from the history and physical examination, but it should be confirmed by the tensilon test.

Edrophonium (Tension) Test

This test is done by intravenous injection of a cholinesterase inhibitor to confirm the diagnosis of myasthenia gravis and to distinguish between myasthenic crisis and cholinergic crisis. As the edrophonium increases airway discharge due to increased muscarinic transmission of acetylcholine, it may make the interpretation of the test difficult in some cases. In that case, it is useful to inject 0.5 mg of atropine sulfate subcutaneously or intramuscularly before the test to prevent excessive airway discharge. As atropine inhibits only muscarinic transmission and not nicotinic transmission, it does not affect neuromuscular transmission (see Chapter 20-1).

To perform the **Tensilon test**, 10 mg of edrophonium is injected intravenously, but it is effective to inject 2 mg over a period of the first 30 seconds, and if the myasthenic symptoms either improve or worsen, the test can be stopped, and it is not necessary to complete the test. If no change occurs with 2 mg, then the remaining 8 mg may be injected over a period of another 30 seconds. If muscle weakness improves by this test, it suggests myasthenic crisis, and if it worsens, it suggests cholinergic crisis.

For the immunotherapy of crisis, plasmapheresis used to be considered superior, but Mandawat et al. (2010) reported that intravenous immunoglobulin (IVIg) was equally effective with less complications and expense compared with plasmapheresis.

BOX 97 ACUTE POISONING CAUSING RESPIRATORY PARALYSIS

As intoxication may occur unexpectedly, it is always important to prepare for the emergency. Among others, intoxications with puffer toxin and botulinum toxin are notorious for causing acute respiratory paralysis. As a result of oral intake of the **puffer toxin (tetrodotoxin)**, which is contained in the liver and testis of the puffer fish, the voltage-gated sodium channel is blocked. Clinically, perioral numbness begins several minutes after intake of the toxin, which spreads to the whole body, and flaccid paralysis rapidly develops causing breathlessness. It can only be treated by artificial support of respiration. Botulism is caused by oral intake of the **botulinum toxin**, which is produced by *Clostridium botulinum*. A typical source of intoxication is a homemade canned food at high altitude where water boils at a lower temperature. Botulinum toxin severs a protein in the presynaptic nerve terminal that is important for the release of neurotransmitters, and thus inhibits acetylcholine release at the neuromuscular junction. Clinically, first the abducens muscle is paralyzed several hours after intake of the toxin, followed by paralysis of other extraocular muscles and bulbar muscles, and finally respiratory paralysis. For treatment, respiration should be supported first, and then gastric lavage and administration of antitoxin are necessary. It is noteworthy that local injection of this toxin is nowadays used for treatment of various movement disorders, pain, and disorders of the autonomic nervous system as well as wrinkles.

In intoxication with insecticides containing **organophosphate**, cholinesterase is inhibited so that the nicotinic as well as muscarinic cholinergic transmission becomes hyperactive, causing respiratory paralysis and increased airway secretion. For treatment of the acute phase, in addition to the support of respiration, atropine sulfate and pralidoxime (PAM) may be administered.

B. GUILLAIN-BARRÉ SYNDROME

In many cases of Guillain-Barré syndrome, muscle weakness begins in the lower extremities and ascends up to the thoracic level, and may cause dyspnea. In some cases, however, dyspnea might predominate from the early clinical stage. Cranial muscles might also be involved. Guillain-Barré syndrome is typically associated with reduction in tendon reflexes. Treatment primarily consists of immunosuppressive therapy, but airway management with a respirator may be needed in severe cases. Intravenous immunoglobulin and plasma exchange have been proven effective (van den Berg et al, 2014 for review). A study of a large number of cases from the United States showed that, even in the acute stage, the use of plasmapheresis is decreasing while IVIg is increasingly used (Alshekhlee et al, 2008).

C. ACUTE ANTERIOR POLIOMYELITIS

In the past, acute anterior poliomyelitis (polio) due to polio virus infection was the most common cause of acute infectious diseases causing motor paralysis. Clinically it is characterized by weakness of either of four extremities (monoplegia), but other extremities may also be involved to a certain extent, and tendon reflexes are diffusely lost. Sensory symptoms may be also seen, although this is rare. Polio has nearly disappeared in most advanced countries as a result of wide use of vaccination, but it may still be encountered in developing regions (see Chapter 16-3C).

D. ACUTE BRAINSTEM LESION

As there is a respiratory center in the brainstem, acute respiratory paralysis may be seen in inflammatory or vascular lesions of the brainstem. A representative form of brainstem encephalitis is **Bickerstaff brainstem encephalitis**. Infarction or hemorrhage of the brainstem might cause sudden dyspnea. Mechanisms of respiratory abnormalities due to brainstem lesions are described in Section 5-C of this chapter.

E. AMYOTROPHIC LATERAL SCLEROSIS

As amyotrophic lateral sclerosis is a slowly progressive disease, possible occurrence of dyspnea can be predicted in most cases. In some cases, however, it might show rapid progression at some point during the clinical course, resulting in acute respiratory paralysis. Although it depends on the patient's circumstance, it is advisable to explain the situation to the patient and his family beforehand and to discuss what to do when respiration becomes very weak.

2. DISORDERS WITH DISTURBANCE OF CONSCIOUSNESS

As discussed in Chapter 4-2, when faced with patients with disturbance of consciousness, it is important to judge whether it is due to a decrease or loss of neuronal excitability of the consciousness center (nonepileptic disorders) or due to its excessive excitation (epileptic disorders). In case of disturbance of consciousness associated with convulsive seizures, the patient should be placed in a safe environment with clothes loosened and the tongue guarded from injury. For adult patients, 10 mg of diazepam can be intravenously injected while watching the respiration. If the seizures still occur repeatedly, more intensive treatment for status epilepticus is warranted.

Nonepileptic Disorders with Disturbance of Consciousness

Patients with nonepileptic disorders presenting with disturbance of consciousness may be examined systematically as shown in Figure 29-1 for an example. First, **vital signs** should be checked, and if necessary, airway support and

TABLE 29-1 CAUSES OF NEUROLOGIC EMERGENCIES

1. Respiratory paralysis
a. Crisis of myasthenia gravis
b. Guillain-Barré syndrome
c. Motor neuron diseases
d. Acute anterior poliomyelitis
e. Brainstem encephalitis
f. Brainstem vascular lesion
g. Acute intoxication: puffer (tetrodotoxin), botulinum, organophosphate, etc.
2. Disturbance of consciousness
a. Status epilepticus
b. Nonepileptic disorders
Metabolic and toxic encephalopathies
Anoxic encephalopathy
Meningoencephalitis
Intracranial hemorrhage
Cerebral herniation
3. Continuous spasm other than epilepsy
a. Tetanus
4. Conditions in which functional recovery is poor unless treated promptly
a. Acute compression of spinal cord
b. Progressive ischemic cerebrovascular diseases
c. Acute meningoencephalitis

other primary care should be provided. At the same time, level of consciousness disturbance (**coma scale**) can be evaluated. Then, the eyes, face, and extremities should be observed, looking for any **asymmetry** between the two sides, including conjugate deviation of eyes, asymmetry of nasolabial lines, and asymmetry of posture, muscle tone, strength, tendon reflexes, and plantar reflex of extremities. If any of the above items is found asymmetric, it highly suggests the presence of a focal organic lesion in the brain parenchyma, and a neuroimaging study with CT or MRI is indicated. In cerebral infarction, the conventional CT or MRI may not show any abnormality within 24 hours after the onset of clinical symptoms. However, special imaging techniques such as diffusion MRI may detect a very early ischemic lesion. If the neuroimaging study does not reveal any abnormality in spite of clinical evidence of asymmetry, blood and cerebrospinal fluid should be examined for possible inflammatory diseases.

In cases where there is no asymmetry in the eyes, face, or extremities, signs suggestive of **meningeal irritation** should be checked, including nuchal stiffness and the Kernig sign (see Chapter 15-1). If nuchal stiffness or the Kernig sign is judged positive, then a neuroimaging study should be done looking for any evidence of intracranial hemorrhage. In this regard, it should be kept in mind that nuchal stiffness may not be detected until 24 hours after subarachnoid hemorrhage. If there is no evidence of hemorrhage on the neuroimaging study in patients with positive meningeal irritation, the cerebrospinal fluid should be examined for possible meningitis.

If there is no sign suggestive of meningeal irritation, the patient may have metabolic or toxic disorders, or anoxic encephalopathy. In these cases, EEG should be obtained, and blood should be tested for electrolytes, glucose level, liver functions including ammonium, renal functions, and various endocrine tests (Box 98). Furthermore, it is extremely important to save a blood sample for possible intoxication with drugs or insecticides.

If EEG shows **triphasic waves**, it most likely suggests metabolic encephalopathy. In particular, when the triphasic waves occur almost continuously, it strongly suggests hepatic encephalopathy (see Figure 22-2). In cases of severe anoxic encephalopathy, periodic synchronous discharges (PSD) as seen in Creutzfeldt-Jakob disease may appear on EEG, but PSD in anoxic encephalopathy does not continue and tends to change rapidly, whereas PSD in Creutzfeldt-Jakob disease is persistent at least for a certain period of the clinical course.

3. STATUS EPILEPTICUS

Frequent occurrence of epileptic seizures associated with continuous disturbance of consciousness even during the intervals is called **status epilepticus**. Complex partial seizure like psychomotor seizure may fall into status, but the status of generalized convulsive seizures, in particular, requires emergency treatment. New-onset status epilepticus in the adult population is often cryptogenic, but among the identified causes, autoimmune encephalitis or paraneoplastic encephalitis is most common (Gaspard et al, 2015).

Treatment of Convulsive Status Epilepticus

The patient with convulsive status epilepticus should be placed in a safe environment, and vital signs should be checked. The airway support, blood pressure maintenance, and intravenous route should be established as necessary. There are a number of pharmacological approaches to treat status epilepticus (Abend et al, 2015, and Betjemann et al, 2015, for review). The pharmacological treatment may start with intravenous injection of 10 mg of diazepam over a period of 30 ~ 60 seconds. If convulsion recurs, another dose of 10 mg diazepam may be added while paying attention to respiration. Furthermore, 15 ~ 20 mg of phenytoin per kilogram of body weight may be infused intravenously with a rate of 50 mg per minute. If convulsions still occur repeatedly, general anesthesia may be needed in an intensive care unit with respiratory support. For anesthetics, midazolam or isoflurane may be used. For laboratory tests, blood should be drawn for complete blood count and chemistry, but EEG and neuroimaging study can be done after the condition is stabilized. During the status, EEG is expected to show marked diffuse abnormality with a lot of movement artifacts, and therefore EEG can be obtained more effectively after the convulsions diminish in their degree and frequency.

Tetanus

From the viewpoint of intensive care, tetanus is clinically similar to generalized convulsive status, although they are caused by different mechanisms (Chapter 16-3E). Patients with tetanus are extremely sensitive to external stimuli, and even a small sound or touch may cause generalized muscle spasm and opisthotonus. Therefore, it is important to place the patient in a dark, quiet room with intensive care just like the case of convulsive status epilepticus. Active treatment for the causative organism, *Clostridium tetani*, should be started with chemotherapy with penicillin G and tetanobulin, which is antitoxin immunoglobulin. As an extremely large dose of tetanobulin has to be injected intramuscularly (3,000 ~ 6,000 unit), intravenous infusion of tetanobulin IH is more practical and recommended.

4. CONDITIONS EXPECTED TO HAVE POOR FUNCTIONAL RECOVERY UNLESS APPROPRIATELY TREATED AT EARLY CLINICAL STAGE

Some conditions, although there may be no respiratory paralysis, no disturbance of consciousness, or no convulsive status epilepticus, may have to be treated appropriately at early clinical stage in order to obtain as good functional recovery as possible. These are **acute compression of spinal cord**, **progressive ischemic brain lesion**, and **acute meningoencephalitis** (Box 99).

ACUTE MENINGOENCEPHALITIS

Acute infectious meningoencephalitis might leave severe neurologic residuals due to internal hydrocephalus and/or cerebral parenchymal lesions unless it is appropriately treated at early stage. In **aseptic meningitis (viral meningitis)** and **purulent meningitis** due to bacterial infection, the meninges are primarily affected rather than the brain parenchyma. In purulent meningitis, it is important to identify the causative bacteria promptly and to give appropriate antibiotics. In adults, *Streptococcus pneumoniae, Neisseria meningitidis,* and *Hemophilus influenzae* commonly cause aute meningitis. Causative viruses for aseptic meningitis include coxackie A and B, echovirus, and mumps. By contrast, subacute meningitis is often caused by tuberculosis and fungus such as Cryptococcus and *Candida albicans.*

   The most common cause of **acute encephalitis** is viral infection, followed by autoimmune encephalitis. In viral encephalitis, the common pathogens are different depending on the geographical region. The most common pathogen in the United States is herpes simplex virus, followed by varicella-zoster virus, West Nile virus, Epstein-Barr virus, and HIV (Singh et al, 2015). Japanese B virus encephalitis is also common in Japan. Advanced age, immunocompromised state, and coma portend a worse prognosis (Singh et al, 2015). It is important to administer antivirus agents from the early stage, combined with symptomatic treatment for brain edema and convulsive seizures.

A. ACUTE COMPRESSION OF SPINAL CORD

If the spinal cord is acutely compressed by a mass or trauma, surgical decompression within 6 hours of compression is considered to be necessary for functional recovery. The degree of compression can be judged clinically, but of course MRI is very useful. In order to detect abnormalities of the vertebral bone itself, plain X-ray of the spine is also useful. Causes of acute extramedullary compression include vertebral trauma, extramedullary tumor, vertebral fracture due to metastatic tumor, and extradural abscess. **Extramedullary tumors** of spinal cord are different depending on the age of patients and site of vertebra, but neurofibroma, meningioma, and metastatic tumor are common. Acute myelogenous leukemia might form a mass and compress the spinal cord (Graff-Radford et al, 2012). As a result of worldwide expansion of human immunodeficiency virus (HIV), tuberculosis is increasing. In those regions, paraplegia might be seen from compression of the spinal cord by abscess or fracture due to vertebral tuberculosis (**Pott paraplegia**).

B. PROGRESSIVE ISCHEMIC CEREBROVASCULAR DISEASES

In contrast with cerebral embolism, in which symptoms develop abruptly, symptoms in cerebral thrombosis usually take a few hours or even longer to reach their peak after the initial symptom develops. Some cases of cerebral thrombosis, however, show progressive course even several hours after the onset, in which case active **thrombolytic therapy** is necessary. In particular, progressive ischemia in the vertebrobasilar artery territory requires special attention and quick approach.

   Recently thrombolytic therapy with **tissue plasminogen activator (tPA)** is widely used for promoting functional recovery. Patients in the acute phase of cerebral infarction are candidates for this therapy, as far as there is no history of hypertension, or mild if any, and no neuroimaging evidence of intracranial hemorrhage. It is important to start this therapy as soon as possible, ideally within 3 hours but practically within 4½ hours, after the onset of the initial symptom (American Academy of Neurology Practice Advisory, 1996; Minematsu et al, 2013).

5. EXAMINATION OF COMA

All cases of coma require an emergency approach. When a patient is brought to an emergency room in comatose state, the first thing to do is to check vital signs. If the patient is not breathing or is only poorly breathing, airway support with artificial respiration should be started. After checking pulse rate and blood pressure, fluid infusion and drugs for maintaining blood pressure may be started as necessary. If no information is available, it is safe to start with intravenous infusion of 5% glucose solution. Thiamine is always given together with the glucose to prevent the precipitation of Wernicke's encephalopathy. If drug use is prevalent in the area, naloxone might be administered as well.

   After vital signs are stabilized, then etiology of coma may be evaluated (Table 29-2). Usually, at least some information is obtained from the family or the accompanying persons, but if no source of information is available, physical examination should be started immediately. Evaluation of comatose patients can be executed according to the general principle shown in Figure 29-1. Practically, it is reasonable

TABLE 29-2 CAUSES OF COMA

1. Associated with meningeal irritation
Subarachnoid hemorrhage
Ventricular rupture of intracerebral hemorrhage
Meningoencephalitis
2. Associated with focal neurologic signs
Intracerebral hemorrhage
Cerebral contusion
Cerebral embolism
Intracranial subdural hematoma
Brain tumor
Brain abscess
Brainstem hemorrhage
Brainstem infarction
3. Associated with neither meningeal irritation nor focal sign
Toxic encephalopathy (ethanol, narcotics, carbon monoxide, etc.)
Metabolic encephalopathy (diabetes mellitus, hypoglycemia, uremia, hepatic failure)
Anoxic encephalopathy
Shock (hemorrhage of organs other than brain)
Cardiac failure
Postictal state

to pursue the examination focusing on the following four points.

A. DEGREE OF COMA (COMA SCALING)

In order to judge whether a patient is in deep coma or not, it is important to apply the most effective painful stimulus. Strong pressure of the supraorbital nerve at the eyebrow by the examiner's thumb, strong pressure of the jaw with the examiner's thumbs from its two sides, or pinching the fingertip with the examiner's thumb and index finger may be adopted. For scaling the degree of coma, Coma Scales shown in Tables 4-2 and 4-3 may be used.

B. PRESENCE OR ABSENCE OF ASYMMETRY IN NEUROLOGIC SIGNS

As described in Section 2 of this chapter, asymmetry of neurologic signs, if present, provides an important clue to the etiology of coma. First, spontaneous position of the eyes should be observed as to whether there is any conjugate

deviation or not (see Chapter 9-2 for detail). Disconjugate deviation is rare, but if present, it highly suggests the presence of a brainstem lesion. The left and right nasolabial lines should be compared for any asymmetry, although this observation is often faced with difficulty because of intubation. Then extremities should be checked for any asymmetry of posture, muscle tone, muscle strength, tendon reflex, and plantar reflex between the two sides. For practical purposes, the patient's arms or legs are lifted by the examiner and then they can let them fall. The paralyzed or more flaccid side will fall earlier than the intact or less affected side. In fact, in comatose patients, motor paralysis is most often of flaccid type. If any of the above signs is found to be asymmetric, it suggests the presence of a gross organic lesion in the contralateral cerebral hemisphere causing the coma.

Conjugate Deviation of Eyes

Conjugate deviation of the eyes, if present, gives an important clue to the anatomical diagnosis. If the frontal lobe is unilaterally affected, eyes deviate to the side of the lesion, because lateral gaze to the contralateral side is paralyzed. An exception to this rule is thalamic hemorrhage, which may be associated with conjugate deviation of eyes to the side contralateral to the lesion at least in the acute phase, which is considered to be a positive neurologic symptom. In contrast, a unilateral lesion of the pontine tegmentum may cause conjugate or disconjugate deviation of the eyes to the side contralateral to the lesion (see Figure 9-5).

C. EXAMINATION OF BRAINSTEM FUNCTIONS

As the brainstem contains important centers for controlling vital signs, the center of consciousness (see Figure 4-1), and many reflex arcs that can be clinically tested in comatose patients, testing of brainstem functions plays a key role in the neurologic examination of comatose patients.

1) Observation of Respiration

The respiratory center is widely distributed in the brainstem, but the medullary respiratory center that is located in the ventral lateral part of medullary reticular formation, and the pontine respiratory center that is located in the pontine reticular formation, play main roles (see Figure 5-4). The **medullary respiratory center** is also called the ventral respiratory group, and receives information about movement of the thorax and lung, and pH and carbon dioxide content of blood, and controls rhythmicity of the motor

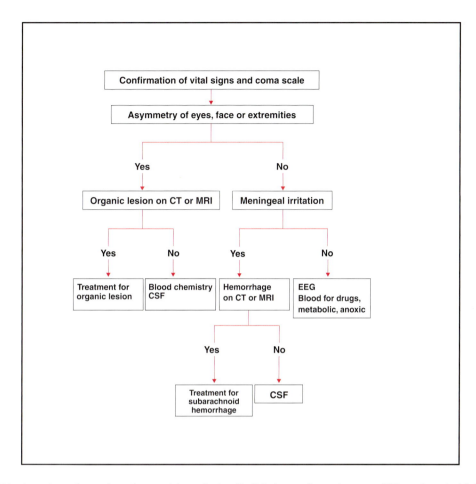

Figure 29-1 Flow chart to show steps of procedures for examining patients with disturbance of consciousness. CSF: cerebrospinal fluid.

neurons innervating the diaphragm and other respiratory muscles. The **pontine respiratory center** is believed to control spontaneous breathing, which is maintained by the medullary respiratory center.

Repetitive occurrence of phases of hyperventilation and apnea is known as **Cheyne-Stokes respiration**. In this case, breathing gradually becomes deeper, and after reaching the peak, it gradually becomes shallower, followed by short apnea, and this cycle is repeated. As a result of these repetitive cycles, it is dominated by hyperventilation and results in respiratory alkalosis. Cheyne-Stokes respiration is seen in association with transtentorial herniation due to a space-occupying hemispheric lesion, with a lesion of the rostral brainstem, or with metabolic encephalopathy.

Continuous hyperventilation, associated with a decrease in partial pressure of carbon dioxide (PCO_2) and with an increase in partial pressure of oxygen (PO_2) and pH in arterial blood, in spite of absence of drug effect or metabolic acidosis, is called **central neurogenic hyperventilation**. This state is commonly seen in association with a pontine

tumor, and is characterized by continuous hyperventilation even during sleep. It is considered to be an excitatory effect of the pontine respiratory center and chemoreceptors (Tarulli et al, 2005).

By contrast with hyperventilation, the condition in which ventilatory volume of each breath is increased (**hyperpnea**) and the respiratory rate per minute is also increased (**tachypnea**) is not necessarily associated with a decrease in PCO_2. Hyperpnea seen in metabolic acidosis is called **Kussmaul respiration**.

Arrest of respiration in the deep inspiratory phase is called **apneustic breathing**. Normally, the apneustic center in the pontine respiratory center is suppressed by the pneumotaxic center so that the inspiratory phase can shift to the expiratory phase, and impairment of this mechanism is considered to cause apneustic breathing (El-Khatib et al, 2003).

Irregular breathing in terms of depth and period is called **ataxic breathing**, and it occurs when the medullary respiratory center is impaired. If spontaneous (automatic) breathing is lost due to a medullary lesion, only voluntary breathing is left intact. In this condition, breathing might stop during sleep or decreased vigilance, the condition called the **Ondine curse**.

As the brainstem respiratory centers are easily inhibited by anesthetics, barbiturates, hunger, and metabolic alkalosis, a possibility of drug effect and of those general systemic conditions has to be taken into account when examining respiration.

2) Brainstem Reflexes

As ordinary motor and sensory functions are impossible to test in comatose patients, reflexes are the only objective signs that can be tested. It is practical to test the brainstem reflexes starting from the midbrain level through the medullary level, namely light reflex, corneal reflex, oculocephalic reflex or doll's eye sign, gag reflex, and cough reflex in this order.

Light Reflex

The neural circuit of the light reflex is composed of the optic nerve as its afferent arc and the oculomotor nerve as its efferent arc with the reflex center in the midbrain (see Figure 7-6). As comatose patients are usually placed in a well-lit room like an intensive care unit, it is better to test the light reflex after dimming the room. That is because the pupils might be already shrunk because of the room light, which might mislead judgment as to the presence or absence of the light reflex. Even in a bright room, however, it may be still possible to detect the pupillary reaction, if any, just after passively opening the eyelids, because it takes a short but recognizable time for pupils to react to light. Namely, if the pupils shrink after opening the eyelids in a bright room, it might be sufficient to confirm the presence of light reflex. At any rate, it is important to use a sufficiently bright light stimulus to test this reflex.

Corneal Reflex

The neural circuit of the corneal reflex is composed of the first branch of the trigeminal nerve (ophthalmic nerve) as its afferent arc and the facial nerve as its efferent arc with the reflex center in the pons (see Figure 10-3). As the eyelids are usually kept closed in comatose patients, the cornea can be stimulated with the tip of a twisted paper string or wisp of cotton while the eye to be tested is kept open by the examiner's hand. As nociceptive receptors are present in the cornea but not in the bulbar conjunctiva, it is important to stimulate the cornea instead of the sclera. As the stimulated eye is kept open by the examiner, the reaction can

be judged by observing contraction of the orbicularis oculi muscle of the nonstimulated side. If the reflex is sufficiently preserved, the reaction of the stimulated eyelids can be felt by the examiner's hand, but when the reaction is weak, it is more easily detected in the contralateral eye.

A similar reflex can be elicited by touching the cilia (ciliary reflex). However, as this reflex is less sensitive than the corneal reflex, the corneal reflex has to be tested even if the ciliary reflex is absent.

Doll's Eye Sign

The neural circuit of the oculocephalic reflex is composed of the vestibulocochlear nerve (receptors in the semicircular canal) and cervical nerve (receptors in the cervical muscles) as the afferent arc and the lateral as well as vertical gaze center as the efferent arc. Thus, this reflex involves a neuronal circuit extending from the cervical cord to the midbrain (see Chapter 9-5C). By holding the head with the examiner's hands from both sides in the supine position, the head is rotated laterally for testing the horizontal reflex and vertically for the vertical reflex, and the response is judged by observing the position of the eyes relative to the head. The presence of this reflex is judged as the **doll's eye sign** positive, and it suggests that this reflex circuit is intact throughout the whole length of brainstem. Doll's eye sign usually appears as a conjugate movement of the two eyes, but in case of brainstem lesions, the reflex may be complicated by extraocular muscle palsy or internuclear ophthalmoplegia. In relation to this, the presence of lateral gaze palsy may be predicted by the presence of conjugate deviation of eyes before testing the oculocephalic reflex.

Gag Reflex and Cough Reflex

Gag reflex and cough reflex have the reflex center in the medulla oblongata, and both reflexes are important for diagnosis of brain death because they represent activities of the most caudal part of brainstem (see Chapter 14-2 for the reflex circuit). However, as comatose patients are usually intubated for artificial respiration, these two reflexes are often difficult to test. In this case, it is possible to judge the presence or absence of these reflexes by observing the reflex vomiting or coughing (bucking) during aspiration of the airway.

Caloric Test

For diagnosis of brain death, the caloric test is necessary in addition to the above reflexes. For the caloric test, while the head is tilted backward by 60 degrees (downward because of supine position), 5 ~ 10 mL of cold water (0 ~ 10°C) is injected into the external auditory meatus and movement of eyes thus evoked is observed (see Chapter 13-2). The reflex circuit of the caloric response is formed of the semicircular canal and vestibular nerve as its afferent arc and the lateral gaze center of the pons as its efferent arc, thus involving the medulla oblongata and the pons. Normal caloric response consists of deviation of both eyes to the stimulated side associated with horizontal nystagmus with its quick phase directed toward the nonstimulated side. If any one of these responses is observed, it suggests that the reflex circuit is functioning. Before doing this test, it is advisable to confirm the intact tympanic membrane by an otoscope.

Ciliospinal Reflex

This is a cutaneous pupillary reflex that is elicited by nociceptive stimulus given to the neck skin, and the response is seen as dilation of the pupils. Its afferent arc is the cervical nerve, and the efferent arc is the sympathetic nervous system originating from the ciliospinal center of Budge at the intermediolateral nucleus of the first thoracic segment (see Figure 8-4). How much this reflex circuit involves the brainstem is not well understood. If this reflex circuit is limited to the cervical cord, preservation of this reflex may not exclude a possibility of brain death. This is because brain death is defined as irreversible death of all neurons in the medulla oblongata and above. However, as long as a possibility of this reflex involving the brainstem structures still remains, preservation of this reflex may reserve the diagnosis of brain death.

If all of the above brainstem reflexes are lost in comatose patients, it suggests that all the brainstem functions are lost. However, a possibility remains that many other neurons not directly related to these reflexes are still preserved. In judgment of brainstem reflexes, it is of utmost importance to keep in mind that all these reflexes may be completely lost by intake of a large dose of narcotics, during general anesthesia, or under hypothermia. If there is any possibility of these conditions, it is useful to follow up the clinical course by repeating these tests. It is needless to say that, in case of coma due to brainstem lesions, loss of these reflexes may also serve for local diagnosis of the lesion.

3) Cerebral Herniation

Secondary compression of the brainstem as a result of gross organic lesion of cerebral hemisphere(s) causes cerebral herniation, which requires quick attention and treatment. **Central transtentorial herniation** is caused by rapid compression of the thalamus from above bilaterally, and it causes coma quickly. **Uncal herniation** is caused by compression of the midbrain unilaterally from above, and causes clouding of consciousness, Cheyne-Stokes respiration, anisocoria and loss or decrease of light reflex, and decerebrate rigidity/posture. Namely, if all or any of the above signs appear in patients with a gross hemispheric lesion or brain edema, it suggests that uncal herniation is taking place. Pathologically, uncal herniation is associated with hemorrhagic lesions of various degrees in the midbrain tegmentum, which affects the brainstem reticular formation, causing disturbance of consciousness, respiratory impairment, and postural abnormality.

Anisocoria

Anisocoria in uncal herniation is considered to be caused not by a direct intramedullary damage of the oculomotor nerve in the midbrain, but by entrapment of the oculomotor nerve between the superior cerebellar artery and the posterior cerebral artery (see Figure 9-3). When the compression is relatively mild in this case, anisocoria and a loss or decrease of the light reflex of the dilated pupil may be seen, but paralysis of the extraocular muscles may not be observed. This is most likely because the autonomic fibers are located in the peripheral part of the oculomotor nerve at this extramedullary site, so that they are easily affected by external compression. Involvement of the oculomotor nerve in uncal herniation is more commonly seen on the side ipsilateral to the hemispheric lesion, but in some cases it may be seen on the contralateral side.

Decerebrate Posture

This abnormal posture consists of tonic extension and internal rotation (pronation) of the upper extremities and extension of the lower extremities, either spontaneously or more often provoked by nociceptive stimulus. It is associated with increased tone of extensor muscles (**decerebrate rigidity**). It is considered that the decerebrate posture/rigidity is caused as a result of interruption of the inhibitory pathway projecting to the vestibular nucleus at the level of the midbrain, which increases tone of the extensor muscles through disinhibition of the vestibulospinal tract (see Chapter 13-1). The presence of this phenomenon suggests either the presence of a severe lesion in the midbrain or the beginning of an uncal herniation.

Tonic Neck Reflex

This is a postural reflex in response to lateral rotation of the neck, consisting of extension of the upper and lower extremities of the side to which the neck is rotated and flexion of the contralateral upper and lower extremities, resembling the posture of a shot-putter. This phenomenon is seen when there is an asymmetric severe lesion in the brainstem rostral to the vestibular nucleus. Furthermore in this case, the passive neck flexion may cause flexion of both upper extremities, and the neck extension may cause their extension.

False Localizing Sign

In some cases of uncal herniation, a Babinski sign and homonymous hemianopsia might be seen on the side of a hemispheric lesion. As these signs are not directly related to the primary hemispheric lesion, they are called the **false localizing sign**. Among the above two signs, the Babinski sign ipsilateral to the hemispheric lesion is caused by impairment of the cerebral peduncle contralateral to the hemispheric lesion as a result of midbrain compression. The peduncular pathology in this case is called a **Kernohan notch**. Therefore, the pyramidal signs may be seen bilaterally in this case.

Homonymous hemianopsia on the side ipsilateral to the primary hemispheric lesion is caused by compression of the contralateral posterior cerebral artery as a result of uncal herniation, which causes an ischemic lesion in the occipital lobe contralateral to the primary hemispheric lesion. This sign, however, is not detectable in comatose patients.

In addition to uncal herniation, pyramidal signs might be also seen bilaterally in some other cases of a unilateral cerebral lesion. An example is thalamic hemorrhage, which will compress the contralateral corticospinal tract, causing the ipsilateral Babinski sign, and another example is the presence of an old vascular lesion in the hemisphere contralateral to the new lesion. In this case, distinction from uncal herniation can be easily done from other accompanying signs.

D. MENINGEAL IRRITATION

Nuchal stiffness is a representative sign of meningeal irritation (see Chapter 15-1). This is tested by flexing the neck (lifting the head) in the supine position and is judged by limitation of the neck flexion. If one of the examiner's hands is placed behind the neck while lifting the head by the other hand, the reflex contraction of the nuchal muscles may be palpated in patients with positive nuchal stiffness. This is considered to result from involvement of the dorsal roots of the cervical nerves or the occipital nerves by hemorrhage or inflammation at the site of meningeal penetration. Positive nuchal stiffness suggests the presence of subarachnoid hemorrhage or meningitis. However, nuchal stiffness may not be seen within 24 hours after the subarachnoid hemorrhage.

6. JUDGMENT OF BRAIN DEATH

Brain death is defined as a condition in which **functions of all neurons in the cerebral hemispheres and brainstem are irreversibly** lost due to organic brain diseases. In patients who are evaluated for possible brain death, the cardiovascular center and the respiratory center in the brainstem (see Figure 5-4) are not functioning at all, interrupting the central innervation of the heart and lung. Even in this condition, however, the heart continues to beat for at least some time as long as oxygen is supplied. Thus, all candidate patients for brain death are under the control of a respirator. In other words, patients who are spontaneously breathing, even a little, should be excluded as candidates of brain death.

The most important prerequisite for diagnosis of brain death is the fact that patients are not under profound hypothermia or anesthetics. Clinical diagnosis is based on the confirmation of deep coma and loss of all reflexes that have reflex centers in the brainstem. Thus, the presence of reflexes having their centers in the spinal cord does not exclude brain death.

There are substantial differences in perceptions and practices of brain death worldwide (Wijdicks et al, 2010; Wahlster et al, 2015). Regarding laboratory tests, implication of an EEG record of electrocerebral inactivity (the so-called flat EEG) differs among diagnostic criteria, but if there is any cortical activity detected on EEG, the patient cannot be diagnosed as brain dead. In addition, the caloric test using ice water and the brainstem auditory evoked potentials (BAEP) (see Chapter 12-1) are important tests. If there is any response in these tests, it can exclude brain death. However, as the peak I of BAEP is known to be generated in the cochlear nerve, its presence alone does not exclude brain death. If all these tests suggest loss of all brainstem functions, it is recommended to repeat all the tests sometime after the first test for reconfirmation, although the time interval varies among different diagnostic criteria.

BIBLIOGRAPHY

Abend NS, Bearden D, Helbig I, McGuire J, Narula S, Panzer JA, et al. Status epilepticus and refractory status epilepticus management. Semin Pediatr Neurol 21:263–274, 2015. (review)

Alshekhlee A, Hussain Z, Sultan B, Katirji B. Immunotherapy for Guillain-Barré syndrome in the US hospitals. J Clin Neuromuscul Dis 10:4–10, 2008.

American Academy of Neurology Clinical Practice Guidelines. Thrombolytic therapy for acute ischemic stroke. Neurology 47:835–839, 1996.

Betjemann JP, Lowenstein DH. Status epilepticus in adults. Lancet Neurol 14:615–624, 2015. (review)

El-Khatib MF, Kiwan RA, Jamaleddine GW. Buspirone treatment for apneustic breathing in brain stem infarct. Respir Care 48:956–958, 2003.

Gaspard N, Foreman BP, Alvarez V, Kang CC, Probasco JC, Jongling AC, et al. New-onset refractory status epilepticus: etiology, clinical features and outcome. Neurology 85:1604–1613, 2015.

Graff-Radford J, Fugate JE, Wijdicks EFM, Lachance DH, Rabinstein AA. Extramedullary tumors and leukemia: a diagnostic pitfall for the neurologist. Neurology 79:85–91, 2012.

Mandawat A, Kaminski HJ, Cutter G, Katirji B, Alshekhlee A. Comparative analysis of therapeutic options used for myasthenia gravis. Ann Neurol 68:797–805, 2010.

Minematsu K, Toyoda K, Hirano T, Kimura K, Kondo R, Mori E, et al. Guidelines for the intravenous application of recombinant tissue-type plasminogen activator (alteplase), the second edition, October 2012: a guideline from the Japan Stroke Society. J Stroke Cerebrovasc Dis 22:571–600, 2013.

Mizuguchi M, Yamanouchi H, Ichiyama T, Shiomi M. Acute encephalopathy associated with influenza and other viral infections. Acta Neurol Scand Suppl 186:45–56, 2007. (review)

Singh TD, Fugate JE, Rabinstein AA. The spectrum of acute encephalitis: causes, management, and predictors of outcome. Neurology 84:359–366, 2015.

Tarulli AW, Lim C, Bui JD, Saper CB, Alexander MP. Central neurogenic hyperventilation: a case report and discussion of pathophysiology. Arch Neurol 62:1632–1634, 2005.

Van den Berg B, Walgaard C, Drenthen J, Fokke C, Jacobs BC, van Doorn PA. Guillain-Barré syndrome: pathogenesis, diagnosis, treatment and prognosis. Nat Rev Neurol 10:469–482, 2014. (review)

Wahlster S, Wijdicks EFM, Patel PV, Greer DM, Hemphill JC, Carone M, et al. Brain death declaration: practices and perceptions worldwide. Neurology 84:1870–1879, 2015.

Wijdicks EFM, Varelas PN, Gronseth GS, Greer DM. Evidence-based guideline update: determining brain death in adults. Report of the Quality Standards Subcommittee of the American Academy of Neurology. 74:1911–1918, 2010.

Yamada S, Yasui K, Hasegawa Y, Tsuzuki T, Yoshida M, Hashidume Y, et al. An autopsy case of pandemic (HINI) 2009 influenza virus-associated encephalopathy. Clin Neurol 52:480–485, 2012. (Abstract in English)

30.

DISABILITY, FUNCTIONAL RECOVERY, AND PROGNOSIS

1. ASSESSMENT OF DISABILITY SCALE

Degree of disability and prospect of functional recovery are the most important matters of concern for patients with neurologic disorders. After completing the neurologic examination, it is important to consider the severity of disability, although detail scaling of each activity of daily living can be assessed later. Disability can be evaluated in terms of neurologic **impairment** found by the physical examination, **disability** expressed as **activities of daily living (ADLs)** and the resulting social **handicap**. Scales of disability have been established for some diseases like Parkinson disease (see Table 16-2) and multiple sclerosis, but for other diseases, it is useful to evaluate each of the specific activities used for daily living, such as brushing teeth, washing face, combing hair, dressing, use of toilet facilities, taking a bath or shower, eating, walking indoors as well as outdoors, and so on.

2. MODE OF TISSUE DAMAGE, FUNCTIONAL DISABILITY, AND ITS RECOVERY

Functional disability due to neurologic impairment and prospect of its recovery depend on how the nervous tissue is damaged. A number of factors influence functional disability and its recovery (Table 30-1). For general factors, the age at disease onset and the present age of the patient, general physical condition, and how much the patient is motivated for recovery are important. In aged subjects, functional recovery is expected to be slower and poorer as compared with young subjects. In children, functional recovery due to plastic restoration is directly related to the developmental state of the nervous system.

For the neurologic factors influencing the disability and functional recovery, the mode of onset of neurologic deficits and the mode of tissue damage should be taken into account (see Figure 1-2). Even for a relatively small lesion, the more acutely the tissue is damaged, the more conspicuous are the resulting neurologic deficits. In contrast, even for a gross lesion, the symptoms/signs are relatively mild if their onset is insidious and followed by a slowly progressive course. A typical example is an intracranial meningioma occupying a huge space of the cranial cavity, in which case the patient may be almost unaware of symptoms. On the other hand, neurodegenerative diseases may progress very slowly, but the disability might be quite severe in the advanced stage. Even a small lesion, if it occurs in a region where multiple important structures are closely located like in the brainstem, might cause various neurologic deficits.

The distribution of lesions shows a characteristic histological pattern that is specific for each disease group (see Figure 1-1). The presence of a lesion even at the same region of brain might show a different clinical picture depending on the mode of tissue damage. The size of the lesion is another important factor, but it depends on where in the brain the lesion is located and how quickly it has evolved.

For predicting the prognosis, it is important to take into account the results of laboratory data, but the results of laboratory tests including neuroimaging are not necessarily correlated with the degree of functional disability. Thus, it is necessary to take the whole clinical picture into consideration for judgment of prognosis.

Gray Matter Lesion Versus White Matter Lesion

When considering functional disability and recovery in patients with an organic lesion of the cerebral hemisphere, whether the lesion primarily affects the gray matter or the white matter is one of the key factors (Table 30-2). Generally speaking, a cortical lesion tends to manifest distinct focal neurologic deficits, whereas focal neurologic deficit is rare and relatively indistinct, if any, in the white

TABLE 30-1 FACTORS INFLUENCING THE DEGREE OF FUNCTIONAL DISABILITY AND ITS RECOVERY IN NEUROLOGIC DISORDERS

1. General factors
1. Age of onset and the present age
2. General physical condition
3. Patient's motivation for recovery
2. Neurologic factors
1. Mode of onset
2. Distribution of lesion at tissue level
3. Size of lesion
4. Number of lesions
5. Gray matter lesion versus white matter lesion
6. Axonal damage versus myelin sheath damage

matter lesion. This is because a large number of neurons are located closely in the narrow cortical area and because neurons recover poorly once they are damaged. In contrast, the white matter is formed of myelinated nerve fibers whose myelin sheath may regenerate to a certain extent. However, a disconnection syndrome due to a lesion of the cerebral white matter may cause focal neurologic deficit due to interruption of functional connectivity between different cortical areas (see Chapter 23-1). Furthermore, a progressive diffuse lesion of the cerebral white matter, such as leukodystrophy and ischemic white matter lesions (see Chapter 22-2C), may cause severe dementia and spastic quadriplegia. Convulsive seizures and involuntary movements, myoclonus in particular, are commonly seen in cortical lesions, whereas they are relatively rare in white matter lesions.

In relation to the above, it is important to note that, in the cerebral hemispheres, the gray matter is in the cortex as well as in the deep structures (thalamus and basal ganglia) while the medullary part is formed of the white matter, but

TABLE 30-2 FEATURES OF CLINICAL SYMPTOMS/SIGNS: COMPARISON BETWEEN THE GRAY MATTER LESION AND THE WHITE MATTER LESION

	Gray matter	White matter
Neurologic deficits	Distinct	Indistinct[*]
Focal sign	Common	Rare
Convulsive seizures	Common	Rare
Myoclonus	Common	Rare

[*] An exception is a diffuse white matter lesion of cerebral hemispheres, which may cause severe dementia and spastic quadriplegia.

in the spinal cord, the gray matter is only present in the central portion and all the peripheral parts are occupied by the fiber tracts, namely the white matter.

Axonal Damage Versus Myelin Damage

In close relationship to the issue of gray matter versus white matter damage, the issue of axonal damage versus myelin sheath damage is an important factor at the cellular level (Table 30-3). Generally speaking, in disorders in which axons are primarily damaged, neurologic deficits tend to be severe and functional recovery is incomplete whereas, in conditions in which the myelin sheath is primarily damaged, neurologic deficits are relatively mild and functional recovery is relatively good. However, in multiple sclerosis, which is a representative form of demyelinating diseases, the clinical course is initially characterized by remissions and relapses, but in the long run a progressive course associated with the secondary axonal damage is common (Filippi et al, 2013). Moreover, in the neuromyelitis optica spectrum disorders, which are relatively common in Asian populations, the spinal cord is severely affected, involving axons with severe functional disability (see Box 35).

In cerebral contusion due to head trauma and spinal cord injury, both axons and myelin sheath are damaged, causing severe disability and poor functional recovery.

3. MECHANISMS OF FUNCTIONAL RECOVERY

Mechanisms by which the impaired neurologic functions improve have not been fully clarified, and its molecular mechanisms are an important topic of modern neuroscience.

If the nervous system is only functionally impaired without structural damage even at the tissue level, the impaired function is expected to recover without leaving any residual. Even if there is some tissue damage, if it is only mildly affected with preserved capacity to recover, then its function is also expected to recover along with the recovery of the tissue

TABLE 30-3 CHARACTERISTICS OF NEUROLOGIC IMPAIRMENT: COMPARISON OF AXONAL DAMAGE AND MYELIN DAMAGE

Lesion	Axon	Myelin sheath	Axon + myelin sheath
Degree of disability	Severe	Relatively mild	Severe
Recovery	Incomplete	Relatively good	Poor
Example	Strokes	Multiple sclerosis	Contusion

damage. In case the nervous system is severely damaged, there are two main hypotheses for possible recovery as follows.

Plastic Reorganization

The nervous system is considered to have some capacity to reorganize its structure, function, and network in response to internal or external stimuli. For example, **collateral sprouting** may grow from the remaining part of the damaged axon or from other intact axons so that it could form synaptic contacts with the target neuron and produce some functional recovery (Figure 30-1). In this case, it is expected to take some time for the synaptic reorganization to occur.

Plastic changes are considered to contribute to the recovery of neurologic deficits, but on the other hand they may also cause positive neurologic symptoms that may be even hazardous to the patients. For example, patients with thalamic infarction involving the distal portion of the cerebellothalamic pathway (superior cerebellar peduncle) may develop tremor in the contralateral hand a few months after the stroke. For another example, patients with a thalamic vascular lesion involving the somatosensory afferent pathway may develop unpleasant pain (**thalamic pain**) and **hyperpathia** in the contralateral upper extremity some time after the stroke (see Chapter 19-2B, Box 65). In relation to the plastic reorganization of fiber tracts, application of diffusion tensor tractography might delineate disruption of fiber tracts in the white matter.

In recent years, clinical attempts have been made to apply the scientific principle of plastic reorganization for promoting the functional recovery in patients with trauma and vascular lesion of the central nervous system, psychiatric disorders, habituation, developmental abnormalities of children, and neurodegenerative disorders. Examples

are brain stimulation therapy, pharmacological approach, learning, and rehabilitation (Cramer et al, 2011, and Grefkes & Fink, 2011, for review).

Mobilization of Reserve Functions

Another hypothesis about recovery of impaired function is mobilization of a nervous system that is not primarily related to that particular function (**reserve functions**). For example, about 85% of fibers of the direct corticospinal tract originating from the motor cortex cross at the pyramidal decussation at the medulla oblongata and innervate the extremities contralateral to the motor cortex as the lateral corticospinal tract, while the remaining 15% of fibers descend through the ipsilateral anterior column as the anterior corticospinal tract (see Chapter 16-1A and Figure 16-2). The mobilization theory assumes that the uncrossed fiber tract is not actively participating in actual movement in the healthy condition, but once the crossed fiber tract is impaired, the uncrossed fiber tract becomes actively involved in the movement of the paralyzed extremities.

Alternatively, a nervous system that is closely related to the lost function but is involved in other functions in the healthy condition may be activated to compensate for the lost function when needed. For example, if the corticospinal tract originating from the primary motor cortex is damaged and causes paralysis of the corresponding part of body, fiber tracts originating from the secondary motor cortices (supplementary motor area and premotor area) and from the primary somatosensory cortex are activated to supplement the function of the damaged tract (see Figure 11-3). These mechanisms are being demonstrated by noninvasive techniques such as transcranial magnetic stimulation and functional MRI.

With recent remarkable advance in the field of cell transplantation techniques, histological replacement of the damaged tissue with embryonic stem cells (ES cells) or induced pluripotent stem cells (iPS cells) may be the way of the future.

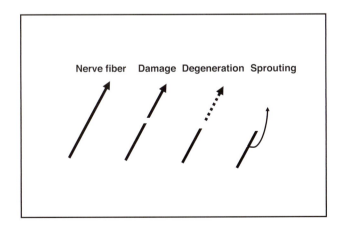

Nerve fiber   Damage   Degeneration   Sprouting

Figure 30-1 Schematic diagram of a nerve fiber showing possible mechanism of damage and regeneration.

BIBLIOGRAPHY

Cramer SC, Sur M, Dobkin BH, O'Brien C, Sanger TD, Trojanowski JQ, et al. Harnessing neuroplasticity for clinical applications. Brain 134:1591–1609, 2011. (review)

Filippi M, Preziosa P, Pagani E, Copetti M, Mesaros S, Colombo B, et al. Microstructural magnetic resonance imaging of cortical lesions in multiple sclerosis. Mult Scler 19:418–426, 2013.

Grefkes C, Fink GR. Reorganization of cerebral networks after stroke: new insights from neuroimaging with connectivity approaches. Brain 134:1264–1276, 2011. (review)

31.

HOW TO PLAN LABORATORY TESTS

t is reasonable and important to plan the necessary laboratory tests after carefully considering the site of lesion, etiology, most likely diagnosis and differential diagnoses based on the history taking and physical examination. For example, when facing with a patient complaining of symptoms suggestive of cerebral lesion, it is a bad practice to immediately obtain a cranial MRI. It is necessary to consider the expected site of lesion and pathogenesis before ordering the MRI in order to reasonably correlate the clinical picture and the neuroimaging data. The quality and size of MRI abnormality may not necessarily be correlated with the severity of neurologic impairment. Moreover, from the viewpoint of limited medical resources and limited size of hospital staff, the number of laboratory tests should be limited to the minimum necessity.

In most neurologic diseases, the sites of lesion and etiology can be diagnosed by the history taking and physical examination, but some special conditions require laboratory tests. For examples, in **primary central nervous system vasculitis** (Salvarani et al, 2007), **primary lymphoma** of the central nervous system (Porter et al, 2008), and **granulomatous inflammation**, there is no specific clinical manifestation or no specific cerebrospinal fluid abnormality. Therefore, cerebral angiography may be needed in the primary vasculitis, and brain biopsy may be needed for the primary lymphoma and granulomatous inflammation. Furthermore, it is needless to say that laboratory tests are necessary to confirm the clinical diagnosis of disorders that might have specific abnormalities such as specific antibodies and causative bacteria or viruses in the blood or cerebrospinal fluid.

1. FUNCTIONAL NEUROIMAGING STUDIES AND ELECTROPHYSIOLOGICAL STUDIES

Functional neuroimaging studies of regional cerebral blood flow with the use of single photon emission computed tomography (SPECT) or positron emission tomography (PET) are commonly used for clinical purposes. A question often addressed is whether a decrease in regional cerebral blood flow is correlated with a decrease in electrical activity of neurons in that area. It has been shown in animal experiments that the hemodynamic response is significantly correlated to neuronal activity, especially local field potential (synaptic activity), within a certain range, but the hemodynamic response tends to be more widespread in space and lasts longer in time as compared with the neuronal activity (Shibasaki, 2008, for review). For example, in patients with a thalamic lesion, blood flow might be found decreased in the ipsilateral frontal cortex as a result of a SPECT study. In this case, however, judgment of frontal hypofunction should be made with caution. This is an example of the neurophysiological changes that occur distant from a focal brain lesion (diaschisis). The concept of **diaschisis**, which was proposed by von Monakow in 1914, nearly disappeared from the mainstream of clinical neuroscience, but with the recent advance of neuroimaging studies of functional connectivity, functional diaschisis has drawn increasing attention of many investigators (Carrera & Tononi, 2014, for review).

By contrast with the central nervous system, electrophysiological studies of the peripheral nerves and muscles provide useful information on their functions. The state of impulse conduction can be directly assessed by various techniques, which will greatly contribute to the clinical diagnosis and evaluation of the treatment effect (Kimura, 2013, for review).

2. LUMBAR PUNCTURE

Lumbar puncture is commonly used for diagnosis of neurologic disorders, but its indication should be carefully considered and its overuse should be avoided. With development of neuroimaging techniques, indications for lumbar puncture are limited to infectious diseases such as meningitis and meningoencephalitis, autoimmune

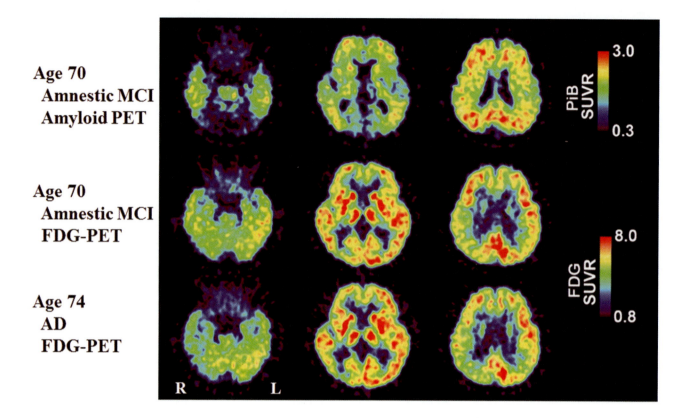

Age 70
Amnestic MCI
Amyloid PET

Age 70
Amnestic MCI
FDG-PET

Age 74
AD
FDG-PET

R   L

PiB SUVR 3.0 – 0.3

FDG SUVR 8.0 – 0.8

Figure 31-1 Amyloid imaging with Pittsburgh Compound B (top) and glucose metabolism imaging with fluoro-deoxy glucose (FDG) (middle) with PET in a 70-year-old patient with amnestic mild cognitive impairment (MCI) who developed Alzheimer disease (AD) at age 74 (bottom). Glucose metabolism was decreased in the right temporoparietal region at age 70, and more so at age 74. Amyloid deposition was seen in bilateral temporoparietal and frontal regions at age 70 (top). (Courtesy of Dr. Kenji Ishii, Tokyo Metropolitan Institute of Gerontology)

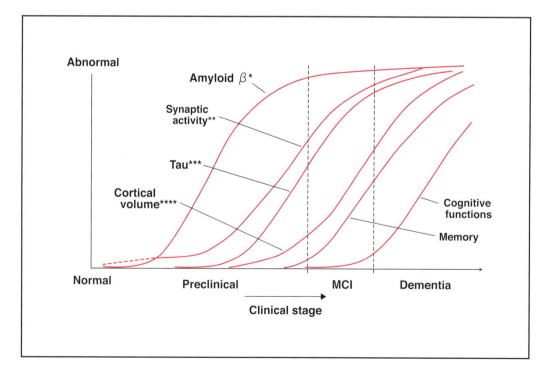

Abnormal

Amyloid β*

Synaptic activity**

Tau***

Cortical volume****

Cognitive functions

Memory

Normal   Preclinical   MCI   Dementia

Clinical stage

Figure 31-2 Time relationship between appearance of various biomarkers and clinical stage of Alzheimer disease. *deposit of amyloid β in brain shown by measurement of Aβ42 in CSF or amyloid imaging with PET, **synaptic activity measured by 18F-deoxyglucose (FDG)-PET or fMRI, ***tau or phosphorylated tau in CSF, ****measured by MRI, MCI: mild cognitive impairment. (Modified from Sperling et al, 2011, with permission)

inflammation of the central nervous system and polyradiculitis, and some metabolic abnormalities.

It is especially important not to abuse the **Queckenstedt test**. This test is used to observe elevation of the cerebrospinal fluid (CSF) pressure measured during the lumbar puncture in response to transient unilateral or bilateral compression of the jugular vein, which is expected to suddenly elevate the intracranial venous pressure in normal condition. If the CSF pressure does not increase by this maneuver, it suggests that there is obstruction of the spinal canal somewhere between the foramen magnum and the level of lumbar puncture (usually the interverbral space L3-L4). Therefore, the only purpose of this test is to prove the presence of a block of the spinal canal, and there is no rationale at all to do this test in patients with intracranial pathology. Furthermore, even in the spinal diseases, mechanical compression of spinal cord can be easily detected by neuroimaging studies. It is especially important to avoid this maneuver in patients with intracranial hypertension, because it might suddenly cause cerebral herniation (see Chapter 29-5C).

3. USE OF LABORATORY TESTS FOR PREVENTION OF DISEASES

If it becomes possible to predict the occurrence of a neurodegenerative disease by laboratory tests before the initial symptom appears, it might be able to prevent its occurrence. For example, it was postulated that the selective inhibitor of monoamine oxidase B, selegiline, might have an effect of **neuroprotection** in Parkinson disease, although this has not been confirmed (Olanow, 2009, for review).

For the purpose of neuroprotection, it is necessary to find a disease-specific abnormality by noninvasive techniques sufficiently far in advance of the clinical onset. One way would be to use functional or chemical imaging of brain. For example, attempts have been made to predict progression of mild cognitive impairment (MCI) to Alzheimer disease by using amyloid imaging with PET (Wolk et al, 2009) (Figure 31-1). Recently, it also became possible to image neurofibrillary pathology in Alzheimer disease by tau imaging with PET (Okamura et al, 2014). Chemically, attempts are extensively being made to measure amyloid β42, tau, and phosphorylated tau in the CSF for differentiating various kinds of dementia and for predicting the prognosis of MCI (Schoonenboom et al,

2012). It was recently shown that amyloid PET and CSF biomarkers equally identified early Alzheimer disease (Palmqvist et al, 2015). In Alzheimer disease, it is known that deposit of amyloid in the brain, abnormality of synaptic functions, and tau-mediated degeneration are seen in advance of the clinical onset (Figure 31-2). If these markers are found elevated in subjects who carry the apolipoprotein E (APOE) ε4 gene, it might suggest a high possibility of those subjects developing dementia in the future (Bateman et al, 2012). It is hoped that these lines of research will advance further and lead to prevention of intractable diseases.

BIBLIOGRAPHY

Bateman RJ, Xiong C, Benzinger TLS, Fagan AM, Goate A, Fox NC, et al. Clinical and biomarker changes in dominantly inherited Alzheimer's disease. N Engl J Med 367:795–804, 2012.

Carrera E, Tononi G. Diaschisis: past, present, future. Brain 137:2408–2422, 2014. (review)

Kimura J. Electrodiagnosis in Diseases of Nerve and Muscle: Principles and Practice. 4th ed. Oxford University Press, New York, 2013.

Okamura N, Furumoto S, Fodero-Tavoletti MT, Mulligan RS, Harada R, Yates P, et al. Non-invasive assessment of Alzheimer's disease neurofibrillary pathology using ^{18}F-THK5105 PET. Brain 137:1762–1771, 2014.

Olanow CW. Can we achieve neuroprotection with currently available anti-parkinsonian interventions? Neurology 72:S59–S64, 2009. (review)

Palmqvist S, Zetterberg H, Mattsson N, Johansson P, Minthon L, Blennow K, et al. Detailed comparison of amyloid PET and CSF biomarkers for identifying early Alzheimer disease. Neurology 85:1240–1249, 2015.

Porter AB, Giannini C, Kaufmann T, Lucchinetti CF, Wu W, Decker Pa, et al. Primary central nervous system lymphoma can be histologically diagnosed after previous corticosteroid use: a pilot study to determine whether corticosteroids prevent the diagnosis of primary central nervous system lymphoma. Ann Neurol 63:662–667, 2008.

Salvarani C, Brown RDJr, Calamia KT, Christianson TJ, Weigand SD, Miller DV, et al. Primary central nervous system vasculitis: analysis of 101 patients. Ann Neurol 62:442–451, 2007.

Schoonenboom NSM, Reesink FE, Verwey NA, Kester MI, Teunissen CE, van de Ven PM, et al. Cerebrospinal fluid markers for differential dementia diagnosis in a large memory clinic cohort. Neurology 78:47–54, 2012.

Shibasaki H. Human brain mapping: hemodynamic response and electrophysiology. Clin Neurophysiol 119:731–743, 2008. (review)

Sperling RA, Aisen PS, Beckett LA, Bennett DA, Craft S, Fagan AM, et al. Toward defining the preclinical stages of Alzheimer's disease: recommendations from the National Institute on Aging-Alzheimer's Association workgroups on diagnostic guidelines for Alzheimer's disease. Alzheimer Dementia 7:280–292, 2011.

Wolk DA, Price JC, Saxton JA, Snitz BE, James JA, Lopez OL, et al. Amyloid imaging in mild cognitive impairment subtypes. Ann Neurol 65:557–568, 2009.

AFTERWORD: FOR THOSE WHO WISH TO STUDY NEUROLOGY

In a video symposium held during the annual congress of American Academy of Neurology in 2007, distinguished neurologists reviewed why they chose neurology for their specialty. The main reasons common to most of the speakers were the diversity and mysteriousness of neurologic symptoms and signs, a thrilling process of thinking about sites of lesion and etiology based on neurologic symptoms and signs, and a close connection with rapidly advancing neuroscience. Basics of clinical neurology are the bedside observation of patients, and in fact many important research endeavors of neurology and neuroscience have originated from careful clinical observation.

Therefore, clinical neurology starts from comprehension of the symptoms and their time course, followed by confirmation of sign(s) found by neurologic examination, and then consideration of the most probable diagnosis based on the symptoms and signs. No matter how laboratory tests are advanced, neglect of symptoms and signs is not effective for clinical practice and research. In this sense, this book was arranged to make a bridge from basic sciences such as anatomy, physiology, pharmacology, and molecular biology to the understanding of clinical symptomatology.

As some of the statements in this book are based on the authors' own thoughts and experiences, different views, if any, are welcomed.

As clinical aspects of neurology are emphasized throughout this book, it might give an impression that the history taking and the neurologic examination are almighty. However, most information on the neurologic symptoms and signs are based on the observation and vast experience of many neurologists over a period of 150 years, and some of the symptoms and signs might have been just handed over from predecessors to successors. Therefore, some of the currently known neurologic signs may not necessarily be meaningful (Johnston & Hauser, 2011, for review). Since the brain is so complex, there is always more to learn about the generating mechanism and diagnostic significance of neurologic signs.

BIBLIOGRAPHY

Johnston SC, Hauser SL. The beautiful and ethereal neurological exam: an appeal for research. Ann Neurol 70:A9–A10, 2011. (review)

INDEX

Page numbers followed by *f* and *t* indicate figures and tables, respectively.

Abducens nerve, 30*f*, 32*f*, 60, 60*f*
Abducens nucleus, 30*f*
Abductor pollicis brevis muscle, 136*t*
Abetalipoproteinemia (Bassen-Kornzweig disease), 130
Acalculia, **215**, 229
Accessory nerve, 33, **105**
Accommodation, 49, 51*f*, **52**, 55
Aceruloplasminemia, 126
Achalasia, 203
Acquired mirror movement, 111
Acquired neuromyotonia (Isaacs syndrome), 146, 253*t*, **254**
Acromegaly, 18, **265**
ACTH-producing pituitary adenoma, 266
Action tremor, 165
Activities of daily living (ADLs), 20, **281**
Acute anterior poliomyelitis, 140, **270**
Acute confusional states, 25
Acute disseminated encephalomyelitis (ADEM), 16, **143**
Acute encephalopathy, 26, 26*t*
Acute meningoencephalitis, 273
Acute polyneuritis, 138
Adamkiewicz artery, 113
Adiadochokinesis, 126, **147**
Adie syndrome, 55
Autosomal dominant nocturnal frontal lobe epilepsy (ADNFLE), 250*t*, 251
Adrenoleukodystrophy (ALD), 143
Adrenomyeloneuropathy (AMN), 143
Adson test, 137
Adult polyglucosan body disease, 143
Ageusia, 88
Agnosia of clock reading, 231, **233**
Agnosia of distance, 231
Agnosia of optic counting, 231
Acquired immunodeficiency syndrome (AIDS), **218**, 219
Akathisia, 172
Akinetic mutism, 27
Alexander disease, 218
Alien hand sign, 228
α motor fibers, 114, 115*f*
ALS/parkinsonism dementia complex, 217
Alzheimer disease
    advanced stage, 26
    clinical features, 216
    functional neuroimaging, 286*f*
    pathological features, 216
Amaurosis fugax, 38
Amnesia, 210
Amusia, 229
Amygdala, 35, 35*f*, 189*f*, 229, **231**
Amyloid angiopathy, 4
Amyotrophic lateral sclerosis, 104, **133**, 134*f*, 217

Analgesia, 190
Andersen-Tawil syndrome, 251*t*, 253
Anesthesia, 190
Anisocoria, 53, **277**
Ankle clonus, 144
Anosmia, 35
Anosognosia, 233
Anterior cerebral artery, 40*f*, 43*f*, 60*f*
Anterior choroidal artery, 40*f*, 43*f*, 60*f*
Anterior communicating artery, 43*f*, 60*f*
Anterior horn cells, 113, 115*f*
Anterior inferior cerebellar artery, 60*f*
Anterior root 114, 115*f*
Anterior spinal artery, 60*f*, 112, 114*f*
Anterior spinal artery syndrome, 113
Anticipation, 129
Antidiuretic hormone (ADH), 266
Aortic receptors (aortic body), 102
Apallic syndrome, 27
Apathy, 27
Ape hand, 135, 138*f*
Aphasia
    Broca/motor, 225, **232**
    classification of, 225
    conduction, 226, **232**
    crossed, 223
    examination, 231
    jargon, 232
    primary progressive, 231
    repetition, 232
    sensory, 225, **232**
    thalamus role, 262
    total, 226
    transcortical motor, 226
    transcortical sensory, 226
    Wernicke, 225
Aphonia, 97, **103**
Apneustic breathing, 275
Apraxia
    callosal, 228
    constructional, 227
    diagonistic, 228
    dressing, **228**, 233
    gait, 233
    ideational, **227**, 233
    ideomotor, **227**, 232
    limb-kinetic, **227**, 232
    reaching, grasping, 227, 228*f*
    sympathetic, 228
    task-specific, 228
Aquaporin-4, 142
Argyll Robertson pupil, 55
Arnold-Chiari malformation (Chiari malformation), 71
Arsenic poisoning, 16
Articulation, 97
Ascending reticular activating system, 23, 23*f*
Aschner eyeball pressure test, 204
Aseptic meningitis (viral meningitis), 273
Asperger syndrome, **179**, 229

Astasia-abasia, 257
Asterixis, **165**, 172, 176
Asterixis, thalamic, 176
Astrocytomas, 131
Asymbolia for pain, 188
Ataxia
    acquired cerebellar, 130
    cerebellar, 126
    episodic, 249, 250*t*
    Friedreich, 129
    gluten-sensitive, 131
    SCA (*see* spinocerebellar ataxia (SCA))
    sensory, **190**, 207
    telangiectasia (Louis-Bar syndrome), 130
    truncal, 127
Ataxic breathing, 275
Atherothrombosis, 4
Athetosis, 160*f*, 167
Atypical acute polyneuritis, 140
Auditory agnosia, 229
Auditory function
    auditory cortex (Heschl gyrus), 89, 90*f*
    auditory input, spatial perception, 89
    brainstem auditory evoked potentials (BAEPs), 89, 91*f*
    cochlear (acoustic) nerve, 89, 90*f*
    cochlear nucleus, dorsal/ventral, 89, 90*f*
    cognitive functions related to, 89
    examination, 90
    inferior colliculus, 89, 90*f*
    lateral lemniscus, 89, 90*f*
    medial geniculate body, 89, 90*f*
    selective attention, **89**, 230
    spiral ganglion, 89, 90*f*
    superior olive, 89, 90*f*
    tinnitus, 91
    tonotopic organization, 89
    vestibulocochlear nerve, 89, 90*f*
Auditory hallucination, 215
Auditory recognition, 229
Auriculotemporal syndrome, 101
Autoimmune autonomic ganglionopathy, 253*t*
Autoimmunity, 16
Autonomic nervous system
    afferent system structure, function, 202
    ciliospinal center of Budge, **51**, 51*f*, 98*f*, 199
    cortical center, 201
    cranial nerves, 31
    gastrointestinal symptoms, 203
    intermediolateral nucleus, 51, 51*f*, 115*f*, **199**, 200*f*
    parasympathetic ganglia, 199, 200*f*
    parasympathetic nervous system, 102*f*, 199
    postganglionic fibers, 199, 200*f*
    preganglionic fibers, 199, 200*f*
    sexual functions, 203
    skin, autonomic symptoms, 202

    sympathetic ganglia, 115*f*, 199, 200*f*
    sympathetic nervous system, 51*f*, 102*f*, 115*f*, 199, 200*f*
    sympathetic tract, 98*f*, 199
    urination (micturition) control, 203
Autosomal recessive dopamine-responsive dystonia with Segawa syndrome, 171, 171*f*
Autosomal recessive spastic paraplegia associated with early baldness, mental retardation, and thinning of the corpus callosum, 143
Autotopagnosia, 231
Axial lateropulsion, 95
Axonal *vs.* myelin damage assessment, 282, 282*t*

Babinski-Nageotte syndrome, 53*t*, 98, 99*f*
Babinski sign, 157, 157*f*
BAFME (benign adult familial myoclonus epilepsy), **175**, 250*t*, 251
Balint syndrome, 234, 234*f*
Ballism (ballismus), 167
Baroesthesia, 189
Baroreceptor of the carotid sinus (carotid body), 101*f*, 102, 103*f*
Barré sign, 134
Basal ganglia
    eye movement role, 64*f*, 65
    mental/cognitive function disorders, 216
    structure and functions, 116
    voluntary movement control, 116*f*
Basilar artery, 60*f*
Basin phenomenon, **190**, 207
Bassen-Kornzweig disease (abetalipoproteinemia), 130
Becker muscular dystrophy, 134
Beevor sign, 142
Behçet disease, 12, 18*f*
Bell palsy, **83**, 86
Bell phenomenon, 69
Benedikt syndrome, 53*t*, 58*f*, 59
Benign paroxysmal positional vertigo, 94
Beriberi, 192
Beta-propeller protein associated neurodegeneration (BPAN), **126**, 171
Biceps brachii muscle, 136*t*
Bielschowsky sign, 67
Bilateral anosmia, 35
Bilateral facial paralysis, 87
Binswanger disease, 218
Bitemporal hemianopsia, **39**, 41*f*, 45
Blepharoptosis (ptosis), 52, **66**
Blepharospasm, **66**, 167
Blindness (ipsilateral), 38, 41*f*
Blink reflex, **78**, 81
Body lateropulsion, 95
Borrelia burgdorferi, **87**, 140
Botulinum toxin, 270, 271*t*
Boule musculaire, 134
Bow hunter's stroke, 95

Brachial plexus, 137, 139*f*
Bradykinesia, 107, **119**
Brain death diagnosis, 278
Brainstem
  acute lesions, 270
  anatomy, 29, 30*f*, 31*f*
  localized lesions, syndromes caused
    by, 53*t*
  medullary respiratory center, 32*f*, 274
  named syndromes related to, 53*t*, 100
  pontine respiratory center, 32*f*, 275
  reflexes, examination, 276
  respiration, examination, 274
  reticular formation, 23, 23*f*
Brainstem auditory evoked potentials
  (BAEPs), 89, 91*f*
Branch atheromatous disease, 7
Brodmann area, 42, 44*f*
Brown-Séquard syndrome, 193, 195*f*
Bulbar muscles, 98, **99**
Bulbar palsy, 98, **104**
Bulbospinal muscular atrophy, 103*f*, 133

CADASIL (Cerebral autosomal dominant
  arteriopathy with subcortical
  infarcts and leukoencephalopa-
  thy), 218
Calculation, **213**, 228, 231
Caloric test, **95**, 276
Camptocormia (bent spine syndrome), 106
CARASIL (cerebral autosomal recessive arte-
  riopathy with subcortical infarcts and
  leukoencephalopathy), 218
Carbon monoxide poisoning, 219
Cardiac syncope, 24*t*, 25
Cardiogenic embolism, 4
Carotid sinus hypersensitivity, 24*t*, 25
Carotid sinus pressure test, 204
Carpal tunnel syndrome, 136, **191**
Cataplexy, 246
Catatonia, 27
Cauda equina, 112, 113*f*
Central core disease, 145, 251*t*, **253**
Central facial paralysis, **86**, 87
Central neurogenic hyperventilation, 275
Central pontine myelinolysis, 212
Central post-stroke pain, 261
Central retinal artery, 38
Central scotoma, 37, **44**, 45
Central transtentorial herniation, 277
Cerebellum
  acquired cerebellar ataxia, 130
  circuit, clinical symptomatology, 126
  corticopontine tract, 125, 127*f*
  cytoarchitecture, 125, 128*f*
  dentatothalamic tract (superior
    cerebellar peduncle), 125, 127*f*
  embryological division, 128*f*
  eye movement role, 64*f*, 65
  granule cells, layer, 125, 128*f*
  inferior olive, 31*f*, 90*f*, 127*f*, 129, **176**
  input/output circuits, 127*f*
  middle cerebellar peduncle, 125, 127*f*
  molecular layer, 125, 128*f*
  mossy fibers, 125, 128*f*
  parallel fibers, 125, 128*f*
  pontine nucleus, 30*f*, 125, 127*f*
  Purkinje cells, 125, 128*f*
  spinocerebellar degeneration, 129
  spinocerebellar tracts, 129, 127*f*
  tumors of, 131, 131*f*
  Voluntary movement control, 116*f*, 126
Cerebral herniation, 277
Cerebral infarction, 4

Cerebral peduncle, **29**, 30*f*, 59, 112, 117*f*
Cerebrotendinous xanthomatosis, 130
Cervical dystonia, **105**, 167
Cervical spondylosis, **106**, 190
Cestan-Chenais syndrome, 53*t*, 98, 99*f*
Chaddock sign, 156
Channelopathies
  autoimmune, 253, 253*t*
  congenital long QT syndrome, 252
  episodic ataxia, 249, 250*t*
  hereditary, 249, 250*t*
  hereditary, muscles, 251*t*, 252
  hereditary, peripheral nervous
    system, 252
  ring chromosome, 250*t*, 251
  transmitter-gated (ligand-gated), 249
  voltage-gated, 249
Character, emotion, 215
Charcot-Marie-Tooth disease, 141
Charcot-Wilbrand syndrome, 231
Charlevoix-Saguenay syndrome, 143
Cherry-red spot, 40*f*, 46
Cheyne-Stokes respiration, 275
Cholinergic crisis, 269
Chorea, 160*f*, 166
Chorea-acanthocytosis, 166
Chronic fatigue syndrome, 135
Chronic inflammatory axonal
    polyneuropathy (CIAP), 141
Chronic inflammatory demyelinating
    polyneuropathy (CIDP), 140
Chronic postradiation leukoencephal-
    opathy, 219
Chronic subdural hematoma, 213
Chronic traumatic encephalopathy, 217
Churg-Strauss syndrome, 140
Chvostek sign, 146
Ciliospinal center of Budge, 51, 51*f*
Circadian rhythm, 39, 267
Cisplatin intoxication, **141**, 192, 193
Citrullinemia, 213
Clasp knife phenomenon, 143
Claude syndrome, 53*t*, 58, 58*f*
Claw hand, 135, 138*f*
Clonus, 144
Clostridium botulinum, 270
Clostridium tetani, 78, **146**, 272
Cockayne disease, 16
Cocktail party effect, 230
Cogan sign, 69
Cognitive functions. *see* mental/cognitive
    functions
Cogwheel phenomenon, **121**, 144
Collateral sprouting, 283, 283*f*
Collet-Sicard syndrome, 99, 99*t*
Color recognition, 230
Color vision, 42
Coma, 25, **273**, 274*t*
Coma scale, **25**, 25*t*, 26*t*, 274
Common knowledge, 215
Complex regional pain syndrome
    (CRPS), 203
Complex tic, 179
Compulsive behavior, 145
Conductive deafness, 91
Cones, 37
Confabulation, 211
Confrontation test, 44
Congenital insensitivity to pain, 188, **252**
Congenital mirror movement, 111
Congenital myasthenic syndrome,
    251*t*, 253
Congenital nystagmus, 70
Conjugate deviation of eyes, 62, **69**, 274

Conjugate nystagmus, 70
Consciousness
  alteration, 25
  anatomical basis, 23
  clouding, 25
  delirium, 25
  disturbance, **24**, 270
  Glasgow Coma Scale, 25*t*
  Japan Coma Scale, 26*t*
  syncope, 24, 24*t*
  transient loss, 24
Conus medullaris, 112
Convergence palsy, 62
Convergence-retraction nystagmus, 71
Coordination, 147
Corneomandibular reflex, 81
Cortical blindness, 230
Cortical sensation examination, 189
Corticobasal degeneration, 218
Corticomuscular coherence, 161
Corticospinal tract
  direct, 109
  laminar structure, 111*f*, 112
  lesions, 111
  structure, 109, 110*f*
Cough syncope, 24*t*, 25
Cranial dystonia, 167
Cranial nerves
  autonomic nervous system, 31
  common structures, 29
  intraocular muscles innervation, 49
  named syndromes related to, 99*t*, 100
  neurologic examination, 33
  nuclei, location in brainstem, 32, 32*f*
  somatosensory function, 31
Craniopharyngioma, 267
Creutzfeldt-Jakob disease, 174*t*, 178*f*, 179
Crocodile tears syndrome, 86
Crossed analgesia, 192
Crow-Fukase syndrome (POEMS), 9,
    14, 16*f*
Crowned dens syndrome, 106
Curtain sign, 97, **103**
Cushing disease, 266
Cushing syndrome, 266

Daily living state, 216
Daytime sleepiness, 245
Deafness, 91. *see also* auditory function
Decerebrate posture, rigidity, **93**, 277
Decorticate state, posture, 27
Deep brain stimulation, **119**, 161, 162,
    169, 261
Deep sleep, 26
Deep tendon reflex. *see* tendon reflex
Deglutition muscles spasm, 103
Degos disease (malignant atrophic
    papulosis), 14
Dejerine-Roussy syndrome, 191, **192**, 261
Dejerine-Sottas disease, 141
Delirium, **25**, 215
Delirium tremens, 26
Deltoideus muscle, 136*t*
Delusion, 215
Dementia, 26, **216**. *see also* Alzheimer
    disease; Lewy body dementia; Par-
    kinson disease
Dementia pugilistica, 217
Dementia with Lewy bodies, 216
Demyelinating diseases, clinical features, 39
Denervation potentials, 134
Denervation supersensitivity, 55
Dentato-rubro-pallido-luysian atrophy
    (DRPLA), **129**, 166, 174*t*

Depression, **119**, 135
Dermatomyositis, **14**, 135
Dermographia, 203
De Sanctis-Cacchione syndrome, 17
Diabetes insipidus, 266
Diabetes mellitus, 6, **7**, 138, 141, 192, 274*t*
Diabetic neuropathy, 255
Diabetic polyneuropathy, 9, **141**, 191
Diadochokinesis, 126
Diagnosis
  acute onset, 3, 3*f*
  anatomical, 1
  clinical, 4
  clinical course, 2, 3*f*
  differential diagnosis, 4
  etiological, 2, 3*f*
  fluctuating clinical course, 3, 3*f*
  improvement, 3, 3*f*
  insidious onset, 3, 3*f*
  lesion distribution, tissue-level, 1, 2*f*
  mode of onset, 2, 3*f*
  negative *vs.* positive symptoms/signs, 2
  paroxysmal clinical course, 3, 3*f*
  polyphasic clinical course, 3, 3*f*
  progressive clinical course, 3, 3*f*
  remissions and exacerbations, 3, 3*f*
  selective vulnerability, 2
  slowly progressive clinical course, 3, 3*f*
  subacute onset, 3, 3*f*
  sudden onset, 3, 3*f*
  system involvement, 2, 2*f*
Diarrhea/constipation, alternating
    occurrence, 201
Diaschisis, 285
Diffuse lesion, 1, 2*f*
Diffuse Lewy body disease, 216
Diffuse thalamocortical projection system,
    23, 23*f*
Diphtheria, 140
Diplopia, causes of, 67, 68*t*
Disability scale assessment, 281
Disconnection syndrome, 223
Disorientation, 209
Disseminated lesion, 1, 2*f*
Dissociated nystagmus, 63, 63*f*
Dissociated sensory loss, **76**, 193, 194*f*
Distal muscular dystrophy, 133
Distal myopathy, 133
Disturbance of optic counting, 233
Disuse atrophy, 142
Divergence, 62
Dizziness, 94, 94*f*. *see also* equilibrium
Doll's eye sign, 69, **276**
Dopamine, 35, 117*f*, **119**, 120*f*, 121*f*,
    145, 171
Dopamine synthesis, 120*f*
Dorsal motor nucleus of the vagus, 31*f*, 32*f*,
    33*f*, 101
Dorsal pathway, primary visual cortex, 42
Dorsal root ganglion, **185**, 186*f*, 187*f*,
    193, 200*f*
Dorsal root ganglion impairment, 193
Dorsal spinocerebellar tract, 127
Down-beat nystagmus, 71
Down syndrome, 18
Dropped head syndrome, 105
Drug intoxication, 2
Duane syndrome, 67
Duchenne muscular dystrophy, 134
Dying-back neuropathy, 193
Dysarthria, 6, **104**
Dysarthria-clumsy hand syndrome, 7
Dysdiadochokinesis, 126, **147**
Dysesthesia, 141, 144, **190**, 191

Dyskinesia, 145, 159, 160*f*, **172**
Dysmetria, 70, **126**, 147
Dysphagia, 53*t*, 78, **97**, 98, 103, 104
Dysphonia, 103
Dysprosody, 225
Dyssynergia, 147
Dystonia, 159, 160*f*, **167**, 170
Dystonia-parkinsonism syndrome, 126, **171**
DYT1, 170

Easy fatigability, 66
Ehlers-Danlos syndrome, 12, 13*f*
Embouchure dystonia, 167
Emery-Dreifuss syndrome, 132
Emotion, character, 215
Encephalitis
   acute, 273
   Bickerstaff brainstem, 270
   limbic, 253*t*, 254, **255**
   paraneoplastic limbic, **254**, 255
   Rasmussen, 253*t*, 254
   subacute sclerosing panencephalitis
     (SSPE), 178, 180*f*
Entrainment, **180**, 258
Entrapment neuropathy, 191
Eosinophilic pituitary adenoma, 265
Ephaptic transmission, **86**, 191
Epilepsia partialis continua (Kojevnikoff
   epilepsy), 146
Epilepsy, epileptic seizures
   absence seizure (petit mal), 237*t*, 238,
     238*f*, **240**, 251
   aura, 240
   automatism, 239
   autosomal dominant lateral temporal
     lobe epilepsy (ADLTLE), 241
   autosomal dominant nocturnal frontal
     lobe epilepsy (ADNFLE), 241, **251**
   cerebrovascular disease, 242
   childhood absence, 250*t*, 251
   classification, 237, 237*t*
   complex partial seizure, 238
   cortical dysplasia, 238
   definition, 237
   déjà vu, 239
   diagnosis, 241
   epigastric rising sensation, 239
   focal, 237*t*, 238
   focal motor seizure, 238
   gelastic (ictal laughter), 240
   generalized, 237, 237*t*, **240**
   generalized tonic-clonic seizures, 240
   gustatory seizure, 239
   hallucinatory seizure, 239
   ictal apnea, 239
   Jacksonian seizure, 238
   jamais vu, 239
   juvenile myoclonic, 250*t*, 251
   medically intractable, 241
   mesial temporal lobe, 239
   painful somatosensory seizures, 238
   photosensitive epilepsy, 241
   postictal paralysis, Todd paralysis, 238
   post-stroke seizures, 242
   posttraumatic, 241
   progressive myoclonus epilepsy (PME),
     174, 174*t*
   pseudoseizure, 241
   psychogenic nonepileptic, 241, **242**
   psychomotor seizure, 239, 240*f*
   secondarily generalized seizure, 238
   simple partial seizure, 238
   SMA seizure, 239*f*
   stimulus-sensitive, 241

   symptomatic, 241
   task-specific, 241
   uncinate fit, 35, **239**
   vertiginous seizure, epileptic vertigo,
     93, 239
Epileptic vertigo, **93**, 239
Episodic memory, 210
Epsilon-sarcoglycan gene mutation, 172
Epstein-Barr virus, **140**, 273
Equilibrium
   caloric test, **95**, 276
   examination of, 94, 94*f*
   pathway structure, function, 90*f*, 93
   saccule, 93
   semicircular canals, 93
   utricle, 93
   vestibular complex, 93
   vestibular ganglion (Scarpa's
     ganglion), 93
   vestibular nerve, 93
Erythema nodosum, *15f*
Erythermalgia, 252
Erythromelalgia, 252
Essential palatal tremor, 176
Essential tremor, 160*f*, 161*f*, 163, 164*f*
Ethanol, involuntary movement
   suppression by, 163
Explosive speech, 104, **126**
Extensor carpi radialis muscle, 136*t*
Extensor carpi ulnaris muscle, 136*t*
Extensor digitorum muscle, 136*t*
Extensor hallucis longus muscle, 136*t*
Extrapontine myelinolysis, 212
Eye-of-the-tiger sign, 125*f*, 126
Eye-tracking test, 70

Fabry disease, 12, **192**
Facial angiofibroma, 11, 10*f*
Facial emotion recognition, 231
Facial nerve
   anatomy, 32*f*
   blink reflex, **78**, 81, 87
   ciliary sign, 87
   functions, examination, 86
   geniculate ganglion, 83, 84*f*
   gustatory (taste) sense, 84*f*, **85**, 88
   lacrimation, 84*f*, **85**, 86, 88
   mimetic muscles, 88
   motor cortex somatotopic organization,
     83, 84*f*
   motor functions, examination, 86
   parasympathetic nervous system, 86
   salivation, **85**, 88
   skin, mucosa, **86**, 88
   solitary nucleus, 31*f*, 32*f*, 84*f*, 85
   somatosensory function testing, 88
   somatosensory nerve, 84, 84*f*
   structures, functions, 83, 84*f*
   taste sense, **85**, 88
Facial paralysis, 86, **87**
Face recognition, **44**, 230
Faciobrachial dystonic seizures, 254
Facioscapulohumeral muscular dystrophy,
   132, 132*f*
False localizing signs, 61, **278**
Falx meningioma, 201
Familial amyloid polyneuropathy, 141, **201**
Fasciculation, 103, **134**, 181
Fatal familial insomnia, 179, **246**
Festination, festinating gait, 119
Fibrillation, 134
Fibromyalgia, 135
Finger agnosia, 231
Finger-nose-finger test, 147

Finger splitting, 191
Finger-to-nose test, 147
Fixed posture dystonia, fixed dystonia,
   168, 169*f*
Flexed posture, 105
Flexor carpi radialis muscle, 136*t*
Flexor carpi ulnaris muscle, 136*t*
Flexor digitorum longus muscle, 136*t*
Flexor digitorum sublimis muscle, 136*t*
Floppy infant, 145
Flutter-like oscillation, 71
Focal dystonia, 105, **167**
Focal hand dystonia, 167
Focal lesion, 2, 2*f*
Focal neurologic deficit, 223
Foot drop, **136**, 207
Forced crying, 104
Forced grasping, 81
Forced groping, 81
Forced laughter (laughing), 104
Fovea centralis, **37**, 38*f*, 46
Foville syndrome, 53*t*, 87
Fragile X associated tremor/ataxia
   syndrome, 166
Freezing phenomenon, freezing of gait,
   121, **206**, 233
Frey syndrome, 101
Froment sign, 136, 138*f*
Frontal eye field, 61, 64*f*, 65*f*, 85*f*
Frontotemporal dementia, 217
Frontotemporal dementia, behavioral
   variant, 217
Frontotemporal lobar degeneration, 217
FTD/Pick complex, 217
Fukuhara disease, 175
Functional localization
   (specialization), 223
Functional neuroimaging, 226, 226*f*,
   228*f*, **285**
Functional recovery assessment, 281, **282**,
   282*t*, 283*f*

Gait
   ataxic, 206
   central control mechanism, 205, 205*f*
   falling, falls, 206, 207
   festinating, 206
   freezing of, **206**, 233
   Parkinsonian, 206
   propulsion, 206
   retropulsion, 206
   scissor, 206
   spastic, 205
   steppage, 207
   tandem, 206
   waddling, 207
   wide-based, 206
Galactorrhea, 265
Galactorrhea-amenorrhea syndrome, 265
Gastrocnemius-soleus muscle, 136*t*
Gaucher disease, 124
Gaze, neural control mechanism, 61, 61*f*,
   64*f*, 65*f*
Gaze nystagmus, 71
Gaze palsy, 69
Gegenhalten (paratonia), 145
Generalized dystonia, **167**, 168
Genetic heterogeneity, 166, **249**
Geniculate zoster, 12, 14*f*
Geniculocalcarine tract, 40
Gerstmann-Sträussler-Scheinker syn-
   drome, 179
Gerstmann syndrome, 215, 228, **231**
Giant axonal neuropathy, 141

Giant evoked potential, 173
Gigantism, 265
Gilles de la Tourette syndrome, 179
Girdle sensation, 193
Give-way weakness, 257
Glasgow Coma Scale, 25, 25*t*
Globus pallidus, 116, 117*f*
Glossopharyngeal nerve, 30*f*, 32*f*, 97, 98*f*
Glossopharyngeal neuralgia, 100
Glove and stocking distribution, 191, 193*f*
Glutamate, 116, 117*f*, 118*f*, 128*f*
Glycogen storage disease, 147
Gowers sign, 142
Gradenigo syndrome, 99*t*
Granulomatous inflammation, 285
Graphesthesia, 186*t*, **189**, 233
Gray *vs.* white matter lesion, 281, 282*t*
Grönblad-Strandberg syndrome. *see*
   pseudoxanthoma elasticum
Guillain-Barré syndrome
   clinical features, 138
   differential diagnosis, 140
   pain in, 191
   respiratory paralysis, 270
Guillain-Mollaret triangle, 129, **176**
Gustatory (taste) sense, **85**, 88, 100

Hallervorden-Spatz syndrome, 126
Hallucination, 215
Hamstrings muscles, 136*t*
HAM (HTLV-I-associated myelopathy)/
   TSP (tropical spastic
   paralysis), 144
Handedness, 7
Handicap, 281
Hashimoto encephalopathy, 255
Hatchet face, 78
Headache
   classification, 242, 242*t*
   cluster 244
   idiopathic intracranial hypertension, 243
   morning headache, 243
   muscle contraction, 244
   post-lumbar puncture, 243
   primary, 242, 242*t*
   pulsating, 244
   secondary, 242, 242*t*
   spontaneous intracranial hypoten-
     sion, 243
   tension, 244
   throbbing, 244
Head thrust, 69
Hearing, *see* auditory function
Heavy metals intoxication, **2**, 16, 130, 141
Heel-knee test, 147
Heerfordt disease, 87
Heine-Medin disease, 140
Hemangioblastoma, 131
Hemianalgesia, 197, **257**
Hemianesthesia without motor
   paralysis, 7
Hemianopsia
   bitemporal, **39**, 41*f*, 45
   homonymous, 39, 40, 41*f*, **45**
Hemiballism, 167
Hemifacial spasm, 66, 83, 86, **146**, 181
Hemiplegia
   abducens crossed, 61
   causes, 112
   crossed, 53*t*, **59**, 87
   hypoglossal crossed, 98
   pure motor, 7, **112**
Hemispatial neglect, 233
Hepatic encephalopathy, 165, 212*f*, **271**

Hereditary diffuse leukoencephalopathy with spheroids (HDLS), 218
Hereditary dystonia, 170
Hereditary motor sensory neuropathy (HMSN), 141
Hereditary paroxysmal dyskinesia, 172
Hereditary polyneuropathy, 141
Hereditary progressive dystonia with marked diurnal fluctuation (Segawa's disease), 171, 171*f*
Hereditary spastic paraplegia, 143
Hereditary startle disease, 249, 250*t*
Herpes zoster, 191
Heschl gyrus, **89**, 90*f*, 229
Hiccup, **172**, 177
Hippocampus, 35*f*, 117*f*, 213, 213*f*
Hippus, 55
Hirayama disease, 135, 137*f*
History taking
    chief complaints, 5
    family history, 8
    history of the present illness, 7
    past medical history, 7
    present age/age at onset, 5, 6*f*
    problem-finding, 5
    sex/gender, 5
    social history, 7
HIV-related neurological disorders, 218
Hoarseness, **97**, 103
Hoffmann syndrome, 134
Homocystinuria, 6
Homonymous hemianopsia, 39, 40, 41*f*, **45**
Homonymous inferior quadrantanopsia, 41*f*, 43
Homonymous scotoma, 41*f*, 42
Homonymous superior quadrantanopsia, 41*f*, 43
Hoover sign, 257, **258**
Horizontal nystagmus, 70
Horner syndrome, **51**, 51*f*, 52, 53, 53*t*, 66, 80, 98, 98*f*, 202
H reflex, 153
Hunt syndrome, see Ramsay Hunt syndrome
Hunter-Russell syndrome, **2**, 45, 130
Huntington disease, 166
Hyperacusis, **83**, 87
Hyperalgesia, 190
Hyperekplexia, **175**, 249, 250*t*
Hypermetria, **70**, 126
Hyperopia, 52
Hyperpathia, **190**, 191, 261, 283
Hyperphagia, 267
Hyperpnea, 275
Hyperthyroidism, **165**, 251
Hypertrichosis, 14, 16*f*
Hypesthesia, 190
Hypnagogic hallucination, 246
Hyp(o)algesia, 190
Hypocretin (orexin), 246
Hypoglossal canal, 50*f*, 97
Hypoglossal nerve, 31*f*, 32*f*, 50*f*, 97, 98*f*
Hypoglossal nucleus, 31*f*, 32*f*, 97
Hypometria, 70
Hypophonia, 121
Hypophysis. *see* pituitary gland
Hypothalamic hamartoma, 240
Hypothalamus
    body temperature control, 267
    circadian rhythm control, 267
    external environment adjustment, 267
    feeding control, 267
    homeostasis, 267

structure, 265, 266*f*
suprachiasmatic nucleus, 266*f*, 267
Hypotonia, 145

Ichthyosis, **11**, 143
Ideational apraxia, **227**, 233
Idiopathic cramp, 146
Idiopathic normal-pressure hydrocephalus, 201, **207**
Iliopsoas muscle, 136*t*
Illusion, 215
Immediate memory, 210
Impairment, 281
Impotence, 203
Impulse control disorders, 145
Inattention, 27
Inclusion body myositis, 133
Incoordination, 126
Indifference to pain, 188
Infection, 16
Inferior colliculus, 28, 29, **89**, 90*f*
Inferior olive, 29, 31*f*, 127*f*, 129, **176**
Inflammatory diseases, 12, **16**
Influenza encephalopathy, 272
Infraspinatus muscle, 136*t*
Inter-areal functional coupling, 223
Intermediate nerve, 84*f*, 85
Intermediolateral nucleus, 51, 51*f*, 52, 115*f*, **199**, 200*f*
Intermittent claudication, 207
Internal auditory artery, 60*f*, 61
Internuclear ophthalmoplegia, 59, 61*f*, **63**, 63*f*
Interossei muscles, 136*t*
Intervertebral foramen, 114
Intracerebral hemorrhage, 4
Involuntary movements
    action tremor, 165
    athetosis, 160*f*, 167
    ballism (ballismus), 160*f*, 167
    chorea, 160*f*, 166
    dyskinesia, 145, 159, 160*f*, **172**
    dystonia, 132, 159, 160*f*, **167**, 169, 170
    essential tremor, 160*f*, 161*f*, 163, 164*f*
    examination, 159, 160*f*
    fragile X associated tremor/ataxia syndrome, 166
    intention tremor, 165
    irregular, 159
    kinetic tremor, 165
    motor stereotypies, 178
    myoclonus (*see* Myoclonus)
    periodic, 159
    peripheral nerve origin, 181
    physiological tremor, 165
    postural tremor, 161*f*, 162
    primary orthostatic tremor, 165
    primary writing tremor, 165
    psychogenic, 180
    re-emergent tremor, 162
    resting tremor, 160, 161*f*
    restless legs syndrome, **180**, 246
    rhythmic, 159
    rhythmicity, 159
    task-specific tremor, 165
    tics, 160*f*, 179
    titubation, 165
    tremor, 159
    voice tremor, 165
Ion channel disorders. *see* channelopathies
Irresistible desire to sleep during the day, 246
Isaacs syndrome, 146, 253*t*

Japan Coma Scale, 25, 26*t*
Jaw-winking phenomenon, 78, **79**
Jendrassik maneuver, 155
Joint position sense, 186*t*, 189
Judgment, 215
Jugular foramen, 50*f*, 97, 99
Juvenile muscular atrophy of unilateral upper extremity (Hirayama disease), 137, 137*f*

Kallmann syndrome, **36**, 111
Kana (syllabogram), 226, 227*f*
Kanji (morphogram), 226, 226*f*
Kearns-Sayre syndrome, 68, 68*t*, 92, 175
Kernig sign, **106**, 271
Kernohan notch, 278
Kinésie paradoxale (paradoxical kinesia), 206
Kinesthesia, 186*t*, 189
Kleine-Levin syndrome, **246**, 267
Klüver-Bucy syndrome, 212
Kocher-Debre-Semelaigne syndrome, 134
Kojevnikoff epilepsy (epilepsia partialis continua), 146
Korsakov (Korsakoff) syndrome, **211**, 212, 267
Krabbe disease, adult form, 143
Kufor-Rakeb disease, 126
Kugelberg-Welander disease, 133
Kussmaul respiration, 275

Laboratory tests, planning, 285
Lacrimal nucleus, 30*f*, 32*f*, **85**, 201
Lacrimation, 84*f*, **85**, 86, 88
Lacunar infarction, 4, **7**
Lagophthalmos, 87
Lambert-Eaton syndrome, 253*t*, 254
Lance-Adams syndrome, 174
Landau-Kleffner syndrome, 232
Language
    alexia, 225
    alexia with agraphia, 226
    alexia without agraphia , 225
    anatomy and functions, 223
    anterior language area, 223, 225*f*
    arcuate fasciculus, 224, 225*f*
    basal temporal language area, 223, 225*f*
    Broca's area, 224, 225*f*
    evaluation, 231
    left angular gyrus, 224, 225*f*
    posterior language area, 223, 225*f*
    repetition, 224
    spoken, 223, **226**
    testing battery, 233, 234*f*
    Wernicke's area, 223, 225*f*
    writing center (Exner's area), 224, 225*f*
    written, 223, **226**
Laryngeal dystonia, 104
Larynx, somatosensory innervation, 100
Lasègue sign, **106**, 140, 191
Lateral geniculate body, 39, 41*f*, 43*f*
Lateral medullary syndrome, 52, 53*t*, 76, 94, 97, **98**, 98*f*, 99*f*
Lateral vestibulospinal tract, 93
L-Dopa, 120*f*, **124**, 126, 145
Leber hereditary optic neuropathy (atrophy), **37**, 175
Left-right disorientation, 231
Leigh syndrome, 175
Lengthening reaction, 143
Lenticulostriate artery, 60*f*
Lesch-Nyhan syndrome, 18
Lethargy, 26
Leukoaraiosis, 218

Leukoencephalopathy, 218
Levine-Critchley syndrome, 18, 19*f*, **166**
Lewy body dementia, 216
Lhermitte-Duclos disease, 131, 131*f*
Lhermitte sign, **106**, 191
Limb-girdle muscular dystrophy, 132
Limbic system, 35, **254**, *255*
Limb-shaking TIA, 167
Line of Gennari, 42
Literal paraphasia, 225
Livedo reticularis (livedo racemosa), 12, 13*f*
Locked-in syndrome, **27**, 28
Lockjaw (trismus), 78, 146
Lumbar puncture, 285
Lumbosacral plexus, 137, 139*f*
Lyme disease, **87**, 138, 140

Machado-Joseph disease, **129**, 171
Macroglossia, 18
Macular sparing, 42
Maculopapillary bundle, 37, 38*f*
Magnocellular layer, 42, 43*f*
Malignant atrophic papulosis (Degos disease), 14
Malignant hyperthermia, **145**, 251*t*, 253
Malignant lymphoma, 219
Malignant syndrome (syndrome malin), 145
Mammillothalamic tract of Vicq d'Azyr, 213
Mandibular nerve, **75**, 76*f*, 79
Marchiafava-Bignami disease, 212
Marcus Gunn phenomenon, 78, 79
Marin Amat syndrome, 79
Marinesco-Sjögren syndrome, 130
Mariotte blind spot, 45
Mask-like face, 88
Maxillary nerve, 75, 76*f*
McArdle disease, 147
Medial lemniscus, 29, 30*f*, 31*f*, 187*f*, **188**
Medial longitudinal fasciculus (MLF), 30*f*, 31*f*, 57, 59, 61*f*, **63**, 90*f*
Medulla oblongata, anatomy, 29, 31*f*
Medulloblastomas, 131
MELAS (mitochondrial encephalomyopathy, lactic acidosis and stroke-like episodes), 6, **175**
Melkersson-Rosenthal syndrome, 88
Membranous lipodystrophy (Nasu-Hakola disease), 219
Memory, **210**, 213*f*, 262
Ménière disease, 94
Meningeal irritation, **106**, 271, 275*f*, 278
Meningoencephalitis, acute, 273
Mental/cognitive functions
    basal ganglia disorders, 217
    calculation, 210*t*, 213
    character, 215
    common knowledge, 215
    daily living state, 216
    delusion, 215
    dementia, 216
    emotion, 215
    examination of, 209
    frontotemporal lobar degeneration, 217
    hallucination, **215**, 239, 246
    illusion, 215
    judgment, 215
    leukoencephalopathy, 218
    memory, **210**, 210*t*, 213*f*, 262
    orientation, 209
    quantitative evaluation, 209, 210*t*
Meralgia paresthetica, 191

MERRF (myoclonus epilepsy associated with ragged-red fibers), 174*t*, 175
Mesencephalic tegmentum, 29
Mesial temporal lobe epilepsy (MTLE), 239
Metabolic encephalopathy, 26*t*, 174*t*, **213**, 271, 274*t*
Metabolic polyneuropathy, 141
Metachromatic leukodystrophy, 143
Metamorphopsia, 230
Meyer's loop, 40
MIBG in myocardium, decreased uptake, 204
Micrographia, 121, 123*f*
Micturition syncope, 24*t*, 25
Midbrain (mesencephalon), 29, 30*f*
Middle cerebral artery, 40*f*, 43*f*, 60*f*
Migraine
  aura, 243
  basilar artery, 243
  clinical features, 243
  familial hemiplegic, **243**, 249, 250*t*
  hemiplegic, 243
  ophthalmoplegic, 243
  retinal, 243
  scintillating scotoma, 243
Migrainous cerebral infarction, 244
Mikulicz syndrome, 88
Millard-Gubler syndrome, 53*t*, 87
Miller Fisher syndrome, 68, 68*t*
Mimetic muscles, 88
Minamata disease, **2**, 45, 130
Mini-Mental State Examination (MMSE), 209, 210*t*
Miosis, **52**, 53
Mirror movements, 111
Mirror neurons, 229
Mirthless laughter, 240
Mitochondrial encephalomyopathy, 68*t*, 174*t*, 175
MNGIE (mitochondrial neurogastrointestinal encephalomyopathy), 175
Möbius syndrome, **67**, 87
Monoplegia, 110*f*, **112**, 135
Monoplegia, site of lesion, 135
Montreal Cognitive Assessment (MoCA), 209, 210*t*
Morvan syndrome, 253*t*, **254**, 255
Motor functions
  anterior corticospinal tract, 110, 110*f*, 111*f*
  anterior horn cells, **113**, 115*f*, 134
  cingulate gyrus, 85*f*, 109
  corticospinal tract, 109, 110*f*, 111*f*
  corticospinal tract laminar structure, 111*f*, 112
  corticospinal tract lesions, 111
  direct corticospinal tract, 109
  end-plate potential, 115
  excitation-contraction coupling (EC coupling), 115
  final common pathway, 109
  giant motor unit potentials, 114
  indirect corticospinal tract, 109
  lateral corticospinal tract, 110, 110*f*, 111*f*
  lateral premotor area, 85*f*, 109
  lower motor neurons, 109, 110*f*
  miniature end-plate potential, 115
  motor cortex, 85*f*, 109, 110*f*, 116*f*, 123*f*, 127*f*
  motor end-plate, 115
  motor nerves, peripheral, **113**, 114, 115*f*
  motor unit, 114
  muscle pain, 135

muscle testing, manual, 135
neuromuscular junction, 68*t*, 110*f*, 115
pre-SMA, 85*f*, **109**, 115
primary motor area (Brodmann area 4; MI), 85*f*, **109**, 115
pyramidal decussation, 110, 110*f*
pyramidal tract, pyramidal signs, 109
reinnervation, 114
SMA proper, 85*f*, 109
spinal cord structure, function, 112, 113*f*, 114*f*
supplementary motor area (SMA), 85*f*, **109**, 115
upper motor neurons, upper motor neuron signs, 109
voluntary movement control (*see* Voluntary movement control)
α motor fibers, 114, 115*f*
γ motor fibers, **114**, 153, 186, 187*t*
Motor functions examination
  acute polyneuritis, polyradiculoneuritis, 138
  atypical acute polyneuritis, 140
  chronic inflammatory demyelinating polyneuropathy (CIDP), 140
  clonus, 144
  coordination, 147
  disuse atrophy, 142
  fasciculation, 103, **134**, 181
  Gowers sign, 142
  hereditary polyneuropathy, 141
  hypotonia, 145
  metabolic polyneuropathy, 141
  monoplegia, site of lesion, 135
  muscle atropy, 132
  muscle hypertrophy, 134
  muscle spasm, cramp, **145**, 146
  muscle strength, 134
  muscle tone, 142
  myotonia, 147, 148*f*
  plexus lesions, 137, 139*f*
  posture, **132**, 205
  rigidity, 121, 142, **144**
  spasticity, 143
  spastic paralysis, 141
  toxic polyneuropathy, 141
Motor impersistence, 233
Motor neuron disease, 109, 271*t*
Motor stereotypies, 178
Motor trick, 168
Motor vision, 42
Moyamoya disease, 6
Müller muscle, 52
Multifocal lesions, 2, 2*f*
Multifocal motor neuropathy with conduction block, 141
Multiple cranial neuritis, 99
Multiple mononeuritis (mononeuritis multiplex), 140
Multiple sclerosis
  ADEM *vs.*, 143
  clinical course, 3, 3*f*
  clinical features, **39**, 46, 63, 68*t*, 106, 130, 142, 143, 146, 282*t*
  immunosuppressive treatment, 219
  lesion distribution, tissue-level, 2, 2*f*
Multiple system atrophy, 122*f*, 124*t*, 145, 203, **204**, 245
Multiple system atrophy predominantly presenting with cerebellar ataxia (MSA-C), 204
Multiple system atrophy predominantly presenting with parkinsonism (MSA-P), 126, **204**

Muscles. *see also specific muscles*
  atrophy, 132
  hypertrophy, 134
  pain, 135
  spasm, cramp, 145
  strength, 134
  stretch reflex (*see* tendon reflex)
  testing, manual, 135
  tone, 142
Music agnosia (amusia), 229
Musician's cramp, 167, 168*f*
Myalgia, 135
Myasthenia gravis, 66, 203, 253*t*, **254**, 269, 271*t*
Myasthenic crisis, 269
Mycoplasma pneumoniae, 140
Mydriasis, **49**, 53
Myerson sign, 81
Myoclonus
  brainstem origin, 175
  classification, 173
  cortical origin, 173, 173*f*, 174*t*
  cortical reflex, 173
  cortical reflex negative, 174
  definition, 172
  epileptic, 174
  hiccup, 172
  negative, 174
  nocturnal, 172
  periodic dystonic, 178, 180*f*
  photic cortical reflex, 174
  positive, 172
  postanoxic, 174
  progressive myoclonus epilepsy, 174, 174*t*
  propriospinal, 178
  reticular reflex, 175, 177*f*
  spinal cord origin, 177
  spinal segmental, 177
  spontaneous cortical, 173
  startle disease, 175
  undetermined origin, 177
Myoclonus-dystonia syndrome, hereditary, 172
Myokymia, **134**, 181
Myopia, 52
Myorhythmia, **176**, 261
Myotonia, 147, 148*f*
Myotonia congenita, 147, 251*t*, **252**
Myotonic dystrophy, 78, **133**, 147, 148*f*

Narcolepsy, 246
Nasal voice (rhinolalia), **97**, 103
Nasu-Hakola disease, 219
Natalizumab, 219
Near point, 52
Neck examination, 105
Neck pain, 106
Neuralgia, **190**, 191
Neuralgic amyotrophy, 137
Neuroacanthocytosis, 18, 19*f*, **166**
Neurodegeneration with brain ion accumulation (NBIA), 126
Neurodegenerative diseases, 2, 2*f*
Neuroendocrinology, 265
Neuroferritinopathy, 126
Neurofibromatosis type 1, 12, 12*f*
Neurofibromatosis type 2, 12
Neurogenic muscle atrophy, 133
Neuroleptic malignant syndrome, 145
Neurologic emergency
  asymmetry of neurologic signs, 274, 275*f*
  brain death diagnosis, 278
  brain lesion, progressive ischemic, 273

  coma, 25, **273**, 274*t*
  coma scale, 25, 25*t*
  conjugate deviation of eyes, 62, 69, **274**
  disturbance of consciousness, 270
  meningeal irritation, 278
  nonepileptic disorders, 271
  poor functional recovery conditions, 272
  respiratory paralysis disorders, 269
  status epilepticus, 272
  tetanus, 78, 81, 146, 271*t*, **272**
Neurologic examination
  activities of daily living, 20, **281**
  cranial nerves, 33
  hypothesis-driven, 20
  steps of, 20
  symmetry of signs, 20
Neuromuscular junction, 110*f*, **115**, 254
Neuromyelitis optica spectrum disorders, 142
Neuroprotection, 287
Neurosecretory cells, 266
Nicotinic acetylcholine receptor antibodies, 254
Night blindness (nyctalopia), 45
Nociceptive cortical areas, 188, 189*f*
Nociceptive pathway, 187, 187*f*
Nonketotic hyperglycemic-state, 167
Nose-finger-nose test, 147
Nuchal stiffness, **106**, 278
Nucleus ambiguus, 31*f*, 32*f*, 97, 98*f*
Nystagmus
  congenital, 70
  conjugate, 70
  convergence-retraction, 71
  dissociated, 63, 63*f*
  down-beat, 71
  gaze, 70, **71**
  horizontal, 70
  optokinetic, 70
  pendular, 70
  periodic alternating, 71
  positional, 95
  rebound, 71
  rotatory, **70**, 95
  spontaneous, 70
  up-beat, 71
  vertical, 70
  vestibular, 95

Obstructive sleep apnea, 244
Ocular bobbing, 71
Ocular dipping, 71
Ocular dysmetria, 69
Ocular flutter, 71
Ocular fundus, 46
Ocular motor apraxia, 69
Ocular muscles
  extraocular, congenital disorders of, 67
  extraocular, examination of, 58*f*, 65,
  extraocular, nerve innervation, 57, 58*f*
  extraocular, paralysis of, 66, 68*t*
  intraocular, examination, 53
  intraocular, nerve innervation, 49, 51*f*
Ocular myoclonus, 71
Ocular myopathy, 68
Oculogyric crisis, 69
Oculomotor nerve
  anatomy, 30*f*, 57, 58*f*, 60*f*
  extramedullary lesion, 59, 60*f*
  functions, 57
  intramedullary lesion, 58, 58*f*
  parasympathetic nervous system, 49, 51*f*
Oculopharyngeal muscular dystrophy, 132
Olfactory bulb, 35, 35*f*

Olfactory groove meningioma, 36
Olfactory nerve, 35, 35*f*
Olfactory sensation, 35
Olfactory tract, 35, 35*f*
Ondine curse, 276
One-and-a-half syndrome, 63, 63*f*
Onion bulb formation, 141
On-off phenomenon, 145
Opalski syndrome, 110
Ophelia syndrome, 255
Ophthalmic artery, **37**, 40*f*, 42
Ophthalmic nerve, 75, 76*f*
Ophthalmoplegia plus, 68
Ophthalmoplegic lipidosis, 62
Opisthotonus, 78, **81**
Opponens pollicis brevis muscle, 136*t*
Opsoclonus, 71, 72*f*, 176
Opsoclonus-myoclonus syndrome, 71
Optic atrophy, 40*f*, 46
Optic chiasm, 38, 41*f*
Optic disc (optic papilla), **37**, 38*f*, 40*f*, 46
Optic foramen, 37
Optic nerve, 38, 38*f*, 41*f*
Optic neuritis, 37, **46**
Optic radiation, 40, 41*f*
Optic tract, 39, 41*f*
Optokinetic nystagmus, 70
Oral festination, **104**, 119
Orbicularis oculi muscle, 86
Orbicularis oris muscle, 86
Orbital apex syndrome, 60
Orexin (hypocretin), 246
Organophosphate poisoning, 270
Organ transplantation, 219
Orolingual, oral dyskinesia, 172
Oromandibular dystonia, 167
Orthostatic hypotension, 24*t*, 25, 94*f*, **102**, 203
Oscillopsia, 70, 94
Osteosclerotic plasmacytoma, 14, 19*f*
Ovarian teratoma, 255
Oxytocin, 266

Pain
  central, **190**, 192, 261
  congenital insensitivity to, 188, **252**
  indifference to, 188
  muscle, 135
Painful dysesthesia, 191
Painful hand and moving fingers syn-
    drome, 181
Painful legs and moving toes syndrome, 181
Painful ophthalmoplegia, 60
Painful tonic spasm, 146
Painless diabetic motor neuropathy, 138
Palatal tremor, 71, **176**
Palinopsia, 231
Palmar grasp, 81
PANDAS (pediatric autoimmune neuro-
    psychiatric disorders associated
    with streptococcal infection), 166
Pantothenate kinase-associated neurode-
    generation (PKAN), 125*f*, **126**, 171
Papez circuit, **212**, 213*f*, 262
Papilledema, 46
Paracentral lobule, 201
Paradoxical kinesia (kinésie paradox-
    ale), 206
Paradoxical pupillary reaction, 54
Parainfectious, 16
Paralysis agitans, 159
Paramedian pontine reticular formation
    (PPRF), 61, 61*f*
Paramyotonia, 147

Paramyotonia congenita, 147, 251*t*, **252**
Paraneoplastic cerebellar degeneration,
    253*t*, 254
Paraneoplastic syndrome, 9, **16**
Paraphasia, 232
Parasympathetic nervous system, 199, 200*f*
Paratrigeminal (Raeder) syndrome, 80
Paresthesia, 190
Parinaud syndrome, 53*t*, 62
Parkinson disease
  bradykinesia, 119
  clinical features, 119
  deep brain stimulation, 119
  with dementia, 216
  disability rating scores, 124, 127*t*
  L-Dopa, 120*f*, 126, **145**, 172
  mask-like face, 88
  MIBG in myocardium, decreased
    uptake, 204
  nonmotor symptoms/signs, 122
  olfactory sensation, 36
  postural abnormalities, 105
  resting tremor, **160**, 161*f*, 163
  rigidity, 121
  saccades, 65
  sleep disorders, 245
  tremor, generating mechanism, 161,
    161*f*, 162*f*
  writing abnormalities, 121, 123*f*
Parkinsonism, **119**, 122. *see also* Parkinson
    disease
Parotid gland, 101
Paroxysmal exercise-induced dyskinesia
    (PED), 172
Paroxysmal kinesigenic dyskinesia
    (PKD), 172
Paroxysmal nonkinesigenic dyskinesia
    (PNKD), 172
Parvocellular layer, 42, 43*f*
Past pointing, 95
Pathological gambling, 145
Pathological tremor, 160
Pedunculopontine nucleus (PPN), 118*f*,
    122, 123*f*, **124**
Pellagra, **18**, 192, 216
Pendular nystagmus, 70
Penetrating arterial branch, 7
Perception, 185
Percussion myotonia, 147, 148*f*
Periodic alternating nystagmus, 71
Periodic limb movement in sleep, 180, **246**
Periodic paralysis, 251*t*, 252
Periodic synchronous discharge, 178,
    178*f*, 180*f*
Peripheral facial paralysis, 87
Peroneus longus, brevis muscles, 136*t*
Perry syndrome, 124
Perseveration, 233
Phantom limb pain, 191
Pharynx, somatosensory innervation, 100
Phenotypic heterogeneity, 166, 218, **249**
Phonation, **97**, 102, 103
Photoreceptor cells, 37, 38*f*
Physical examination
  findings, describing, 19
  general, **9**, 19
  inflammatory diseases, 16
  initial clinical evaluation, 9
  oral cavity abnormalities, 17
  skin abnormalities, **9**, 12, 16
  sunlight photosensitivity, 16, 18*f*
Physiological tremor, 160
Pickwickian syndrome, 245
Pilomotor reflex, 203

Pituitary gland
  anterior lobe, 265
  hypophysial portal vascular
    system, 265
  hypothalamohypophysial tract, 266
  posterior lobe, 266
Plantar grasp, 81
Plastic reorganization, 283
Plexus lesions, 137, 139*f*
POEMS (Crow-Fukase syndrome), 9,
    14, 16*f*
Poikilothermia, 212, **267**
Polio (acute anterior poliomyelitis), 270
Polyarteritis nodosa, 140
Polyganglionitis, 140
Polymyalgia rheumatica, 38, **135**
Polymyositis, 14, **135**
Polyneuropathy
  alcohol vitamin deficiency, 141
  chronic inflammatory axonal, 141
  chronic inflammatory demyelinat-
    ing, 140
  diabetic, **141**, 191
  examination of, 191
  familial amyloid, 141, **201**
  hereditary, 141
  metabolic, 141
  painful sensory, 138
  sensory predominant, 192
  toxic, 141
Polyopia, 68, **231**
Polyradiculoneuritis, 138
Polysensory areas, 230
Polysomnography (PSG), 244
Pons, 29, 30*f*
Pontine artery, 60*f*
Pontine basis, 29
Pontine tegmentum, 29
Portal-systemic encephalopathy, 213
Positional nystagmus, 95
Positive sharp waves, 134
Posterior cerebral artery, 40*f*, 43*f*, 60*f*
Posterior choroidal artery, 43*f*
Posterior communicating artery, 40*f*,
    43*f*, 60*f*
Posterior inferior cerebellar artery, 60*f*, 97
Postherpetic myelitis, 7
Postherpetic neuralgia, 79, **191**
Postinfectious, 16
Posttetanic potentiation, 254
Posture, **132**, 205
Pott paraplegia, 273
Pourfour du Petit syndrome, 52
Praxis, **227**, 232
Precentral gyrus, 85*f*
Pressure sensitive neuropathy, 141
Pretectal nucleus, 39, 41*f*
Priapism, 203
Primary amyloidosis, 18
Primary central nervous system vasculi-
    tis, 285
Primary lateral sclerosis, 143
Primary lymphoma, 285
Primary motor area (Brodmann area 4;
    MI), 85*f*, **109**, 115
Primary somatosensory cortex (SI), 76, 77*f*,
    85*f*, 168*f*, **188**, 188*f*, 189
Primary visual cortex, 42, 44*f*, 65*f*
Prion disease, 179
Procedural memory, 210
Prognosis assessment, 281, 282*t*
Progressive encephalomyelitis with rigidity
    and myoclonus (PERM), 146
Progressive external ophthalmoplegia, 68

Progressive multifocal leukoencephalopathy
    (PML), 219
Progressive muscular dystrophy, 132
Progressive nonfluent aphasia, 217
Progressive ophthalmoplegia, 175
Progressive supranuclear palsy (PSP), 62,
    69, 105, 122*f*, 124*t*, 178, 206, **218**
Pronator teres muscle, 136*t*
Proprioceptive pathway, 75, 187*f*, **188**, 188*f*
Prosopagnosia, **44**, 230
Pseudoathetosis, 181, **190**
Pseudobulbar palsy, 80, **99**, 104
Pseudohypertrophy, 134
Pseudoxanthoma elasticum, 11, 11*f*
Psychogenic neurologic diseases
  classification, 257
  common features, 258
  conversion disorders, 257
  factitious disease, 257
  malingering, 257
  motor paralysis, 257
  sensory loss, 257
Ptosis (blepharoptosis), 52, **66**
Puffer toxin (tetrodotoxin), 270
Pull test, 127*t*, 206
Punch-drunk encephalopathy, 217
Punding, 145
Pupillary dilator, 51, 51*f*
Pupillary sphincter, 49, 51*f*
Pupillotonia, 55
Pupils
  convergence reflex, **49**, 55
  examination, 53
  light reflex, 39, 41*f*, **49**, 54, 54*f*, 276
  special abnormal findings, 55
  sympathetic nervous system control,
    51, 51*f*
Pure akinesia, 206
Pure autonomic failure, 203
Pure word deafness, 226
Pure word dumbness, 226
Purulent meningitis, 273
Pyramid, 29, 31*f*
Pyramidal tract, 29, **109**, 110

Quadriceps femoris muscle, 136*t*
Quadrigeminal bodies, 29
Queckenstedt test, 287

Rabbit syndrome, 161
Radicular arteries, 113, 114*f*
Raeder (paratrigeminal) syndrome,
    80, 99*t*
Ramsay Hunt syndrome, 12, 14*f*, **85**, 88
Rapid alternating movement, 147
Raymond-Cestan syndrome, 53*t*
Rebound nystagmus, 71
Rebound phenomenon, 147
Recent memory, **210**, 211
Recognition, 223, **229**
Recognition of faces, 44
Recurrent laryngeal nerve, 97
Referred pain, 202, 202*f*
Reflexes
  abdominal, abdominal wall/muscle,
    157, 158
  anal sphincter, 203
  ankle jerk (Achilles tendon), **154**, 155,
    155*f*, 156
  Babinski sign, **156**, 157, 157*f*
  biceps brachii, 154, 155*f*
  bulbocavernous, 203
  ciliary, **80**, 276
  ciliospinal, 277

convergence, **49**, 55
corneal (blink), 77f, **78**, 80, 276
cough, 276
cremasteric, 158
extensor plantar, 156, 157f
finger flexor, 154, **156**
flexor withdrawal, **156**, 157
head retraction, 81
Hoffmann, **154**, 156
inverted biceps, 153
inverted triceps, 153
jaw jerk, 77, 77f, **80**, 154, 155f
light, 39, 41f, **49**, 54, 54f, 276
masseter reflex (jaw jerk), 77, 77f, **80**, 154, 155f
Mendel-Bechterew, **154**, 156
oculocephalic, **69**, 276
palmomental, 81
patellar tendon (knee jerk), 154, 155f
pathological, 156
pharyngeal (gag), **100**, 103, 276
pilomotor, 203
plantar, 156
primitive, 81
quadriceps femoris (knee jerk), 154, 155f
rooting, 81
Rossolimo, **154**, 156
snout, 81
startle, **175**, 178
sucking, 81
toe flexor, 154
tonic neck, 277
triceps brachii, 155f
Wartenberg, **154**, 156
Refsum disease, 12, 46, 92, **130**
Relapsing polychondritis, **12**, 255
Remote memory, 210
Reserve functions, 283
Resonance, 119
Respiration, examination of, 274
Restless legs syndrome, **180**, 246
Retina
  blood vessel observation, 46
  ganglion cells, 37, 38f
  migraine, 38, **243**
  pigment degeneration, 12, 17, **45**, 46
  structure, 37, 38f
Retinotopic organization, **42**, 230
Retrobulbar neuritis, **37**, 46
Retrocollis, **105**, 218
Retrograde amnesia, **210**, 211
Rett syndrome, 174t, 179
Reversible cerebral vasoconstriction syndrome, 244
Reversible posterior leukoencephalopathy, 244
Reye syndrome, 272
Rigidity, 121, 142, **144**
Rinne test, 91
Risus sardonicus, 78
Rods, 37, 38f
Romberg sign, **190**, 190f, 207
Root pain, 106, **190**
Ross syndrome, 55
Rostral interstitial nucleus of MLF, 62, 64f
Rotatory nystagmus, **70**, 95
Round and isocoric (pupils), 53
Roussy-Lévy syndrome, 141
R-R interval, 203

Saccades
  catch-up, 70
  control mechanism, 64, 64f
  definition, 63

hypermetric, 70
hypometric, 70
memory-guided, 64, 64f
  in Parkinson disease, 65
visually-guided, 64, 64f
Saccadic lateropulsion, 95
Saccadic pursuit, 70
Sacral sparing, 188
Salivation, **85**, 88, 101
Sarcoidosis, 68t, **87**, 142
Satiety center, 267
Savant syndrome, 230
Scanning speech, **104**, 126
Scapula alata, winged scapula, 132, 132f
Schirmer test, 88
Secondary somatosensory cortex (SII), 76, **188**, 189f, 260
Segawa's disease, 171, 171f
Segmental dissociated sensory loss, 193, 194f
Segmental sensory impairment, 192, 194f
Selective attention, 89, **230**
Semantic dementia, 217
Semantic memory, 210
Semicoma, 25
Semilunar (gasserian) ganglion, 50f, 75, 76f
SENDA (static encephalopathy of childhood with neurodegeneration in adulthood), 126
Sensation (sense), 185
Sensorineural deafness, 91
Sensory trick, 105, **168**
Sepiapterin reductase deficiency, 171
Serotonin syndrome, 26
Serotonin synthesis, 120f
Sexual functions, 203
Shy-Drager syndrome, 203
SIADH (syndrome of inappropriate secretion of ADH), 266
Sicca syndrome, 88
Simple tic, 179
Simultanagnosia, **231**, 233
Simultanapraxia, 233
Sjögren-Larsson syndrome, 11, **143**
Sjögren syndrome, 88, **140**, 142, 193
Skew deviation, 67
Skin
  autonomic symptoms, 202
  congenital/hereditary diseases, 9
  heavy metals intoxication, 16, 17f
  inflammatory diseases, 12
Sleep disorders
  central sleep apnea-hypopnea syndrome, 245
  classification, 244
  cognitive disturbance in, 245
  non-REM sleep, 244
  obstructive sleep apnea-hypopnea syndrome, 244
  periodic limb movement in, 180, **246**
  polysomnography (PSG), 244
  REM sleep, 244, 245t
  REM sleep behavior disorders, 245
  stages of sleep, 244, 245t
Sleep paralysis, 246
Slurred speech, **104**, 126
SMON (subacute myelo-optico-neuropathy), 144
Smooth pursuit eye movement, 63, 65f
Sneddon syndrome, 12, 13f
Soft palate examination, 103
Somatic sensation, 185
Somatosensory system
  Burdach column, 187

cortical receptive areas, 77f, 188
cortical sensation examination, 189
cuneate fascicle, 186
cuneate nucleus, 187
deep/proprioceptive, **185**, 186, 186t, 187f, 260
dorsal column, 111f, 186
dorsal root ganglion, 76f, 84f, 144, **185**, 186f, 187f, 193, 200f
examination, 189
Goll column, **186**, 193
gracile fascicle, 186
gracile nucleus, **186**, 188
impairment, symptom distribution, 191
medial lemniscus, 29, 30f, 31f, 90f, 187f, **188**
modality specificity, 185
nociceptive pathway, 187, 187f, 189f
peripheral nerves, 185, 186f, 187t
proprioceptive pathway, 186t, 187f, 188
rapidly adapting receptors, 185
receptor/generator potential, 185
receptors, 185
sensation, modalities of, 185, 186t
slowly adapting receptors, 185
somatotopic organization, 77f, 188
in spinal cord, 111f, 186, 187f
superficial sensation, 185, 186t
symptoms/signs, 190
third sensory neuron, 188
Somnolence, 25
Spasmodic dysphagia, **103**, 167
Spasmodic dysphonia, **104**, 166, 167
Spasmodic torticollis, 167
Spasticity, 142, **143**
Spastic paralysis, 141
Spinal cord
  acute compression, 273
  autonomic nervous system, 199, 200f
  blood supply, 112, 114f
  laminar structure, 111f
  motor system, 112
  nociceptive impairment, 196
  root lesions of, 137
  somatosensory system, 111f, 186
  structure, function, 112, 111f, 113f
  subacute combined degeneration, 131
  transverse, sensory impairment, 193, 195f
Spinal nerve, 113f, 200f
Spinal shock, **145**, 157
Spinocerebellar ataxia (SCA)
  definition and classification, 129
  SCA1, 129
  SCA2, 124t, 126, **129**
  SCA3, **129**, 171
  SCA5, 129
  SCA6, 126, **129**, 243, 249
  SCA7, 129
  SCA8, **126**, 129
  SCA10, 129
  SCA12, 129
  SCA13, 129
  SCA14, 129
  SCA17, **126**, 129
  SCA27, 129
Spongiform encephalopathy, 179
Spontaneous nystagmus, 70
Spurling sign, **106**, 190
Square-wave jerks, 69
SSRIs (selective serotonin reuptake inhibitors), 26
Stapedius muscle paralysis, 87
Start hesitation, 121
Startle disease, 175

Status epilepticus, 271t, 272
Steal phenomenon, **24**, 207
Steele-Richardson-Olszewski syndrome, **62**, 218
Stellate ganglion, 51, 51f
Stereognosis, 186t, **189**, 260
Sternocleidomastoid muscle, 105
Stiff-person syndrome, 146
Stokes-Adams syndrome, 25
Straight leg raising test, 106
Striate area, 42
Stroke, **6**, 7, 242
Stupor, 25
Sturge-Weber syndrome, 10f, 11
Subacute cerebellar degeneration, 130
Subacute combined degeneration of the spinal cord, 131
Subacute sclerosing panencephalitis (SSPE), 178, 180f
Subarachnoid hemorrhage, 3, **4**, 6, 106, 244, 271, 274t
Subclavian steal syndrome, 24
Subdural hematoma, 213, 274t
Sunlight photosensitivity, 16, 18f
Superficial siderosis, 4, **92**
Superior cerebellar artery, 60f
Superior colliculus, 29, 30f, **39**, 41f, 64f
Superior oblique muscle, unilateral paralysis, 67
Superior oblique myokymia, 71
Superior salivatory nucleus, 30f, 32f, 84f, 85
Supinator muscle, 136t
Supplementary eye field (SEF), 61, 64f, 65f, 85f
Supplementary motor area (SMA), 85f, **109**, 115
Suprachiasmatic nucleus, 39, **267**
Supranuclear paralysis, 69
Supraspinatus muscle, 136t
Susac syndrome, 92
Swallowing, 97
Sweet disease, 12, 15f
Sydenham chorea, 166
Sylvian aqueduct syndrome, 71
Sympathetic nervous system, 51f, 98f, 102f, 115f, 199, 200f
Symptomatic oculopalatal tremor, 71
Synchronization of basal ganglia activities, 119
Syncope, 24, 24t
Syndrome of Alice in Wonderland, 229
Synesthesia, 231
Synkinesis, 86
Syringomyelia, 193, 194f
Systemic amyloidosis, 201
Systemic lupus erythematosus (SLE), 6, 16, **140**, 241

Tabes dorsalis, 55, **145**
Tachypnea, 275
Tactile sense, 186t, 189
Tardive dyskinesia, 172
Tardive dystonia, 169
Task specificity, **167**, 241
Taste sense, **85**, 88, 100, 101f
Tectum, **29**, 39
Telegraphic speech, 225
Temperature sense, 185, **189**, 192, 195f, 196f, 201
Temporal arteritis, **38**, 135
Temporal information processing hypothesis, 119
Temporal lobe epilepsy, 93, 215, 238, **239**

Temporal lobe lesion, character change due to, 215, 214*f*
Temporal pallor, 37, 40*f*, 46
Tendon reflex
  distal extremity muscles, **154**, 156
  examination, 153, 155*f*
  hyperactive, significance of, 155
  Ia fibers, 144*f*, 153
  Ib fibers, 144*f*, 153
  Jendrassik maneuver, 155
  muscle spindle, 144*f*, 153
  physiological mechanism, 144*f*, 153
  reinforcement technique, 155
  Renshaw cell, 153, 154*f*
  stretch receptor, 143, 144*f*, **153**
  tendon hammers, 154
  tendon organ, 143, 144*f*, **153**
Tensilon test, 66, 254, **269**
Tetanus, 78, 81, **146**, 271*t*, 272
Tetany, 146
Thalamic asterixis, 174, **176**
Thalamic hemorrhage, 62, **259**, 274, 278
Thalamic infarction, 214*f*, **259**, 283
Thalamic pain, 191, **192**, 283
Thalamic syndrome, 191, **192**, 261
Thalamus
  anterior thalamic nucleus, 259, 260*f*, **262**
  CM-Pf complex, 262
  dorsal medial nucleus, 213, 260*f*
  internal medullary lamina, **259**, 260*f*, 262
  intralaminar nucleus, 260*f*, 262
  lateral geniculate body, 30*f*, 39, 40, 43*f*, 260*f*, **262**
  lateral nuclear group, 259, 260*f*
  massa intermedia, 259, 260*f*
  medial dorsal (mediodorsal) nucleus, 260*f*, 261
  medial geniculate body, 30*f*, 89, 90*f*, 260*f*, **262**
  medial nuclear group, 259
  motor thalamus, 261
  nociceptive afferents, 260
  paramedian thalamic artery, 262
  pulvinar, 30*f*, 179, 259, 260*f*, **262**
  structure, 259, 260*f*
  tactile, deep/proprioceptive afferents, 260
  thalamic hand, 261
  thalamogeniculate artery, 260
  tuberothalamic artery, 261
  ventral intermediate nucleus, 125, **261**
  ventral posterolateral nucleus, **187**, 187*f*, 260, 260*f*
  ventral posteromedial nucleus, 75, 76*f*, **187**, 187*f*, 260, 260*f*
Thallium poisoning, 16, 17*f*
Thoracic outlet syndrome, 137
Thrombolytic therapy, 273
Thymoma, 66, **254**
Thyrotoxic myopathy, 68
Tibialis anterior muscle, 136*t*
Tibialis posterior muscle, 136*t*
Tic douloureux (trigeminal neuralgia), 79
Tics, 160*f*, 179
Tinel sign, 191
Tinnitus, 91

Tissue damage assessment, 281, 282*t*
Tissue plasminogen activator (tPA), 273
Titubation, 165
Toes, motor paralysis, 157
Tolosa-Hunt syndrome, 60
Tongue, 97
Tongue atrophy, 103*f*
Tongue bite, 18, 19*f*
Tonotopic organization, **89**, 229
Top of the basilar artery syndrome, 60
Topographic disorientation, 231
Torsion dystonia, 170
Torticollis, 105
Touch localization, 160*t*, 190
Toxic cerebellar diseases, 130
Toxic polyneuropathy, 141
Toxic sensory ganglionopathy, 193
Transcortical reflex, 173
Transient global amnesia, 210, **211**
Transient myoclonic state with asterixis in elderly patients, 176
Trapezius muscle, 106
T reflex, 153
Tremor
  central, 165
  clinical features and classification, 159
  enhanced physiological, 165
  essential, 160*f*, 161*f*, 163, 164*f*
  essential palatal, **176**, 177
  fragile X associated, 129, **166**
  intention, 165
  kinetic, 165
  mechanical, 165
  midbrain lesion etiology, 165
  palatal, 175, **176**
  physiological, 165
  postural, 162
  primary orthostatic, 165
  primary writing, **165**, 167
  re-emergent, 162
  resting, 160, 161*f*
  symptomatic palatal, 176
  task-specific, 165
  voice tremor, 165
Triceps brachii muscle, 136*t*
Trigeminal autonomic cephalalgia, 242*t*, 244
Trigeminal nerve
  anatomy, 50*f*, 75, 76*f*
  corneal reflex, 77*f*, **78**, 80, 276
  examination of functions related to, 78
  extramedullary lesions, 76
  intramedullary lesions, 76
  jaw jerk (masseter reflex), **77**, 77*f*, 80
  main sensory nucleus, 75, 76*f*
  masticatory muscles innervation, 76
  mesencephalic nucleus, 76*f*, 77
  motor nucleus, 76, 76*f*, 77*f*
  primary sensory neuron, 75
  primitive reflexes, 81
  semilunar (gasserian) ganglion, 50*f*, 75, 76*f*
  somatosensory input, cortical reception, 76
  somatosensory pathway, 75, 76*f*
  spinal nucleus, 30*f*, 31*f*, 32*f*, 75, 76*f*
  spinal tract, 30*f*, 31*f*, 75, 76*f*, 98*f*

trigeminothalamic tract, **75**, 76*f*, 80, 84
Trigeminal neuralgia (tic douloureux), 79
Trigger zone, 79
Triphasic waves (EEG), 212*f*, 271
Trismus (lockjaw), **78**, 146
Trochlear nerve, 29, 32*f*, 50*f*, **60**
Trousseau sign, 147
Trunk examination, 106
Tuberous sclerosis, **11**, 10*f*, 241
Tumors, 2, 2*f*, **3**, 131, 267, 273
Tunnel (tubular) vision, **45**, 258
Two-point discrimination, 186*t*, 189
Tyrosine hydroxylase deficiency, **126**, 172

Uncal herniation, 277
Uncinate fit, 35, **239**
Unconsciousness, 24. *see also* consciousness
Uncus, 35, 35*f*
Unified Parkinson's Disease Rating Scale (UPDRS), 124
Unilateral anosmia, 36
Unverricht-Lundborg disease, 174, 174*t*
Up-beat nystagmus, 71
Urge incontinence, 203
Urinary frequency, 203
Urinary retention, 203
Urination (micturition) control, 203
Utilization behavior, 81, **228**

Vagus nerve
  anatomy, 32*f*, 50*f*, 97
  dorsal motor nucleus, 31*f*, 32*f*, **101**, 122
  nucleus ambiguus, 31*f*, 32*f*, 97, 98*f*
Vanishing white matter disease, 219
Variant Creutzfeldt-Jakob disease, **179**, 262
Varicella zoster virus, 7, **12**, 14*f*, 84, 273
Vascular dementia, 216, **218**
Vascular disease, **6**, 7
Vascular parkinsonism, 122. *see also* Parkinson disease
Vasopressin, 266
Vasovagal syncope, 24*t*, 25
Venous sinus thrombosis, **4**, 243
Ventral pathway, primary visual cortex, 42
Ventral spinocerebellar tract, 31*f*, 129
Ventriloquist effect, 230
Verbal paraphasia, 225
Verbal perseveration, 232
Vernet syndrome (jugular foramen syndrome), 99, 99*t*
Vertebral artery, 24, 60*f*, 95
Vertebrobasilar artery territory, 24, **60**, 60*f*, 94, 273
Vertical gaze palsy, 53*t*, **62**, 69, 218
Vertical nystagmus, 70
Vertiginous seizure, 93, **239**
Vertigo, **94**, 94*f*, 127. *see also* equilibrium
Vertigo and loss of equilibrium, 98
Very long chain fatty acid, 143
Vestibular nystagmus, 95
Vestibulocochlear nerve, 30*f*, 32*f*, 89, 90*f*
Vibration sense, 101, 186*t*, **189**
Villaret syndrome, 99*t*, 100
Visceral efferent/visceromotor nerve, 101, 102*f*

Visceral organ, **101**, 102, 102*f*
Visceral pain, 202, 202*f*
Visceral sensation, 102, **185**, 202, 204
Visual field, psychogenic constriction, 258
Visual field defects, 41*f*, 44
Visual function examination
  accommodation, 49, 51*f*, **52**, 55, 80
  acuity, 44
  field, 44
  higher functions, symptoms/signs, 229
  ocular fundus, 46
  peripheral visual field constriction, 45
  retinal blood vessel observation, 46
  retinal pigment degeneration, 46
Visual hallucination, 215
Visual motion, 230
Visual object agnosia, 230
Visual recognition, 233
Visual system
  anatomy and functions, 37
  blood supply to, 42
  cytoarchitecture, 42
  lateral geniculate body, 39, 41*f*, 43*f*
  retina, 37, 38*f*
  special functions, 42
  visual cortex, 42
Visuospatial agnosia, 231
Vitamin B12 deficiency, 131
Vitamin E deficiency, 130
Vocal tic, 179
Voluntary movement control
  basal ganglia, 116
  cerebellum, 125
  corticospinal tract, 109
  feedforward control, 115
  final common pathway, 115
  motor cortices, higher functions, 115
  motor selection, 118
  motor thalamus, 261
  nigrostriatal system, 119
Von Hippel-Lindau disease, 131
Von Recklinghausen disease. *see* neurofibromatosis type 1

Waddling gait, 142
Wallenberg syndrome, 53*t*, 76, 94, 97, **98**, 98*f*, 99*f*
Waning, 66
Warm-up phenomenon, **147**, 252
Wearing-off phenomenon, 145
Weber syndrome, 53*t*, 58*f*, 59
Weber test, 90
Wernicke encephalopathy, 68*t*, 211, 211*f*, **212**, 267
Wernicke-Mann posture, 132
Wernicke's area, 223
Williams syndrome, 230
Wilson disease, **164**, 165, 168, 169, 170*f*
Wing beating tremor, 164
Wolfram syndrome, 267
Wrist drop, 136, 138*f*
Writer's cramp, **167**, 169

Xeroderma pigmentosum, 16, 18*f*
X-kinked recessive dystonia-parkinsonism (DYT3), 126, **171**